Innovations in Ayurvedic Nutrition

Anil Kumar • Manoj Kumar Tripathi
Nidhi V. Maheshwari • Sanjay Kumar
Editors

Innovations in Ayurvedic Nutrition

Principles and Concepts

Springer

Editors
Anil Kumar
Rani Lakshmi Bai Central Agricultural University
Jhansi, Uttar Pradesh, India

Manoj Kumar Tripathi
ICAR Central Institute of Agricultural Engineering
Bhopal, Madhya Pradesh, India

Nidhi V. Maheshwari
Somaiya Vidyavihar University
Mumbai, Maharashtra, India

Sanjay Kumar
Agricultural Scientists Recruitment Board (ASRB)
Indian Council of Agricultural Research (ICAR)
Pusa, Delhi, India

ISBN 978-981-95-1212-6 ISBN 978-981-95-1213-3 (eBook)
https://doi.org/10.1007/978-981-95-1213-3

This Springer imprint is published by the registered company Springer Nature Singapore Pte Ltd.
The registered company address is: 152 Beach Road, #21-01/04 Gateway East, Singapore 189721, Singapore

Foreword

The rapid pace of urbanization and technological progress has transformed dietary habits, often leading to nutrient deficiencies and a surge in lifestyle diseases such as diabetes, obesity, hypertension, cancer, and cardiovascular disorders. Traditional reliance on pharmaceutical interventions frequently poses adverse effects, highlighting the need for alternative, holistic approaches. Nutrition-based strategies, which fortify the body's natural defenses, are increasingly recognized as pivotal in disease prevention and management. This paradigm shift emphasizes the integration of food and medicine, giving rise to nutraceuticals—natural compounds like omega-3 fatty acids, probiotics, β-glucans, vitamins, minerals, and plant extracts. These not only boost immunity but also have potential in therapeutic advancements. The ancient principles of Ayurveda further enrich this field by advocating harmony between diet, lifestyle, and natural remedies. Its focus on *Ahara* (diet) and *Vihara* (lifestyle) underlines the importance of personalized health management, rooted in the *Panchamahabhutas* (five elements) and *Tridoshas* (*Vata*, *Pitta*, *Kapha*).

Modern science complements these traditional insights with cutting-edge "omics" technologies, such as genomics, proteomics, and metabolomics. Together, they form the foundation of Nutri-Ayurgenomics, a transformative approach to personalized nutrition. This integration enables the creation of functional foods and nutraceuticals tailored to individual genetic and *prakriti* (constitutional) profiles, offering precise solutions for health challenges.

This comprehensive book bridges the gap between traditional knowledge and scientific innovation. With a focus on global health issues, Ayurvedic principles, and omics technologies, it serves as an invaluable resource for researchers, students, and professionals alike, fostering advancements in personalized nutrition and functional food development. Ideal for students, researchers, dietitians, and industry professionals, this book serves as both a foundational and advanced resource, fostering a deeper understanding of Nutri-Ayurgenomics and its transformative potential in health and nutrition.

It is a privilege and honor to write the foreword for this remarkable book edited by Dr. Anil Kumar, Dr Manoj Kumar Tripathi, Dr Nidhi V. Maheshwari, and Dr. Sanjay Kumar. Comprising 17 well-crafted chapters, this book promises to be an invaluable resource for research and teaching. It stands as a milestone for academic and research institutions, scientists, professors, students, and health-conscious consumers alike, offering profound insights and practical knowledge across diverse platforms.

Swami Ramdev
Maharshi Dayanand Gram,
Delhi-Haridwar National Highway,
Haridwar, Uttarakhand, India

Preamble

In today's fast-paced world, the pursuit of holistic health has become more essential than ever. Ayurveda, a 5000-year-old tradition, emphasizes the interconnectedness of body, mind, and spirit, with *Ahara* (nutrition) as one of its cornerstones. Together with *Nidra* (sleep) and *Brahmacharya* (regulated lifestyle and self-discipline), *Ahara* is recognized as one of the three *Upastambhas* (pillars of life) that sustain health, vitality, and longevity and serve as the core pillars that support and maintain the physical, mental, and spiritual well-being of an individual, as stated in the *Charaka Samhita*: *Trayopastambha ityahurahridyaṃ satvasamshrayaḥ* | *Aharaḥ swapnaḥ brahmacharyam, ayuh sthitih karanam*.

This book, *Innovations in Ayurvedic Nutrition: Principles and Concepts*, curated by Dr. Anil Kumar, Dr. Manoj Kumar Tripathi, Dr. Nidhi V. Maheshwari, and Dr. Sanjay Kumar, bridges the time-honored wisdom of Ayurveda with modern advancements in nutrition science. It presents a pioneering framework, Nutri-Ayur Innovation, that integrates ancient principles with contemporary insights to empower readers on their journey toward holistic wellness.

Spanning foundational concepts of diet, balanced nutrition, and Ayurvedic biology, the book advances into modern themes such as nutrigenomics, foodomics, and nutraceuticals. Chapters explore the use of millets, spices, herbs, fruits, vegetables, and forest products in Ayurvedic nutrition, while also addressing pharmacological principles, drug delivery systems, and Ayurveda-inspired innovations for developing sustainable and reliable treatments. The text underscores the revolutionary potential of "green drug" modalities, merging nutrition with the pharmacological properties of medicinal plants to enhance immunity and mitigate chronic illnesses.

In Ayurveda, food is not just sustenance but a vital force influencing every aspect of well-being. Food is the essential foundation for life and sustenance of all living beings, as highlighted in the *Charaka Samhita*: *Ahara-sambhavaḥ sthitiḥ sarvabhutanam*.

By blending Ayurvedic wisdom with the transformative power of mindful nutrition, this book offers readers a path to holistic health. May it inspire and empower you to align dietary choices with Ayurveda's principles, cultivating a life of balance, vitality, and lasting wellness.

Prof. Vaidya Rabinarayana Acharya

Preface

The modern era, characterized by urbanization and technological advancements, has led to significant shifts in dietary habits, resulting in nutrient deficiencies and an increased prevalence of lifestyle diseases such as diabetes, obesity, hypertension, cancer, and cardiovascular disorders. Traditional reliance on pharmaceutical interventions often brings adverse effects, underscoring the need for alternative strategies. Strengthening the body's natural defense system, primarily through nutrition, emerges as a vital approach to disease prevention and management. This calls for a focus on dietary innovations with medicinal properties, bridging the gap between food and medicine. The emerging field of nutraceuticals embodies this paradigm shift, blending nutrition and medicine. Nutraceuticals include natural compounds like omega-3 fatty acids, β-glucans, probiotics, vitamins, minerals, and plant-derived extracts, which not only enhance immunity but may also contribute to drug development. Rooted in ancient Ayurvedic practices, the concept of nutraceuticals emphasizes harmony between diet, lifestyle, and natural remedies, advocating for holistic health management. Ayurveda, often regarded as the "Science of Life," promotes balance through proper nutrition, sleep, and lifestyle choices. Its principles of *Ahara* (diet) and *Vihara* (lifestyle) are instrumental in disease prevention and health maintenance.

A balanced diet in Ayurveda considers the *Panchamahabhutas* (five elements: air, water, space, earth, and fire) and Tridoshas (*Vata*, *Pitta*, and *Kapha*), tailoring nutritional intake to an individual's constitution. Modern science complements these traditional principles through advancements in genomics, proteomics, and metabolomics, collectively termed "omics" technologies. These tools provide insights into the interaction between diet, genes, and health, enabling personalized nutrition tailored to an individual's genetic makeup and *prakriti* (constitution).

This integration of Ayurveda and modern science, termed "Nutri-Ayurgenomics," represents a transformative approach to personalized nutrition and health. By studying genetic variations and their influence on dietary responses, Nutri-Ayurgenomics aims to develop functional foods and nutraceuticals that align with individual needs. This innovative approach leverages bioinformatics tools to identify dietary signals, genetic targets, and the interplay of nutrients and genes, facilitating the creation of customized dietary solutions to prevent and manage nutrition-related disorders.

In response to these developments, a comprehensive two-volume book is being assembled to serve as an instructional and reference material. Volume 1 explores foundational concepts of Nutri-Ayur innovations, while Volume 2 delves into translational research and product formulation. The book addresses global health concerns, nutraceutical advancements, Ayurvedic principles, and the integration of omics technologies in nutrition research. It offers detailed insights into gene-diet interactions, molecular biology techniques, and the development of herbal products targeting specific ailments like cancer and diabetes.

The introductory chapters provide an overview of global health challenges, their causes, and treatment strategies, emphasizing the role of a balanced diet and nutraceuticals. Subsequent sections elaborate on Ayurvedic science, omics advancements, and their applications in nutrition. The final chapters highlight R&D efforts, policy implications, and the demand for Nutri-Ayur products in addressing disease-specific nutritional needs. The book is designed to cater to a diverse audience, including students, researchers, dietetic practitioners, and industry professionals. It aligns with the curricula of research institutions in Ayurveda, food technology, and biotechnology, offering a robust resource for understanding the intersection of traditional knowledge and modern science. By synthesizing fundamental and advanced concepts, this book aims to foster innovation in personalized nutrition and functional food development, bridging the gap between tradition and technology.

This book comprises 17 chapters covering the basic concepts of translational research and the development and role of Nutri-Ayur products in disease prevention and treatment. Chapter 1 introduces diet and nutrition. Chapter 2 focuses on human nutrition and the concept of a balanced diet. Chapter 3 explores nutrition biology as a new paradigm for human health. Chapter 4 emphasizes the impact of nutrigenomics on human health. Chapter 5 discusses food-drug interactions. Chapter 6 highlights foodomics as a new field for the modern food era. Chapter 7 explains nutraceuticals and nutritionally functional foods. Chapter 8 discusses Nutri-Ayur components, including millets, fruits and vegetables, spices, pulses, cereals, nuts and seeds, and herbs. Chapter 9 explores the utilization of forest products for developing Nutri-Ayur components. Chapter 10 provides a detailed account of Indian traditional medicine as a medical inheritance, focusing on adaptogenic and rejuvenating properties. Chapter 11 delves into innovative strides in Ayurvedic biology for holistic healing.

Chapter 12 narrates the basic principles of Ayurvedic nutrition for wellness. Chapter 13 addresses Ayurvedic drugs, covering pharmacological and pharmaceutical principles and delivery systems. Chapter 14 elaborates on medicinal plants and their role in sustainable human health in the context of Nutri-Ayur products. Chapter 15 discusses Ayur-nutrigenomics, an integration of Ayurveda-inspired nutrition and omics platforms, from inception to evidence. Chapter 16 elaborates on integrated approaches for developing herbal medicine. Finally, Chap. 17 provides insights into Ayurveda's opportunities for developing safe and effective treatment options for the future.

This book is conceptualized to provide our esteemed readers with insights into the diverse nature of nutraceuticals, functional foods, and medical foods, along with the challenges and opportunities in their development, characterization, and marketing. It explores the rationale for these products, rooted in their long history of application, while highlighting the demand for Nutri-Ayur innovations, the role of molecular biology tools, product development, R&D efforts, current status, and policy focus on their use for disease-specific treatments tailored to individual *prakriti*. Authored by experts, the chapters align with the syllabi of Ayurvedic, food technology, and related institutions, catering to researchers, students, and industry professionals. This book serves as instructional material for researchers in Ayurveda, food and nutrition, and related fields, as well as a reference for industry and R&D labs. We thank the contributors for their cooperation and our families for their support during the editing process.

We extend our heartfelt gratitude to all the contributors of the 17 chapters for their invaluable efforts and unwavering cooperation, from the initial submission of drafts to incorporating the revisions suggested by the editors. We also express our deep appreciation to our family members for their patience and support throughout the process of editing this book.

Jhansi, Uttar Pradesh, India — Anil Kumar
Bhopal, Madhya Pradesh, India — Manoj Kumar Tripathi
Mumbai, Maharashtra, India — Nidhi V. Maheshwari
Delhi, India — Sanjay Kumar

Contents

Editors and Contributors

About the Editors

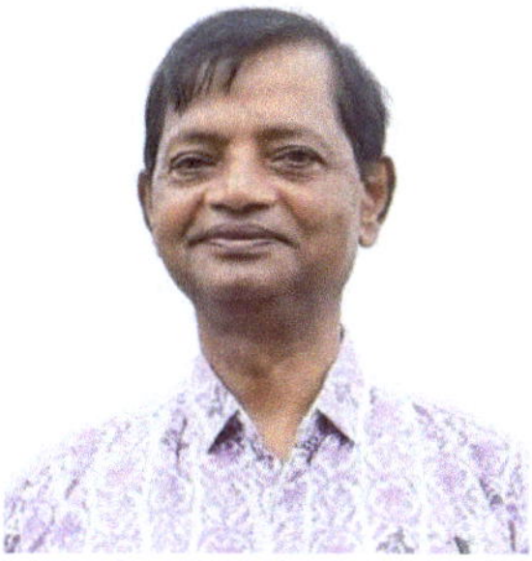

Anil Kumar is an eminent teacher, outstanding educationist, and scientist of international repute. He joined GB Pant University of Agriculture and Technology as Assistant Professor in 1993 and served for 25 years in different capacities. After successful completion of three tenures (~12 years) as Professor and Head, Department of Molecular Biology and Genetic Engineering, CBS&H, he joined as Director Education at the Rani Lakshmi Bai Central Agricultural University, Jhansi, in 2018. His current responsibilities include establishing new colleges/campus, functional research, and teaching labs and initiating various teaching and research programs in agriculture and allied sectors. He has made outstanding research contributions in the area of Genomics for Crop Improvement, especially in resolving the complexity of agriculturally important traits such as the biotic stresses (fungal biology) and mineral nutrition. For the first time, he has identified several gene regulatory networks controlling agriculturally important traits using multi-pronged OMICS approaches. He has filed 11 patents (out of which 2 were granted). He has developed a sound center on agricultural biotechnology which is nationally recognized for its R&D in Biotechnology, now known as "Pantnagar Biotechnology Programme." His pioneering research has been highlighted by several magazines like *Nature* and published in international journals of repute. He has published more than 275 research papers both in national and internationally reputed peer-reviewed journals, 20 books and manuals besides around 80 popular articles, 75 book chapters, etc. The impact of Dr. Anil's work can be judged by >7775 citations with H-index 46 and i10 index 163. He is editor-in-chief of Agri-Life and Krishi Jeevan (The RLBCAU publications). He has guided 53 students for their PhD, MSc, and MVSc degree program in molecular biology and biotechnology besides 28 students of BTech (Biotech) for their project research guidance. He has successfully handled several DBT, DST, CSIR, and DRDO funded projects as principal investigator and program co-coordinator. During his long career, Dr. Kumar contributed to the development of modern agriculture at national and international level. He has been an outstanding teacher and researcher who is credited with many awards and recognitions from different organizations including ICAR, INSA, and DBT. He got recognition in the university, state, and at national level in the form of Dr. Sarvepalli Radhakrishnan University Best Teacher Award 2015; Uttarakhand Governor's Award three times in the year 2015, 2016, and 2018 for Best Research Paper; Bharat Ratna Dr. C. Subramaniam outstanding Teacher Award 2015; and INSA Teacher's Award 2014. Besides, he was also recipient of Regional Service Award (IFCC and APACC, 1993), Financial Award (IFCC, 1990), International Bursary Award (UK, 1996), and Food and Agricultural Organization Fellowship Award under ICAR-AHRD scheme from FAO (Rome, 2000–2001). He is a member of National Academy of Sciences, India, and executive member and Fellow of National Academy of Biological Sciences, Chennai, for his scientific contributions in the field of biological sciences. Dr. Anil has also been awarded the "Shiksha Rattan" and "Scientist of Excellence Award" and latest in the series Dr. Norman Borlaug Memorial Award-2025 for his meritorious services to the cause of Biotechnology education and research.

He is a widely travelled scientist and was visiting scientist/professor at several universities/institutes. He scintillated young minds and inculcated scientific temperament among his students who are serving on important positions at the national and international level. He is the most revered teacher who made modern biology look so simple and elegant at conceptual level.

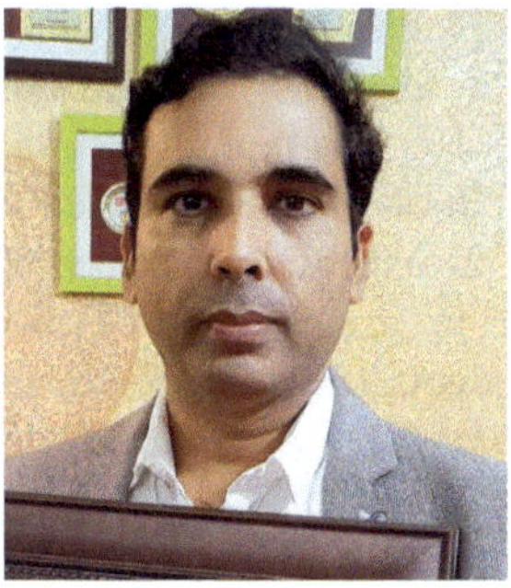

Manoj K. Tripathi is a postgraduate of Biochemistry from Dr. RMLA University and obtained PhD in Biochemistry from GB Pant University of Agriculture and Technology, Pantnagar. He is currently working as principal scientist (Biochemistry) at APPD, ICAR-CIAE (Govt. of India), Bhopal. His major areas of professional interest include medicinal compounds, functional and nutraceutical food, and fermented and probiotic food. He has guided more than 50 PG students and advisory member of 20 PHD students. He has published more than 105 research papers in international and national journal of repute, 93 abstracts, 60 book chapters, 55 popular articles, and 97 abstracts. He has authored/edited 15 books and 6 technical books in areas of food biochemistry, food processing, and food biotechnology. Two books received awards for Book of the Year and bestseller book. He has developed more than 34 process/technologies, worked on 22 national projects as PI and Co-PI, group leader of PMO-based activities on fruit-based carbonated beverage development, patent granted (Patent no. 435233), patents apply for 4 products, commercialized many process technologies, and registered genes in NCBI. He received several research grants from global network project on millet, NASF, ICAR, DST, and Ministry of Environment.

He has qualified for prestigious CSIR-Shyama Prasad Mukherjee fellowship (SPM, CSIR-2002. He has enlisted in the top 2% scientists of world—2021, 2022, 2023, and 2024 compiled by Stanford University, published by Elsevier. He has been elected as a Member of the National Academy of Sciences, India (NASI). He has been recipient of several prestigious awards and honors such as Established Scientist Award 2014, ISAE Team Award 2020, SAAR Distinguished Scientist Award in Crop Science 2021, Best Scientist Award 2017, Young Scientist Award, Recognition Award 2016, 16 best presentation awards in international and national conferences, honored as Marvellous Personality of India Award 2016 in Science, Lifetime Achievement Award 2017 by Innovative Research, Chennai, for outstanding achievements in the field of food processing research and publications. He has been conferred for Innovative Food Product Development (IFPD) Award, Certificate of Excellence-2012 by Science being Journal Publishing Group, Dehradun, India. He has been recognized as a Fellow of the Scientific Planet Society (FSPS), awards for Swachhta Abhiyan Mission and National Productivity Mission. His biography was published in Marvellous Records Book of India in science chapter, 2016. He is serving as executive member of Scientific Panel of DST WISE program, FSSAI: Fruits and Vegetables and their Products (FSSAI), Govt. of India, executive member of *BIS: FAD 10* and FAD 19 (Vegetables and Allied Products Sectional Committee, FAD 10 Products, Sectional committee Indian Standards on Infant Foods) Sectional Committee, BIS, Govt. of India. He is working as an editor-in-chief of *Octa Journal of Bioscience* (international peer-reviewed land NAAS rated), editor-in-chief of *Krishi Abhiyantriki Darpan* (ICAR-CIAE), editor of *Frontier Journal of Horticulture*, Switzerland, associate editor of *Scientific India*, and member of editorial board of more than 10 reputed national and international journals. He is a life member of Indian Society of Analytical Scientist, BARC, India; Society of Biological Scientists of India; the Indian Science Congress Association; Scientific Planet Society (SPS); AFSTI, India; and Society for Agriculture and Allied Research (SAAR), India. He served as nodal scientist for SMD- Agricultural Engineering for G20 Meeting of Agricultural Chief Scientists (MACS) at Varanasi, 2023. He has served as chairman, invited speaker, convener, organizing secretary, and members in more than 123 international and national symposium, conferences, and trainings. He established NABL accredited laboratory for food testing as lab head/quality manager and five others research labs in food technology, biotechnology, and instrumental methods of analysis.

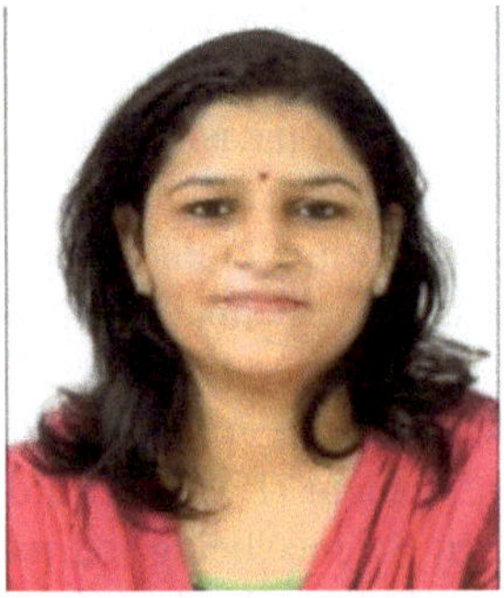

Nidhi V. Maheshwari, a Postgraduate in Microbiology (2005) and obtained PhD in Molecular Biology and Biotechnology (2010) from GB Pant University of Agriculture and Technology, Pantnagar. She has immensely contributed in the area of deciphering the molecular and regulatory networks associated with nitrogen use efficiency in finger millet using genomics, transcriptomics, and proteomics approaches for crop improvement. Understanding the role of plant-specific Dof transcription factors in regulation of NUE and accumulation of grain protein was her main area of interest. She started her career as temporary teaching assistant in 2010 from Department of Microbiology and Biotechnology, Maharaja Sayajirao (MS) University, Vadodara. During this tenure, she got DBT RA Fellowship 2011. Thereafter, in 2012, she received DBT BioCARe Women Scientist Fellowship, India. She is currently working as Assistant professor in Life Science Department, Somaiya Vidyavihar University, Mumbai, and as DST women scientist, a project based on molecular marker studies associated with grain calcium content in finger millet. She is presently also working on bioprospecting of mangroves and their endophytes for their pharmaceutical importance. Her major area of professional interest includes molecular biology, nutraceuticals, microbial biotransformation, and secondary metabolite production from medicinal plants. She has published 10 research papers and review articles, 15 book chapters, and 10 popular articles in national and international repute.

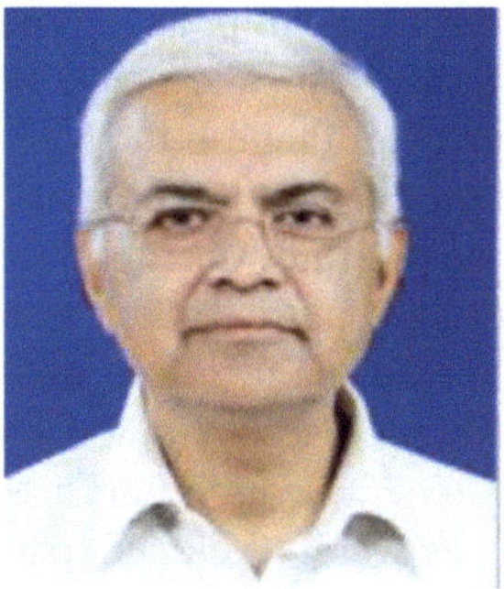

Sanjay Kumar obtained Master's and PhD degrees from GB Pant University of Agriculture and Technology, Pantnagar, and Indian Agricultural Research Institute, New Delhi, respectively. He joined CSIR-IHBT as "Scientist B" in 1990 and received post-doctoral training at Texas Tech University (USA), Rothamsted Research (UK), and Kansas State University (USA).

His major contributions include discovery of a novel carbon fixation pathway and its transplantation in a heterologous system to reduce photorespiratory losses leading to photosynthetic gain and yield enhancement (work lauded by international fraternity), discovery of autoclavable superoxide dismutase from high altitude plant, its characterization and modification, plant adaption mechanism at high altitude, cloning of genes for secondary metabolite synthesis and imparting stress tolerance, deciphering the mechanisms of winter dormancy and drought stress in tea, and enumerating molecular aspects of secondary metabolism in medicinal plants for catechins, picrosides, steviosides, shikonins, and podophyllotoxin biosynthesis. Significant contributions on transcriptome and genome sequencing of Himalayan plants and development of nutraceuticals using traditional/Ayurvedic knowledge. He guided 26 MSc/PhD students, holds several international patents, and has >190 peer-reviewed research/review articles/

edited book/book chapters, etc. Some of his key contributions have percolated to major reviews and books also.

He is Fellow of the National Academy of Sciences, National Academy of Agricultural Sciences and Crop Improvement Society of India. He was bestowed with prestigious VASVIK Industrial Research Award 2013 for Agricultural Science and Technology; R.D. Asana Endowment Lecture Award; Professor G.V. Joshi Memorial Lecture Award; Ultra International Team Award for contribution in Essential Oil Industry; Certificate of Merit in CSIR Leadership Programme and Young Scientist Award by Indian National Science Academy. He has been chairman/member of several professional committees and task forces, and has served on editorial boards of several international journals.

He is serving as Chairman, ASRB, New Delhi, and as Director of CSIR-IHBT since 11th June 2015 vitalized several initiatives for empowering the farmers, which include successful procurement and introduction of Heeng (asafoetida) and Monk fruit in the country, and introduction of saffron, cinnamon, tulip, and apple in non- traditional areas. Promoted aromatic plants in mountain farming, making Himachal Pradesh the leading state in the country for the production of wild marigold essential oil. Coordinated multi-institutional projects of CSIR as director of agri, nutri, and biotech theme, as well as nutraceuticals and nutritionals missions, for delivery of envisaged outcomes. With a keen focus on sustainable bioresource utilization for bioeconomy, a range of technologies were developed, patented, and transferred on priority, for products availability in the market. These efforts lead to brisk increase in MoUs/agreements/MTAs singed by the institute with entrepreneurs (from 9, during 2011–2015 to 650, during 2015–2022). Dr. Kumar catalyzed inclusive development of the institute by mobilizing financial resources from varied agencies and linking with relevant state, national, and international department(s)/agency (ies)/institute(s). With relentless approach for quality science and technology development, he led CSIR-IHBT to attain top position in the state and among top 10 of 37 institutes of CSIR as per the SCImago rating.

Contributors

Ghan Shyam Abrol Rani Lakshmi Bai Central Agricultural University, Jhansi, Uttar Pradesh, India
Manoj S. Aroor Food and Nutraceutical Laboratory, Dietetics and Nutrition Technology Division, CSIR-Institute of Himalayan Bioresource Technology, Palampur, Himachal Pradesh, India

S. S. Barve KET's Scientific Research Centre, Mumbai, India

Prashant Bhatt State Forensic Science Laboratory, Sagar, Madhya Pradesh, India

Riya Chouhan ICAR- Central Institute of Agricultural Engineering, Bhopal, Madhya Pradesh, India

Rahul Dev Food and Nutraceutical Laboratory, Dietetics and Nutrition Technology Division, CSIR-Institute of Himalayan Bioresource Technology, Palampur, Himachal Pradesh, India

Vineeta Dixit Department of Botany, Nilamber-Pitamber University, Garhwa, Jharkhand, India

Rashmi Dubey Department of Chemistry, Lal Bahadur Shastri College, Shaheed Nandkumar Patel Vishwavidyalaya, Raigarh, Chhattisgarh, India

Gayathiri Ekambaram Department of Plant Biology and Plant Biotechnology, Guru Nanak College (Autonomous), Velachery, Chennai, Tamil Nadu, India

Mahesh Gupta Food and Nutraceutical Laboratory, Dietetics and Nutrition Technology Division, CSIR-Institute of Himalayan Bioresource Technology, Palampur, Himachal Pradesh, India

Rajpal Singh Jadam ICAR- Central Institute of Agricultural Engineering, Bhopal, Madhya Pradesh, India

Chandrashekhar Y. Jagtap Central Ayurveda Research Institute, Jhansi, Uttar Pradesh, India

Department of Rasashastra and Bhaishajya Kalpana, All India Institute of Ayurveda, New Delhi, India

Preeti Jain Somaiya Vidyavihar University, Mumbai, Maharashtra, India

Smita Jain Department of Pharmacology, School of Pharmacy and Technology Management, SVKM's NMIMS Deemed-to-be University, Shirpur, Dhule, Maharashtra, India

Sandeep Kumar Jhade Department of Biological Science and Engineering, Maulana Azad National Institute of Technology, Bhopal, Madhya Pradesh, India

Shiny Punalur John Department of Medical Research, Faculty of Medicine and Health Sciences, SRM Institute of Science and Technology, Kattankulathur, Tamil Nadu, India

Swapnil Kadam KET's Scientific Research Centre, Mumbai, India

Shruti Kakodkar Somaiya Vidyavihar University, Mumbai, Maharashtra, India

Karthik Kalidoss Department of Biological Science and Engineering, Maulana Azad National Institute of Technology, Bhopal, Madhya Pradesh, India

Adinath Kate ICAR- Central Institute of Agricultural Engineering, Bhopal, Madhya Pradesh, India

Rishabh Kaundal Chemical Technology Division, CSIR-Institute of Himalayan Bioresource Technology, Palampur, Himachal Pradesh, India

Academy of Scientific and Innovative Research, (AcSIR), Ghaziabad, Uttar Pradesh, India

Samreen Khan ICAR- Central Institute of Agricultural Engineering, Bhopal, Madhya Pradesh, India

Aman Kumar ICAR- Central Institute of Agricultural Engineering, Bhopal, Madhya Pradesh, India

Anil Kumar Rani Lakshmi Bai Central Agricultural University, Jhansi, Uttar Pradesh, India

Ashwani Kumar Institute of Food Technology, Bundelkhand University, Jhansi, Uttar Pradesh, India

Dinesh Kumar Chemical Technology Division, CSIR-Institute of Himalayan Bioresource Technology, Palampur, Himachal Pradesh, India

Academy of Scientific and Innovative Research, (AcSIR), Ghaziabad, Uttar Pradesh, India

Elumalai Kuppusamy Department of Advanced Zoology & Biotechnology, Government Arts College (Autonomous), Nandanam, Chennai, Tamil Nadu, India

Nidhi V. Maheshwari Somaiya Vidyavihar University, Mumbai, Maharashtra, India

Mahendrakumar Mani Department of Biotechnology, Guru Nanak College (Autonomous), Velachery, Chennai, Tamil Nadu, India

Rahul Maurya Central Ayurveda Research Institute, Jhansi, Uttar Pradesh, India

Ashwini Kumar Mishra Department of Pharmaceutics, School of Pharmacy and Technology Management, SVKM's NMIMS Deemed-to-be University, Shirpur, Dhule, Maharashtra, India

Deepankar Mondal Department of Biotechnology, Guru Ghasidas Vishwavidyalaya, Bilaspur, Chhattisgarh, India

A. Nisha VIT School of Agricultural Innovations and Advanced Learning (VAIAL), Vellore Institute of Technology, Vellore, Tamil Nadu, India

Mohineeta Pandey Department of Botany, Guru Ghasidas Vishwavidyalaya, (A Central University) Koni, Bilaspur, Chhattisgarh, India

Sharad Pandey School of Agriculture, Uttaranchal University, Dehradun, Uttarakhand, India

Sudhir Kumar Pandey Department of Botany, Guru Ghasidas Vishwavidyalaya, (A Central University) Koni, Bilaspur, Chhattisgarh, India

Poonam Kumari Pathak Department of Biological Science and Engineering, Maulana Azad National Institute of Technology, Bhopal, Madhya Pradesh, India

Tanvi Phull Food and Nutraceutical Laboratory, Dietetics and Nutrition Technology Division, CSIR-Institute of Himalayan Bioresource Technology, Palampur, Himachal Pradesh, India

Chetna Porwal ICAR- Central Institute of Agricultural Engineering, Bhopal, Madhya Pradesh, India

Roshan Lal Sahu Department of Botany, Government Naveen College, Mainpat, Chhattisgarh, India

Deepa Sharma Central Ayurveda Research Institute, Jhansi, Uttar Pradesh, India

Divya Sharma School of Pharmaceutical Sciences, Delhi Pharmaceutical Sciences and Research University, Delhi, India

Sapnita Shinde Department of Biotechnology, Guru Ghasidas Vishwavidyalaya, Bilaspur, Chhattisgarh, India

Rahul Shrivastava Department of Biological Science and Engineering, Maulana Azad National Institute of Technology, Bhopal, Madhya Pradesh, India

Dhananjay Shukla Department of Biotechnology, Guru Ghasidas Vishwavidyalaya, Bilaspur, Chhattisgarh, India

Vibha Sinha Department of Biotechnology, Guru Ghasidas Vishwavidyalaya, Bilaspur, Chhattisgarh, India

Vigneshwaran Subramani VIT School of Agricultural Innovations and Advanced Learning (VAIAL), Vellore Institute of Technology, Vellore, Tamil Nadu, India

Astha Tirkey Department of Botany, Government Sant Rameshwar Gahira Guruji Mahavidyalaya, Jashpur, Chhattisgarh, India

Ankesh Tiwari Department of Botany, Guru Ghasidas Vishwavidyalaya, (A Central University) Koni, Bilaspur, Chhattisgarh, India

Department of Botany, Government Naveen College, Kabeerdham, Chhattisgarh, India

Atul Kumar Tiwari Department of Environmental Biology, Awadhesh Pratap Singh University, Rewa, Madhya Pradesh, India

Gauvrav Tiwari Department of Biotechnology, Guru Ghasidas Vishwavidyalaya, Bilaspur, Chhattisgarh, India

Vidisha Tomer VIT School of Agricultural Innovations and Advanced Learning (VAIAL), Vellore Institute of Technology, Vellore, Tamil Nadu, India

Manoj Kumar Tripathi ICAR- Central Institute of Agricultural Engineering, Bhopal, Madhya Pradesh, India

Soumya Tripathi Atal Bihari Vajpayee Govt Medical College, Vidisha, Madhya Pradesh, India

Nikitha Susan Varghese VIT School of Agricultural Innovations and Advanced Learning (VAIAL), Vellore Institute of Technology, Vellore, Tamil Nadu, India

Poonam Verma Department of Biotechnology and Microbiology, ISBM University, Gariyaband, Chhattisgarh, India

Naveen Kumar Vishvakarma Department of Biotechnology, Guru Ghasidas Vishwavidyalaya, Bilaspur, Chhattisgarh, India

Introduction: Diet and Nutrition 1

Manoj Kumar Tripathi, Nidhi V. Maheshwari, Anil Kumar, Aman Kumar, Rajpal Singh Jadam, and Adinath Kate

Abstract

Diet and nutrition are essential for maintaining health and well-being. A balanced diet offers the essential fuel for body's everyday activities. Our bodies need critical elements from food to execute efficiently. Consuming proper ratios of different nutrients provides individual requirements for nutrition. To keep a healthy balance, portion control and moderation are crucial. A balanced diet is having necessary nutrients which are crucial for preserving health and lowering the risk of chronic diseases. Attaining proper health conditions which covers body system, brain, and soul must be the key aim in human life. This is able only by proper routine such as concentrating on nutritious food and diet options, regular physical action, and also keeping and managing proper body weight by regular consumption of nutritious diet. Food is mainly governed by human health, and its components' cumulative effects on well-being. Noble diet is usually reflected with healthy life. Poor food and nutrition conditions add to atherosclerosis, osteoporosis, obesity, and some kinds of cancers.

Keywords

Health claims · Diet · Dietary pattern · Energy balance · Caloric intake · Dietary supplements

M. K. Tripathi (✉) · A. Kumar · R. S. Jadam · A. Kate
ICAR- Central Institute of Agricultural Engineering, Bhopal, Madhya Pradesh, India

N. V. Maheshwari
Somaiya Vidyavihar University, Mumbai, Maharashtra, India

A. Kumar
Rani Lakshmi Bai Central Agricultural University, Jhansi, Uttar Pradesh, India

A. Kumar et al. (eds.), *Innovations in Ayurvedic Nutrition*,
https://doi.org/10.1007/978-981-95-1213-3_1

1.1 Introduction

Diet and nutrition refer to the foods and nutrients that a person consumes and the effects those foods and nutrients have on their health and well-being. It contains the types of foods selected, the portion sizes, frequency of eating, and the complete dietary balance. Cultural, societal, economic, and individual aspects can have a major impact on a person's diet (Cenaand Calder 2020). The term nutrients states that *the method by which the body obtains and makes use of the nutrients present in food.* It requires the examination of the physiological and biochemical procedures that are influenced by the nutrition the body eats, absorbs, transports, metabolizes, and excretes. Carbohydrates, proteins, lipids, vitamins, minerals, and water are some of the food components that are important for well development and maintenance. The human system is responsible for the production of some nutrients. A majority of other nutrients are essentially taken from food sources to fulfil the human body's requirements. The nutrient categories which are fulfilled merely from diet are categorized as essential (Table 1.1). Proteins' molecules are involved in building and repairing of body tissues with the support of other biomolecules, especially of vitamins and minerals. These biomolecules are involved in the regulatory function of several human physiological processes.

A majority of people find liking eating of food, and eating allows connecting with people and families in pleasing atmospheres. This gathering always makes enjoyable celebrations. Starvation always indicates the requirement for diet. Hunger is a need for food-centred pleasant memories. At the time of hunger, the body provides some nerve indications, which, if ignored, may become strong, and it is possible to make poor food selection. Diet and nutritional requirement is the consequence of different biological routes by which our body consumes and utilizes for different biological process. When nutrients are extremely absent in the diet for a long period, some nutrient and other deficiency diseases can occur (Table 1.2).

1.2 Classification of Food

Food varies broadly with respect to nutrient contents and is categorized basically into three major categories based on its role as energy source, growth and development, and defensive process for body.

Table 1.1 Important biomolecules and their biological roles

S. No.	Organic nutrients	Biological functions
1.	Carbohydrates	Provide energy
2.	Proteins	Build and repair body tissue Provide energy
3.	Fats	Provide energy
	Inorganic nutrients	
4.	Minerals	Control body regulatory functions
5.	Water	Control body regulatory functions

Table 1.2 Nutrient deficiency conditions and promising reasons

S. No.	Illnesses	Deficiency
1.	Iron insufficiency	Iron
2.	Iron insufficiency anemia	Iron
3.	Night blindness	Vitamin A
4.	Beriberi	Thiamine
5.	Goiter	Iodine
6.	Marasmus	All nutrients
7.	All nutrients	Protein
8.	Osteomalacia	Vitamin D and calcium
9.	Osteoporosis	Calcium and vitamin D, P, Mn
10.	Pellagra	Niacin
11.	Rickets	Ca and vitamin D
12.	Scurvy	Vitamin C
13.	Xerophthalmia	Vitamin A

1.2.1 Energy Food

Energy source foods are mainly rich in carbohydrates and fats, which mainly provide the energy/fuel to preform major body functions, help in nutrient absorption, and also support in daily routine activities. The above food categories derive energy by the oxidation process of intake of foods and food ingredients. Major sources are cereals, dried fruits, several roots and tubers, fat sources, etc.

1.2.2 Growth-Promoting Foods

Protein-rich foods are mainly categorized in this group. They play a very essential role in development, support growth, and also provide energy to the body. Some high-quality protein sources are eggs, milk, meat, pulses, and nuts which provide good sources of protein. These diets are vital for many biological functions as tissue repair, muscular activities and development, and also overall body role.

1.2.3 Regulatory Food

These groups of foods are very rich in proteins, minerals, and vitamins. They play a very essential function in overall health and regulation, some important biological activities such as temperature regulation, muscle contraction, water balance, and cardiovascular activities. The major sources of protective foods include fruits, vegetables, milk, and eggs. Foods rich in proteins, minerals, and vitamins are also known as protective and regulatory foods. This food groups are further categorized into two major classes:

1. Rich in vitamins, minerals, and proteins with high biological value (BV). Example: milk, eggs, and liver.
2. Food rich in some specific vitamins and mineral molecules. Example: green leafy vegetables and fruits.

1.3 Food Group Plan

A majority of foods are classified on the basis of the presence of specific nutrients, and their class varies depending on several factors such as dietary habits, nutritional priorities, cultural aspects, and economic conditions. The nutrient-based classification helps in ensuring satisfactory nutrient intake in maintaining a diverse variety in food (Table 1.3).

1.4 Diet and Health

Proper nutrition is important for optimal human health. Poor food conditions increase the rate and risk of several chronic conditions such as cardiovascular, hypertension conditions, cancer conditions, and diabetic conditions. The intake of

Table 1.3 Food group, major nutrients, and sources

Food group	Key nutrients	Food sources
Cereal and millets	Carbohydrates, partially complete proteins, fibre (except rice), B-complex vitamins, some are rich in iron or calcium	All cereal and their products such as wheat, rice, maize, millets such as jowar, bajra, ragi (Nagali), semolina, poha, bread, noodles, pizza, puffed cereals
Protein body building foods	All pulses, bengal gram, green gram, red gram, black gram, lentil, soybeans, sprouts, groundnuts, sesame, almonds, oilseeds and nut	Moderately complete proteins, carbohydrates, iron, B-complex, niacin
	Protein, fat, iron, vitamins A, vit B complex	Milk and milk products.
	Protein, iron, fat, cholesterol, vitamins. A, B1, B2, B12, niacin.	Meat, fish, poultry, egg
Protective foods	Rich source of vitamins, minerals and fibre	Yellow, orange and red fruits and vegetables
	Ascorbic acid rich source	All citrus fruits, guava, tomato, pineapple etc.
Fats and oils, sugar and jaggery	Calories, oils provide vitamin E and essential fatty acids	Fat rich sources such as Vanaspati, margarine, shortenings, fresh cream, non-dairy cream, butter, clarified butter
	Vitamins A and D, fats rich sources	Plant based, fish oils
	Provide calories	Sugar sources
Secondary protective group	Carbohydrates, fibre, small amounts of vitamins and minerals	Banana, apple, chikoo, grapes, melons, pears

balanced food along with proper proteins, minerals, and protective food ingredients is always helpful in proper health. Several health surveys on food indicate that sufficient protein intake always contributed to proper growth and overall nutrition status.

1.4.1 Importance of Diet

Importance of diet is a concern for:

(a) *Overall Health Management*
A complete diet and appropriate food are vital for keeping general well-being. Energy, growth and development support, body function regulation, and chronic disorders for example cardiovascular disease, obesity, diabetic conditions, and several forms of cancer are all supported by the nutrients included in food.

(b) *Weight Management*
Diet and nutrition are essential for the management of weight. Persons who want to keep a healthy weight or lose weight might do so by having a clear understanding of the notion of calorie intake vs. calorie expenditure. People can make more up-to-date food selection if they are alert of portion size, macronutrients, and the value of balanced meals.

(c) *Disease Prevention and Management*
Consuming a healthy diet is vital for reducing and treating a number of illnesses. A healthy diet is useful in reduction of chronic environments. Some nutrients and eating habits may support in managing of pre-existing medical illnesses and augment general health consequences.

(d) *Energy and Performance*
A healthy diet provides energy as per need for physical activity. To recover, speed up recovery, and decrease the risk of injury, people frequently workout essentials to learn properly before, during, and after physical effort.

(e) *Cognitive Function*
The brain desires a healthy diet to function properly. For the healthy and proper operation of the brain organs, some important nutrients such as omega-3 fatty acids, vitamin B complex, important minerals, and antioxidant molecules are very vital. Diet affects brain health in concentration, memory, and general mental wellness.

(f) *Life Span*
Food has a high impact on long life and healthy ageing of human body. A healthy eating plan is effective to decrease the possibility of several age-related illnesses, recover bone problems, reduces the chance for ageing process, and hold muscle mass.

(g) *Sustainable and Ethical Food Choices*
Making supportable and proper food selection is vital for better understanding of diet and nutrition. It involves taking into account how food production affects the environment, promoting organic and local farming methods, and minimizing food waste.

1.5 Nutrients

Combination and proper quantity of nutrients present in diet are essential for health. The nutritive aspects should include:

The people eat food, not nutrients; though, it is the combination and quantities of nutrients in consumed foods that govern health. The study of nutrients, the ABC and numeric calculations of nutrition, will form a major part of the student's nutrition journey, and should include:

(a) Structure and features.
(b) Food sources, food composition, harvesting conditions, processing steps and formulation, and preparation step.
(c) Cell physiology uptake of the nutrient.
(d) Metabolic reaction.
(e) Nutrient supplies in some conditions such as lactation, pregnancy, and sport occasions.
(f) Nutrient–nutrient, nutrient–non-nutrients, nutrient–anti-nutrients interaction.

1.5.1 Basic Nutrients

The process through which organisms absorb and use nutrients from foodstuff for the body growth, improvement, and keep cell in proper biological functional form is referred to as nutrition. Intake, digestion, absorption, transport, and metabolism of nutrients are all part of it (Gush et al. 2021). Diet is the fundamental requirement of cell and life having nutrients in different forms which is necessary for the nourishment of cells. Food after eating gets digested and broken into different nutrients in absorbable form and then are transported to various parts of the body for daily physiological functions.

1.5.2 Nutritional Types

Carbohydrates, proteins, and fats are macronutrients, which our body requires in higher extent. They deliver energy for the growth and development and repair of human body tissues (Fogelholm et al. 2012). Micronutrients comprise vitamins and several minerals needed very small quantities for cell. They are important for many physiological processes and help in maintaining good health (Godswill et al. 2020). Water is not a nutrient, but essential for optimal hydration and plays many essential roles in the biological process (Camp 2013).

1.5.2.1 Benefits of a Good Nutrition

Optimal Health: A nutritious and balanced diet improves general health and reduces the possibility of chronic conditions in human body.

(a) *Energy and Vitality*: A balanced diet gives the energy need for daily tasks, improves physical performance, and sharpens mind.
(b) *Weight Management*: Keeping healthy body weight avoids obesity and the associated health issues.
(c) *Strong Immune System*: Suitable nutrition care for an immunity, which lowers the possibility of infections.
(d) *Better Mental Health*: Maintaining mental health, enlightening brain function, and lowering the danger of mental health issues are all supported by good nutrition (Nwankwoala and Ekenedo 2021).

1.5.2.2 Negative Effects of Poor Nutrition

Insufficient nutrient consumption and excessive nutrient consumption are two forms of malnutrition that can occur from improper eating of important nutrients. Immune systems that are compromised by poor nutrition are more susceptible to infections and chronic infections. Insufficient nutritional consumption, mainly during childhood and adolescence, can harm healthy growth of the body and brain. Poor nutrition can cause weariness, lower energy levels, and lower productivity in daily tasks. Bone health is compromised when nutrients like calcium and vitamin D are not properly consumed in appropriate amounts, which can result in illnesses like osteoporosis (Posner et al. 1993).

1.5.2.3 Nutritional Needs

Nutritional desires depend on age, sex, body size, physical activity, and general health. Guidelines like dietary consumptions and suggested dietary allowances provide the recommended daily intake of macronutrients, micronutrients, and water. Define specific dietary supplies based on individual circumstances by healthcare supplier or trained dietitian (Scrimshaw and Young 1976).

The human body wants these essential nutrients in order to maintain body function effectively. These nutrients, which a person obtains from diets, can be categorized into six different classes (Table 1.4):

I. *Carbohydrates*: The body utilizes carbohydrates as a chief source of energy. Foods like grains, fruits, vegetables, legumes, and other related things comprise them. Glucose, which is formed after carbohydrates' digestion, is required by cells to produce energy.
II. *Proteins*: Protein molecules are vital for the body growth and development and maintenance of biological tissues of human body. These are made of basic unit

Table 1.4 Basic nutrients and pharmaceutical formulation

S. No	Basic nutrients	Pharmaceutical formulation
1	Carbohydrates	Carbohydrate molecules are regularly used as receivers, fillers, and stabilizers in many pharmaceuticals formulations. Examples: Dextrose, cellulose, and lactose
2	Proteins	Protein molecules such as insulin and growth factors are mainly used as therapeutic agents in medicine industry. These molecules can serve as stabilizers in drug formulations in drug industries
3	Lipids	Lipids are largely utilized in pharmaceutical formulations as lubricants in tablets, emulsifiers, or solubilizers and better carriers in drug delivery systems. Some examples are triglycerides, phospholipids like lecithin and cholesterol
4	Vitamins	Vitamins are incorporated into several medicinal formulations as supplements or active ingredients to enhance nutritional value. They are mainly included in the preparation of several formulations and preparation of pills and capsules
5	Minerals	Minerals are used as medicinal agents and dietary supplements and commonly incorporated into liquid formulations, pills, and capsules
6	Water	Water is a very essential component in many pharmaceuticals formulations and widely used as a source of solvents and diluents in the drug delivery process in many pharmaceutical applications

amino acids, which function as the foundation for tissues and cells. Examples: meat, fish, poultry, dairy products, nuts, and legumes.

III. *Fats*: Fats are also utilized as a good source of energy and for assimilation of vitamins that are fat-soluble. Additionally, they shield and safeguard organs. Avocados, almonds, seeds, olive oil, and fatty seafood are all good sources of fat.

IV. *Vitamins*: Vitamins are important micronutrients and are essential for several biological processes. They classified into two major groups: First group constitutes fat-soluble vitamins A, D, E, and K and second group constitutes water soluble vitamins as; vitamin C and all the B vitamins: Thiamin (B1), Riboflavin (B2), Niacin (B3), Pantothenic Acid (B5), Pyridoxine (B6), Biotin (B7), Folate (B9), and Cobalamin (B12.

V. *Minerals*: Minerals play an important role in many biological processes such as energy metabolic pathways, bone growth and development, nervous system, and signalling pathway. Examples of good food sources of minerals are leafy greens, nuts, seeds, dairy products, and seafood.

VI. *Water*: Water is not categorized as a nutrient but very crucial for hydration of body and its involvement in many physiological functions. It helps in digestion process, nutrient transport, excretion, temperature regulation, and many more biological functions. For better health and staying healthy, our body requires consuming an adequate amount of water daily.

These nutrients are crucial for human health; however, their pharmaceutical applications may vary depending upon situations and formulation requirements. The above given examples are not exhaustive but exemplify common medicinal uses of certain nutrients (Maurya et al. 2021).

1.5.2.4 Energy Equilibrium

Energy equilibrium in food and nutrition states is the connection between calories ingested via diet (energy intake) and calories used in physical activity and biological processes (energy expenditure). It is an important idea for handling weight and maintaining general health. The balance between energy consumption and outflow in humans is known as the energy balance. It is a basis idea in the study of cell metabolism, nutrition, and weight control (Thomas et al. 2014). Energy intake surpasses energy outflow, meaning more calories are taken in than are burned in case the body is in a positive energy balance. In this case, the extra energy is deposited as body fat, which eventually causes weight gain. In contrast, when intake exceeds expenditure, then negative energy balance, which causes weight loss as the body uses up its supplies of stored energy. For overall health and well-being, it is necessary to keep a healthy energy balance. Prolonged negative energy balance can cause undernourishment, a poor immune system, and muscular loss. Keeping energy balance needs depends upon the quality and quantity of the diet. The energy content of per gram of various macronutrients is as follows: Proteins and carbohydrates each provide approximately 4 calories per gram and fat provides about 9 calories per gram.

In order to keep suitable energy balance, following calories are crucial. Consuming extra calories than the body requirements over time can lead to weight gain. Contrarily, eating fewer calories than necessary might result in weight loss. When energy consumption surpasses energy outflow, the human body stores the surplus as fat and leads to increase in body weight gain. Equally, if energy consumption is less than energy outflow, the body uses energy reserves, causing body weight loss. Body weight remains stable when energy intake and consumption are in balance. Achieving energy balance where energy input and output are equal ensures steady weight without any net gain or loss. Energy expenditure primarily consists of three components:

(a) *Basal Metabolic Rate (BMR)*: The amount of energy consumed by body to keep important functions in rest conditions such as breathing, circulation, and cell growth.
(b) *Physical Exercise*: This includes both formalized workouts and everyday chores like walking, gardening, and cleaning.
(c) *Thermal Effect of Food (TEF)*: The energy used during the physiological functions such as digestion, processing, and absorption of nutrients from food.

These food groups offer necessary nutrients while serving to limit calorie intake. Maintaining a healthy balance of energy requires good portion control. Even when choosing nutritious foods, eating greater quantities can result in higher energy intake. Effective portion control is key to keeping a healthy energy balance. Regular exercise increases the number of calories burned, promoting a negative energy balance and potentially aiding in weight loss. To achieve and sustain a healthy energy balance, it is beneficial to combine a balanced diet with regular physical activity.

1.6 Biological Significance of Macronutrients in Human Body

Macronutrients are essential nutrients which are required in large amounts by human body for growth, development, energy production, and overall body well-being. The three crucial macronutrients are carbohydrates, proteins, and lipids (Scholtens et al. 2020).

1.6.1 Carbohydrates

The carbohydrates offer major energy and each gram of carbohydrate provides 4 calories. To keep a constant energy supply, the body stocks carbohydrates in the liver and muscle cells in the form of glycogen, which the body uses when required. The major sources of carbohydrates are included in Table 1.5. Some sources provide significant vitamins, minerals, and some protein molecules. Though, in processing steps, some of these nutrients are gone. To maintain these nutrients, food manufacturers frequently add vitamin B complex such as thiamine, riboflavin, and niacin along with some important minerals. When a nutrient originally is not found in the grain and is added during processing, the product is categorized as fortified.

1.6.1.1 Energy Source

Glucose is utilized as the primary energy source and is formed after hydrolysis of carbohydrates. It fuels important bodily processes such as metabolism, brain function, and muscle contraction. Excess glucose is stored in body in liver and muscles as glycogen, which can be quickly converted back into glucose when energy is needed.

1.6.2 Carbohydrate Types

The major groups of carbohydrates are classified as simple and complex (Ortiz et al. 2022).

1.6.2.1 Simple Carbohydrates

These are grouped as sugars which are rapidly digested and absorbed. Excessive eating of simple carbohydrates causes fast spike in blood sugar levels and diabetic conditions. Examples include table sugar, honey, candies, and sweetened beverages.

Table 1.5 Brief descriptions of carbohydrate molecules

Types of carbohydrates	Functions	Source of carbohydrates	Deficiency symptoms
Monosaccharides			
Glucose	Furnish energy	Berries, Grapes	Fatigue
	Spare proteins Prevent ketoacidosis	Sweet corn syrup	Weight loss
Fructose	Provide minerals, vitamins, and dietary fibre	Ripe fruits, honey	
Galactose		Lactose molecules	
Disaccharides			
Sucrose	Energy source Protein sources Prevent ketoacidosis	Sugar cane Sugar beets Molasses Maple syrup Jams and jellies	Fatigue Weight loss
Maltose	Energy source	Digestion of starch	
Lactose	Support for gut health Calcium absorption	Milk	
Polysaccharides			
Starch	Energy source Prevent ketoacidosis	Cereal grains and their products	Fatigue Weight loss
Dextrins	Provide fibre	Hydrolyzed starch	
Glycogen	Provide fibre	Stored glucose in liver and muscles	
Cellulose	Provide fibre	Whole-grain cereals, leafy vegetables, and fruits	Constipation Colon cancer Diverticulosis

1.6.2.2 Complex Carbohydrates

Complex carbohydrates require longer time for hydrolysis and slow release of glucose into the bloodstream. Additionally, they are rich in fibre molecules, which help in regulation of blood sugar levels. Examples: whole grains, legumes, vegetables, and fruits, and consist of longer chains of sugar molecules.

1.6.2.3 Fibre

Fibre molecule is a category of complex carbohydrate which the body cannot completely digest and is found mainly in foods with plant origin like whole grains, legumes, fruits, vegetables, and offers several health benefits, including:

(a) *Improved Digestive Health*: Dietary fibre improves steady bowel movements and decreases the possibility of constipation. It also helps to prevent several digestive disorders such as diverticulitis and haemorrhoids.
(b) *Blood Sugar Control*: Soluble fibre reduces the absorption of glucose molecules and also supports in controlling blood sugar levels and decreases the occurrence of the possibility of type 2 diabetes conditions.

(c) *Management of Body Weight*: Fibre-rich foods promote satiety and help in reduction of starvation and are frequently make them more filling. This can support in maintaining an improved body weight.
(d) *Management of Heart Health*: Soluble fibre, which is found in legumes and oats, helps in reducing the cholesterol levels, which decreases the risk of cardiovascular diseases.

1.6.2.4 Recommended Intake

The recommended carbohydrate consumption depends on person's health conditions Usually, carbohydrates should make up 45–65% of the regular caloric consumption. It is significant to prioritize complex carbohydrates from whole, unprocessed foods and reducing the intake of refined grains and additional sugars.

The glycaemic index (GI) value shows how rapidly a carbohydrate-containing food increases blood sugar levels. Low GI diets, such as whole grains and legumes, cause blood sugar levels to increase more gradually and progressively than foods with a high GI, such as white bread and sugary food items that cause quicker and higher spikes in blood sugar (Atkinson et al. 2008).

1.6.3 Proteins

Proteins are essential to maintain structural and functional properties of every cell. By the age of four, the protein content in the body stabilizes at approximately 18% of total body weight equivalent to the levels found in adults. An acceptable supply of proteins in the everyday diet is important for human health. The term *protein* is derived from the Greek word *proteios*, meaning "of first importance." Proteins build and repair body tissue, play key roles in regulating many body functions, and provide energy if there is inadequate carbohydrate and fat in the diet.

Proteins are found in both animal and plant foods. The animal food sources deliver the top quality of complete proteins. They comprise meats, fish, poultry, eggs, milk, and cheese. In spite of the high biologic value of proteins from animal food sources, they also provide saturated fats and cholesterol. Accordingly, complete proteins should be carefully selected from low-fat animal foods such as fish, lean meats, and low-fat dairy products. Proteins originating from plant foods are incomplete proteins and are of a lower biologic quality than those found in animal foods. Examples of plant foods containing protein are corn, grains, nuts, sunflower seeds, sesame seeds, and legumes such as soybeans, navy beans, pinto beans, split peas, chickpeas, and peanuts. Plant proteins can be used to produce textured soy protein and tofu, also called analogues. Meat alternatives (analogues) made from soybeans contain soy protein and other ingredients mixed together to simulate various kinds of meat. Meat alternatives may be canned, dried, or frozen. Analogues are excellent sources of protein, iron, and B vitamins. Tofu is a soft cheese-like food made from soy milk. Tofu is a bland product that easily absorbs the flavours of other ingredients with which it is cooked. Tofu is rich in high-quality proteins and B vitamins, and low in sodium. Textured soy protein and tofu are both economical and nutritious meat replacements. Because of their inclusion of either dairy products and eggs or dairy products alone, most individuals who follow lacto-ovo vegetarian or lacto-vegetarian diets will be able to meet their protein requirements through a balanced diet that includes milk and milk products, enriched grains, nuts, and legumes. Strict vegetarians who consume no animal products will need to be more careful to include other protein-rich food sources such as soybeans, soy milk, and tofu.

The quality and value of protein molecules is determined by the number and kinds of amino acids present in proteins. Out of the 20 amino acids, only 10 are grouped as essential to humans (Table.1.6).

Human health, diet, and nutrition depend greatly on proteins, which are important macronutrients. Proteins are important for the growth, repair, and involve in many bodily functions (Cianci 2021).

1.6.3.1 Building Blocks

Amino acids are the smallest units that make up proteins. Our bodies need each of the 20 different amino acids for optimum operation. Nine of these amino acids are regarded as essential since our bodies are unable to manufacture them, necessitating dietary intake. One or more necessary amino acids are missing from incomplete proteins, which are found in plant-based food sources.

(a) Proteins serve as the basis for the growth, development, and repair of human body. Protein supplies are significant for healthy development. Protein molecules are also essential for tissue regeneration and repair following injuries or strenuous activity.
(b) Proteins function as enzymes, which act as catalysts for biological reactions within the body. Likewise, some proteins also function as hormones, as chemical messengers that control many biological processes. Enzymes help several critical roles in the human body such as digestion, metabolism, and body molecular physiology as DNA replication, while hormones control and manage many important physiological activities.
(c) Proteins are necessary for proper immune system functioning. Antibodies, which are proteins formed by the immune system, play a crucial role in the

Table 1.6 Types of amino acids

Essential		Nonessential	
Arginine[a]	Phenylalanine	Alanine	Glutamine
Histidine[a]	Threonine	Arginine[a]	Glycine
Isoleucine	Tryptophan	Asparagine	Histidine[a]
Leucine	Valine	Aspartic acid	Proline
Lysine		Cysteine	Serine
Methionine		Glutamic acid	Tyrosine

[a]Essential in childhood only

defensive system of the body against illnesses and other invaders. Insufficient quantity of protein consumption directly affects immune response, and body cell become more sensitive for infections and illnesses.

(d) Foods rich in protein are commonly more satisfying than those high in carbohydrates or lipids. Containing a sufficient quantity of protein in diets and snacks can be advantageous in controlling hunger by reducing hungers and encouraging weight management by avoiding overdosing.

(e) Protein requirements might vary with person, differ in age, sex, body weight, and overall health prospects. Common recommendations are 0.8 grams of protein per kilogram of body weight that usually accounts for 10–35% of daily caloric intake. However, certain cases such as athletes, pregnant women, patients recovering from illness or injury may need higher protein consumption.

(f) The value of protein indicates composition and digestibility of amino acid present in protein. Animal-based proteins are high-quality proteins as they are simply digested and rich in all essential amino acids in the correct amounts. In comparison, plant-derived proteins have fewer amounts of digestible quantities of certain essential amino acids. By consuming a diversity of plant-derived protein with appropriate level, one can achieve a complete amino acid profile.

1.6.3.2 Biological Value of some Important Proteins

Biological value (BV) of food is an indication of food quality in terms of proteins and defined as the quantity of absorbed nitrogen which is reserved in the body. A high BV has more nitrogen than a protein with low BV (Table 1.7). Perfect protein shows a biological value of 100 (Schaafsma 2005).

Animal-based proteins (e.g., eggs, milk, meat, and fish) commonly have higher BV because they comprise almost totally essential amino acids in ideal quantities. Plant-based proteins (e.g., soy, legumes, rice, and wheat) have lesser BV as they may be deficient in one or more essential amino acids (as limiting amino acids) and have inferior digestibility due to the presence of fibre and some anti-nutritional factors (Layman and Rodriguez 2009). Whey protein has the maximum BV, and the value reported is beyond 100; due to its rapid digestibility and excellent amino acid profile, it is the popular choice for muscle repair and growth. Whole eggs are reported as gold standard for protein quality, with a BV of 100 which provides total essential amino acids in the maximum bioavailable form.

Table 1.7 Biological values of important foods

Foodstuff	Biological value (BV)	Foodstuff	Biological value (BV)
Gelatin	00	Soy protein	78
Groundnuts	55	Fish	83
Wheat	66	Milk	85
Rice	73	Egg	100 (reference standard)
Meat	75	Whey protein	104

1.6.4 Lipids or Fats

Fats are hydrophobic in nature which do not dissolve in water molecules and soluble in organic solvents. Fat-rich foods are generally more expensive than carbohydrate-based alternatives. Like carbohydrates, fats are composed of carbon, hydrogen, and oxygen, but they contain significantly less oxygen.

Our health, diet, and nutrition depend greatly on fats and essential macronutrients. It is true that fats have frequently been linked to bad health outcomes (Chen et al. 2013). The intense form of energy arises from fats. They deal more than double as many calories per grams proteins and carbohydrates. Adipose tissue in body stores fat and is utilized as a basic source of energy during fasting period or when body calorie consumption is deficient. There are various kinds of fat, and each one has a particular effect on health:

Saturated Fats: Mainly originate from animal-based foods like butter, full-fat dairy products, and fatty meats. Saturated fats should be consumed in moderation since a high intake has been reported to cause a risk of heart disease.

Unsaturated Fats: Classified into two kinds, and reported to be healthier substitutes.

Monounsaturated Fats: Foods like olive oil, avocados, and almonds are rich in these fats. They involve in lowering the levels of LDL (bad fat) cholesterol although increases levels of HDL (good fat) cholesterol, which has been associated with boosted heart health.

Omega-3 and Omega-6 Fatty Acids: Omega-3 and omega-6 fatty acids are essential polyunsaturated fats which our body cannot produce. Omega-3 sources comprise fatty fish, flaxseeds, and walnuts, while omega-6 is present in vegetable oils and seeds. Keeping a proper and balance intake is key for heart health, inflammation regulation, and brain function.

Trans Fats: Trans fats are produced during the process of hydrogenation. They are reported in fried, processed, and baked goods as well as in margarine and several fast food items. Trans fats should be avoided as much as possible because they are strongly associated with heart problems (Gurr et al. 2008).

Fat molecules plays an essential role in the absorption of all fat-soluble vitamins. For efficient absorption and proper utilization of fat-soluble vitamins, the presence of fat is essential. Addition of fats (healthy) in food helps in possible absorption of above fat-soluble vitamins. Fats are also involved in the production of some hormones. Many hormones, comprising sex hormones and adrenal hormones derived from the fat named cholesterol.

Fats are necessary parts of cell membranes, giving them structure and supporting in the cellular functions. For the health and brain biological functions, omega-3 fatty acids play a very vital role (Bloomer et al. 2009). Depending on a person's necessities and health objectives, different amounts of fats are advised which differ according to individuals. Though, it is mostly recommended that fats used 20 and 35 percent of our daily caloric intake. Consuming mainly unsaturated fats from plant-derived food sources should be a priority. Trans fats and saturated fats must be minimum in the diet. The focus should be on ingesting healthy sources of fats in moderation rather than altogether avoiding them.

1.6.4.1 Utilities

Many important roles of fats and oil in biological reactions are:

1. Energy source for many tissues.
2. Protein function.
3. Body thermal insulation and supports in holding body heat.
4. Guarding of vital organs from much external mechanical damage.
5. Involved in absorption of fat-soluble vitamins.
6. Essential for linoleic and linolenic acids requirement in body.
7. Enhance the flavour of food.
8. Involved in cell membranes synthesis.
9. Involved in synthesis of some important hormones.

1.7 Micronutrients

Micronutrients are essential nutrients which is required in very minimal amounts for the body to maintain good health and proper action. Micronutrients comprise of minerals and vitamins, which are crucial to several biological roles. Micronutrients are commonly defined in milligrams (mg) or micrograms (g), which are required in minor quantities in comparison to macronutrients. Vitamins and minerals are the two core groups of micronutrients. The following sections summarize the several micronutrient varieties found in these groups:

1.7.1 Vitamins

Vitamin molecules are important compounds which are required in lesser quantities and involved in many biochemical and physiological reactions in cells. Vitamin molecules not only provide energy but also play an important role in the body by using the energy provided by major macronutrients. The term vitamin highlights vitamins' crucial role, with word "vita" meaning life in Latin. They should be used in moderation, as using more does not necessarily yield better results. Excessive consumption of vitamins can cause human toxicity. They are categorized on the basis of their solubility property (Table 1.8).

Vitamin deficiencies in human bodies can cause various diseases and health issues. Several persons are in high risk due to vitamin deficiencies caused by several reasons such as imbalanced intake includes alcohol, low income, patients with severe illnesses which affect hunger, with intellectual disabilities, and inadequate care by children.

Vitamins are heat sensitive and reported to lost or reduce during processing. In some processing industries, it is replaced with other synthetic sources for

Table 1.8 Essential vitamins for human health

Vitamin types	Vitamins	Key functions
Fat-soluble	Vit A	Helps in eye vision, immunity development, and skin issue
	Vit D	Calcium and phosphorus absorption for bone and immune function
	Vit E	Antioxidant function supports skin and eye health
	Vit K	In blood clotting and bone strengthening.
Water-soluble vitamins	Thiamine (Vitamin B1)	Role in energy metabolism and nerve function
	Riboflavin (Vitamin B2)	Key for energy production and skin health.
	Niacin (Vitamin B3)	Role in transforming food into energy and supports skin and nerve health
	Pantothenic acid (Vit B5)	Supports in metabolic energy control and in synthesis of hormone
	Pyridoxine (Vitamin B6)	Vital for brain development and function, energy conversion
	Biotin (Vitamin B7)	Essential in metabolic process
	Folic acid (Vitamin B9)	In synthesis of DNA and cellular division, important during pregnancy process
	Cobalamin (Vit B12)	In nervous system, synthesis of RBC and DNA
	Ascorbic acid (Vit C)	Boosts immune function, helps in wound healing, acts as an antioxidant

maintaining the nutritional conditions of processed food as unprocessed food materials. The presence of light, air, heat, and water simply damage the biological properties of some vitamins. Therefore, it is crucial to minimize the vitamin loss during preparation/cooking stage. These damage can be minimized as:

- Use of fresh vegetables and fruits.
- Formulating fresh vegetables and fruits products.
- Steaming vegetables preserves more vitamins compared to boiling.
- Avoid excess of cutting. Keep them in larger pieces if possible.
- Store cooked foods in airtight containers.
- Avoid overcooking to minimize vitamins destroy.
- Use frozen forms.
- Minimize the use of water.
- Stored in cool and dark place.
- Preserve with minimal processing.

1.7.2 Importance of Vitamins

Retinol (Vit A): Retinol is important for eye health. It also supports the immunological reaction, cell division and growth, and protects mucous membranes and skin.

Cholecalciferol (Vit D): Vit D is crucial for healthy bones and absorption of calcium. It upkeeps perfect bone mineralization by regulating the body's calcium and phosphorus levels. Vitamin D may play additional roles in cell development and differentiation, beyond its well-known role of immune system function (Holick 2007).

Tocopherols (Vit E): Vit E also categorizes as an antioxidant which helps in preventing free radical generation and detoxification from damaging cells. Vitamin E is useful in maintaining healthy skin, enhances immune function, and also benefits in cardiovascular health (Bertone-Johnson 2009).

Phylloquinone (*Vit K)*: Vitamin K is needed during blood clotting in human body. It involves in making of clotting factors. It also helps bone health by facilitating proper calcium deposition in bones (Shea and Booth 2011).

Ascorbic Acid (Vit C): Vit C acts as a strong antioxidant which is very helpful in avoiding cellular damage. It supports immune system, boosts collagen synthesis, improves iron absorption, and serves in various enzymatic processes as a cofactor (Carr and Maggini 2017).

B-complex Vitamins: B-complex vitamins play an important role in the process of energy metabolism. They support in the metabolism of major biomolecules to produce energy. These vitamins are also play crucial roles in DNA synthesis, red blood cell formation, and appropriate neuronal function (Harrison and Johnson 2006). Vitamins are usually found in balanced diet. Since different foods deliver different vitamins, therefore, consuming a variety of foods (plant and animal sources) helps in maintaining the vitamin level in the body.

1.7.3 Minerals

Minerals are inorganic matters important for many physiological processes in the body. They are important for keeping complete health and essential to be consumed in appropriate amounts to safeguard best nutrition (Miller and Farber 2006). Highly processed or refined foods contain minimal to no minerals. To balance this shortage, nutrients like iron, thiamine, riboflavin, niacin, and folate are often supplemented, which are then branded as "enriched foods."

Maximum amount of minerals in food occurs as soluble salts, and the probability of loss during cooking with water is very high. To reduce this loss, foods should be prepared with least water or, ideally, steamed. Any remaining cooking liquid should be preserved and repurposed in soups, gravies, or sauces. This workout not only increases the flavour of this food but also boosts their nutrient content.

1.7.3.1 Calcium

Calcium molecule is important for the growth and development to maintain healthy bones, nerves' communication, blood clotting, and hormones' metabolism.

1.7.3.2 Magnesium

Magnesium is a crucial element involved in many biochemical and physiological reactions in the body system such as synthesis of protein, control of blood glucose level, nervous system, muscular function, and blood pressure regulation (Rude 2010, Dickinson et al. 2006; Del Gobbo et al. 2013). Magnesium is also important in vitamin D conversion into active form for calcium absorption and metabolism, parathyroid hormone function (Medalle et al. 1976).

1.7.3.3 Iron

Iron (Fe) is found abundantly in all body cells and plays a major role in myoglobin and haemoglobin structure and also works as an oxygen carrier in the blood and muscles. Iron quantities in body should essentially be controlled because extreme iron concentration causes tissue damage because of free radical generation in the body (Imam et al. 2017).

1.7.3.4 Zinc (Zn)

Zinc participates in structure, catalytic, and regulatory actions in the body (Kawamura et al. 2012) and is one of the important trace element in the human body. It plays an important role in many molecular, cellular, metabolic, and immunological processes in the human body as an antioxidative agent, anti-inflammatory agent, and anti-apoptotic agent (Haase and Rink 2014). Zinc participates in a variety of enzymatic reactions and is necessary for DNA synthesis, protein synthesis, immune system activity, and wound healing. It affects how taste and smell are perceived as well.

1.7.3.5 Selenium

Selenium (Se) is found in minor amounts in the human body (Attar et al. 2015). A suitable amount is significant for numerous human biological activities such as immunity, reproductive system, thyroid gland working, nervous system, cardiovascular, endocrine, and muscle function (Roman et al. 2014; Rayman 2012). It helps as a defensive molecule to inactivate the free radical molecules with the help of enzymatic activity (Fang et al. 2017, Bellinger et al. 2009). As an antioxidant, selenium shields the body cells from injury with free radicals. It affects the metabolism of thyroid hormones, immunological system, and reproductive system.

1.7.3.6 Potassium

It is an electrolyte that supports healthy neuron and muscle function, blood pressure regulation, and fluid balance. Additionally, it affects how the heart works and how the body communicates electrical signals.

Another electrolyte that contributes to fluid equilibrium and is essential for nerve and muscle contractions is sodium. It is essential for preserving healthy cellular activity.

1.7.3.7 Iodine

Iodine (I) is an important trace element for regular growth and development process and is also involved in protein, carbohydrates and lipid synthesis, and physiological functions and coordinates the metabolic processes. Iodine deficiency causes hypothyroidism, goitre, foetal defects, and higher frequency of neonatal death (Führer et al. 2014; Pearce 2014). Iodine controls metabolism, growth, and development.

1.7.3.8 Copper

Copper (Cu) plays a crucial role in biological functions in humans as a cofactor of several enzymes and proteins (La Fontaine et al. 2002; Attar et al. 2014). It is associated with certain defence enzymes as superoxide dismutase and also with red blood cells formation (Attar et al. 2013).

1.7.3.9 Manganese

Manganese is a critical element associated with enzyme synthesis, protein synthesis, vitamin B, and vitamin C synthesis, regulation of the blood sugar levels, immune system, and haematopoiesis It also plays an antioxidative function ((Deng et al. 2013; Lee et al. 2015).

A balanced food including a range of foods such as whole grains, fruits, vegetables, legumes, nuts, seeds, and lean proteins is usually how these minerals are obtained. For preserving the overall health and avoiding shortages or imbalances that could cause health problems, it is crucial to consume enough minerals. Under the direction of a healthcare practitioner, dietary supplements could occasionally be suggested to address particular deficits.

1.8 Common Diet Patterns

Common dietary patterns are those which populations constantly monitor when it comes to eating habits and dietary practices. These trends frequently reflect social, geographic, and cultural variables.

1.8.1 Mediterranean Eating

The Mediterranean diet (MedDiet), abundant in minimally processed plant-based foods, rich in monounsaturated fat from olive oil, but lesser in saturated fat, meats, and dairy products, appears an ideal nutritional model for cardiovascular health.

The traditional eating practices of the residents of Mediterranean Sea-bordering nations including Greece, Italy, Spain, and Morocco are the motivation for the Mediterranean diet, a dietary style. It has gained attention for its possible health benefits and is usually suggested as a healthy eating strategy (Martínez-González and Martín-Calvo 2016). The Mediterranean diet strongly emphasizes on plant-based foods and encourages the consumption of fruits, vegetables, whole grains, legumes, nuts, and seeds. These foods are a good source of fibre, antioxidants, vitamins, and minerals. The diet emphasizes the consumption of healthy fats, mainly olive oil. Olive oil is rich in monounsaturated fats (MUFA), a good fat group for the heart health. Some additional sources of healthy fats include nuts, seeds, and fatty fish such as salmon and sardines, all of which contribute to overall heart health and well-being.

The Mediterranean diet contains moderate intake of dairy food products like yogurt and cheese, along with poultry and eggs. Dietary habits and practices reflect common patterns that persons or peoples regularly follow. These patterns are usually affected by geographical, cultural, and societal factors (Sacks 2001).

The Mediterranean food is encouraged by the old consumption practices of individuals in nations nearby the Mediterranean Sea, such as Greece, Italy, Spain, and Morocco. Well known for its possible health benefits, it is frequently suggested as a fit and supportable food plan. The diet confines red meat intake and highlighting protein sources like fish and seafood, which are rich in heart-favourable omega-3 fatty acids.

1.8.2 The Mediterranean Diet Has Many Advantages

1.8.2.1 Management of Heart Health

The Mediterranean food is linked with lesser amounts of LDL (bad) cholesterol having reduced possibility of heart disease. It highlights heart-healthy fats, fibre-rich foods, and minimally treated constituents although restricts the eating of saturated fats and processed foods.

1.8.2.2 Management of Body Weight

Mediterranean food does not enforce strict calorie constraints, its stress on total, nutrient-dense diets and needful portion control can help in keeping a healthy weight (Paoli et al. 2013).

1.8.2.3 Management of Diabetes

Accepting a Mediterranean-style consumption arrangement has been shown to help in control of blood sugar levels in diabetic patients and can also decrease the threat of emerging type 2 diabetes.

1.8.2.4 Management of Brain Health

According to some research, the Mediterranean diet may protect against cognitive decline and lower the risk of neurodegenerative disorders like Alzheimer's.

1.8.2.5 Management of Certain Cancers

Several studies reported that intake of a Mediterranean-style diet, which is higher in fruits, vegetables, and antioxidants, can decrease the case of increasing certain cancers, including colorectal and breast cancers.

1.9 Plant-Based Diet

A plant-based food highlights the intake of foods derived from fruits, vegetables, whole grains, legumes, nuts, and seeds (Tham et al. 1998). This methodology places plant-based foods as the base of a healthy eating pattern. Numerous studies have established that a plant-based diet deals with health benefits and is helpful in minimizing the threat of several chronic conditions. Plant-derived diets are generally concentrated with fibre, phytochemical molecules, antioxidant molecules, vitamins, minerals and several phytonutrients, and ultimately improve healthy conditions.

1.10 Ayurveda Principles of Food Preparation and Intake

Ashta ahara vidhi vishesha yatana, or eight principles of diet development and consumption, is an important aid of Ayurveda to healthy consumption. These eight constituents involve in food making, arrangement, packing, and intake.

1.10.1 Role of Prakriti

The nature of a food indicates the basic types which are observed with the help of complementary quality named gurvadiguna, which mainly signifies the fundamental power of diet. Therefore, the critical life belongings of food mainly indicate the nature of nutrition.

1.10.2 Qualitative Attributes of Food

Ayurveda categorizes diet by many important qualitative aspects. Foods are mainly classified into three categories: Sattvic, Rajasic, and Tamasic, each aligning with different temperaments and dispositions.

Sattvic foods are satisfying in nature with respect to flavour and appearance and support good health, mental clarity, and overall well-being. They are supposed to involve in nourishing mind and body. Many processed, junk, and preserved foods usually consumed currently fall into this category, having harmful effects on health. Tamasic foods are spoiled, dried, or contaminated, and are supposed to cloud the mind, harming its proper functioning. These foods are unfavourable for both physical health and mental clarity, delaying a person's ability to think and act efficiently.

Despite several valuable components of the Ayurvedic viewpoint on food and nutrition, the issues lies in interpreting these concepts into practical applications. The one key issue is the lack of objective, evidence-based approaches to express and measure an individual's *prakriti* (unique composition). A customized food plan, which is central to Ayurveda, needs a thorough understanding of a person's *prakriti*. Recently, there are very limited validated methods to reliably conclude the *prakriti* of healthy individuals. This limitation has made it difficult to implement Ayurvedic principles in a consistent and measurable way (Rastogi 2012a, b; Rastogi and Chiappelli 2010).

The Prototype Prakriti Analysis Tool (PPAT) offer the potential for evidence-based assessment of personal prakriti (Rastogi 2012a, b). The biological system of humans may vary slightly with respect to these functions (Lurie 2012; Bhalerao et al. 2012). Exploring the prospective of prakriti analysis to interpret human genome necessities is now very fascinating. If confirmed, it will be helpful in broad use in classifying substrates that modify specific gene functions, allowing targeted promotion or suppression of these functions for enhanced health outcomes (Rizzo-Sierra 2011; Sethi et al. 2011).

1.11 Dietary Guidelines and Recommendations

Government agency and several health organizations publish evidence-based nutritional guidelines to support persons for suitable dietary choices. These guidelines encourage maintaining overall health, body weight, and preventing chronic diseases. Dietary guidelines and recommendations are developed by expert committees, based on inclusive reviews of the latest research findings in nutrition and health (Camara et al. 2021). The following are brief descriptions:

1.11.1 Intake of Macronutrients

Dietary guidelines frequently include approvals for the ideal ratio of consuming foods and biomolecules in a balanced diet. These ratios are personalized and based on some important factors such as sex, age, overall health, physical conditions, confirming they see personal dietary requirements during health and well-being.

1.11.2 Consumption of Fruits and Vegetables

Majority of guidelines highlighted the significance of consumption of diversity of commodity of fruits and vegetables daily for proper health and well-being. These foods provide many antioxidants, fibre, and micronutrients, which help in overall health and disease prevention.

1.11.3 Intake of Whole Grains

Selecting whole grains than refined grains is usually suggested for good health. Whole grains have very high fibre and nutrients. Whole grains unlike refined grains have high nutritional value because they do not undergo processing, which eliminates several valuable components.

1.11.4 Intake of Good Protein Sources

Some good protein sources generally recommended to be consumed are legumes, nuts, seeds, poultry, and fish. These meals offer the essential amino acid sources required for the body growth, maintenance, and repair.

1.11.5 Intake of Healthy Fats

As per guidelines, it is always advisable to have a combination of healthy fats from some common sources such as nuts, avocados, seeds, and seafood. These fats deliver essential fatty acids which enhance in keeping healthy cholesterol levels. Strategies commonly endorse to reduce the consumption of added sugars and salt in diet. Consumption of excess sodium can raise blood pressure issues and cause cardiovascular problems.

1.11.6 Body Hydration and Portion Control

Recommended guidelines regularly highlight the significance of intake of appropriate amount of water for optimal body hydration. Water is the best choice, although sweat drinks should be limited or avoided. To support individuals in keeping a healthy body weight, guidelines may also be suggested for proper serving sizes.

1.12 Gene–Nutrient Interactions and Genetic Susceptibility

Several evidences indicate that nutrient conditions impact gene expression. Environmental factors play a very crucial role in gene expression and ultimately in disease protection/illness. Varying socio-economic circumstances in several countries may affect the exposure of fundamental genetic disposition to chronic diseases. The dynamics of the relationship of environment and nutrient interaction impact on disease prevention. Several studies explain the role and impact of nutrients in the process of gene expression (Simopoulos and Pavlow 2001; Wald et al. 2002).

1.13 Conclusion

Diet and nutrition comprise the foods and nutrients individual eats and their effect on healthiness and well-being of human body. For ideal health, a balanced/complete food that contains a diversity of food items from several nutrient categories is important. Consulting an experienced and qualified dietitian or healthcare professional can be advantageous to make a personalized diet strategy tailored to specific requirements and preferences. Energy necessities for metabolic activity differ for each individual which depends on numerous aspects like age, sexual status, body composition, and metabolic activity levels. Individually, each person may have different carbohydrate requirements which depend upon physical activity, metabolism, and medical conditions. Protein supplies also differ depending on factors such as exercise, goals, and health issues. Fat molecules are vital for the absorption of fat-soluble vitamins. Healthy fat-rich diet assures the effective absorption and use of these vitamins. However, it is key to address those dietary styles as the mediterranean diet does not fit for all solutions. A well-organized, balanced plant-based food gives many health benefits. In comparison, the western food strategy frequently contains small amounts of whole grains, fruits, vegetables, and high amounts of processed foods, animal products, and added sugars. The Palaeolithic diet highlights whole, natural foods, approaching those eaten by early humans, and has high recognition for its health benefits.

References

Atkinson FS, Foster-Powell K, Brand-Miller JC (2008) International tables of glycemic index and glycemic load values. Diabetes Care 31(12):2281–2283

Attar T, Harek Y, Larabi L (2013) Determination of ultra trace levels of copper in whole blood by adsorptive stripping voltammetry. Bull Korean Chem Soc 57(5):568–573

Attar T, Harek Y, Larabi LL (2014) Determination of copper in whole blood by differential pulse adsorptive stripping voltammetry. Mediterr J Chem 2(6):691–700

Attar T, Ferrah N, Dennouni N, Reguig A, Harek Y, Larabi L (2015) Serum concentration of selenium among healthy adult in the west of Algeria. Der Pharma Chemica 7:102–104

Bellinger FP, Raman AV, Reeves MA, Berry MJ (2009) Regulation and function of selenoproteins in human disease. Biochem J 422(1):11–22

Bertone-Johnson ER (2009) Vitamin E and skin health: a review. J Clin Dermatol 37(5):493–501

Bhalerao S, Deshpande T, Thatte U (2012) Prakriti (Ayurvedic concept of constitution) and variations in platelet aggregation. BMC Complement Altern Med 12:1–5

Bloomer RJ, Larson DE, Fisher-Wellman KH, Galpin AJ, Schilling BK (2009) Effect of eicosapentaenoic and docosahexaenoic acid on resting and exercise-induced inflammatory and oxidative stress biomarkers: a randomized, placebo controlled, cross-over study. Lipids Health Dis 8:1–12

Camara M, Giner RM, González-Fandos E, López-García E, Mañes J, Portillo MP, Martínez JA (2021) Food-based dietary guidelines around the world: a comparative analysis to update AESAN scientific committee dietary recommendations. Nutrients 13(9):3131

Camp S (2013) Nutrition and diet therapy. J Nutr Educ Behav 45(6):806–8e1

Chen B, McClements DJ, Decker EA (2013) Design of foods with bioactive lipids for improved health. Annu Rev Food Sci Technol 4(1):35–56

Cianci M (2021) Introduction to proteins: structure, function, and motion. In: Kessel A, Ben-Tal N (eds). CRC Press/Taylor & Francis Group, Abingdon, 2020, 932 pp., GBP 63.99 (hardback), ISBN 978-1-4987-4717-2

Del Gobbo LC, Imamura F, Wu JH, de Oliveira Otto MC, Chiuve SE, Mozaffarian D (2013) Circulating and dietary magnesium and risk of cardiovascular disease: a systematic review and meta-analysis of prospective studies. Am J Clin Nutr 98:160–173

Deng Q, Liu J, Li Q, Chen K, Liu Z, Shen Y, Yang X (2013) Interaction of occupational manganese exposure and alcohol drinking aggravates the increase of liver enzyme concentrations from a cross-sectional study in China. Environ Health 12:1–6

Fang X, Wu X, Zhou B, Chen X, Chen T, Yang F (2017) Targeting selenium nanoparticles combined with baicalin to treat HBV-infected liver cancer. RSC Adv 7(14):8178–8185

Führer D, Mann K, Feldkamp J, Krude H, Spitzweg C, Kratzsch J, Schott M (2014) Thyroid dysfunction in pregnancy. Dtsch Med Wochenschr (1946) 139(42):2148–2152
Godswill AG, Somtochukwu IV, Ikechukwu AO, Kate EC (2020) Health benefits of micronutrients (vitamins and minerals) and their associated deficiency diseases: a systematic review. Int J Food Sci 3(1):1–32
Haase H, Rink L (2014) Multiple impacts of zinc on immune function. Metallomics 6(7):1175–1180
Harrison GG, Johnson AB (2006) The role of vitamins in maintaining health. J Am Diet Assoc 106(7):1131–1139
Holick MF (2007) Vitamin D deficiency. N Engl J Med 357(3):266–281
Kawamura T, Ogawa Y, Nakamura Y, Nakamizo S, Ohta Y, Nakano H, Shimada S (2012) Severe dermatitis with loss of epidermal Langerhans cells in human and mouse zinc deficiency. J Clin Invest 122(2):722–732
La Fontaine S, Quinn JM, Nakamoto SS, Page MD, Göhre V, Moseley JL, Merchant S (2002) Copper-dependent iron assimilation pathway in the model photosynthetic eukaryote Chlamydomonas reinhardtii. Eukaryot Cell 1(5):736–757
Layman DK, Rodriguez NR (2009) Egg protein as a source of power, strength, and energy. Nutr Today 44(1):43–48
Lee YK, Lyu ES, Oh SY, Park HR, Ro HK, Heo YR, Choi MK (2015) Daily copper and manganese intakes and their relation to blood pressure in normotensive adults. Clin Nutr Res 4(4):259–266
Lurie D (2012) Ayurveda and pharmacogenomics. Ann Ayurvedic Med 1(4):126–128
Martínez-González MA, Martín-Calvo N (2016) Mediterranean diet and life expectancy; beyond olive oil, fruits, and vegetables. Curr Opin Clin Nutr Metab Care 19(6):401–407
Maurya AP, Chauhan J, Yadav DK, Gangwar R, Maurya VK (2021) Nutraceuticals and their impact on human health. In: Preparation of phytopharmaceuticals for the management of disorders. Academic, pp 229–254
Medalle R, Waterhouse C, Hahn TJ (1976) Vitamin D resistance in magnesium deficiency. Am J Clin Nutr 29:854–858
Miller LG, Farber MD (2006) Minerals in human health: their functions, benefits, and toxicology. J Nutr Health 58(2):25–30
Ortiz MS, Alvarado JG, Zambrano F, Marquez R (2022) Surfactants produced from carbohydrate derivatives: a review of the biobased building blocks used in their synthesis. J Surfactant Deterg 25(2):147–183
Paoli A, Rubini A, Volek JS, Grimaldi KA (2013) Beyond weight loss: a review of the therapeutic uses of very-low-carbohydrate (ketogenic) diets. Eur J Clin Nutr 67(8):789–796
Pearce EN (2014) Iodine deficiency in children. Paediatr Thyroidol 26:130–138
Posner BM, Jette AM, Smith KW, Miller DR (1993) Nutrition and health risks in the elderly: the nutrition screening initiative. Am J Public Health 83(7):972–978
Rastogi S (2012a) Development and validation of a prototype Prakriti analysis tool (PPAT): inferences from a pilot study. AYU (Int Q J Res Ayurveda) 33(2):209–218
Rastogi S (2012b) Prakriti analysis in Ayurveda: envisaging the need of better diagnostic tools. In: Evidence-based practice in complementary and alternative medicine: perspectives, protocols, problems and potential in Ayurveda, pp 99–111
Rastogi S, Chiappelli F (2010) Bringing evidence basis to decision making in complementary and alternative medicine (CAM): prakriti (constitution) analysis in Ayurveda. In: Evidence-based practice: toward optimizing clinical outcomes, pp 91–106
Rayman MP (2012) Selenium and human health. Lancet 379(9822):1256–1268
Rizzo-Sierra CV (2011) Ayurvedic genomics, constitutional psychology, and endocrinology: the missing connection. J Altern Complement Med 17(5):465–468
Roman M, Jitaru P, Barbante C (2014) Selenium biochemistry and its role for human health. Metallomics 6(1):25–54
Rude RK (2010) Magnesium. In: Coates PM, Betz JM, Blackman MR, Cragg GM, Levine M, Moss J, White JD (eds) Encyclopedia of dietary supplements, 2nd edn. Informa Healthcare, New York, pp 527–537

Sacks FM (2001) Effects on blood pressure of reduced dietary sodium and the Dietary Approaches to Stop Hypertension (DASH) diet. N Engl J Med 344:3–10

Schaafsma G (2005) The protein digestibility-corrected amino acid score (PDCAAS)—a concept for describing protein quality in foods and food ingredients: a critical review. J AOAC Int 88(3):988–994

Scholtens EL, Krebs JD, Corley BT, Hall RM (2020) Intermittent fasting 5: 2 diet: what is the macronutrient and micronutrient intake and composition. Clin Nutr 39(11):3354–3360

Scrimshaw NS, Young VR (1976) The requirements of human nutrition. Sci Am 235(3):50–65

Sethi TP, Prasher B, Mukerjie M (2011) Ayurgenomics: a new way of threading molecular variability for stratified medicine. ACS Chem Biol 6:875–880

Shea MK, Booth SL (2011) Molecular mechanisms by which vitamin K regulates bone health. Curr Opin Clin Nutr Metab Care 14(1):22–29

Tham DM, Gardner CD, Haskell WL (1998) Potential health benefits of dietary phytoestrogens: a review of the clinical, epidemiological, and mechanistic evidence. J Clin Endocrinol Metabol 83(7):2223–2235

Human Nutrition: The Concept of a Balanced Diet

2

Vibha Sinha, Deepankar Mondal, Gauvrav Tiwari, Sapnita Shinde, Naveen Kumar Vishvakarma, Atul Kumar Tiwari, Prashant Bhatt, Vineeta Dixit, and Dhananjay Shukla

Abstract

Diet is one of the important factors that influence health and fitness. Depending upon a person's culture, geography, and fondness, diet is often considered as subjective choice. However, parameters of healthy living are not subjective enough. Therefore, it is very essential to define what constitutes a healthy diet and to balance various nutritional components of a person's diet in a way that it balances person's subjective choices and considers science of nutrition. A balanced diet gives a person all the nutrients they need without exceeding the daily calorie allowance. By eating a balanced diet and limiting foods that have low nutritive benefits like unhealthy snacks, people may receive all the calories and nutrients they require and avoid diseases. A varied, balanced, and nutritious diet will take on different compositions based on individual attributes (such as age, gender, lifestyle, and amount of physical activity), cultural context, geographically accessible foods, and dietary preferences. However, the core principles of what constitutes a healthy diet remain the same. In this respect, this chapter addresses various dietary practices that are advised globally as well as elements of a balanced diet and their health benefits. Many diseases like type 2 diabetes, obesity, metabolic syndrome, chronic kidney disease, cancer, persistent respira-

V. Sinha · D. Mondal · G. Tiwari · S. Shinde · N. K. Vishvakarma · D. Shukla (✉)
Department of Biotechnology, Guru Ghasidas Vishwavidyalaya, Bilaspur, Chhattisgarh, India

A. K. Tiwari
Department of Environmental Biology, Awadhesh Pratap Singh University, Rewa, Madhya Pradesh, India

P. Bhatt
State Forensic Science Laboratory, Sagar, Madhya Pradesh, India

V. Dixit (✉)
Department of Botany, Nilamber-Pitamber University, Garhwa, Jharkhand, India

A. Kumar et al. (eds.), *Innovations in Ayurvedic Nutrition*,
https://doi.org/10.1007/978-981-95-1213-3_2

tory conditions, and cardiovascular conditions are among the most common in urban population. Additionally, due to population aging, urbanization, and lifestyle changes, their prevalence is rising with time. Numerous studies have shown a direct link between socioeconomic status and health in industrialized and high-income countries. Adopting a healthy lifestyle and eating habits may have preventive effects that lengthen the average lifespan.

Keywords

Non-communicable diseases · Balanced diet · Socioeconomic status · Healthy lifestyle · Dietary habits

2.1 Introduction

Diet represents significant modifiable lifestyle factors that contribute to the management of non-communicable diseases like type 2 diabetes, heart disease, cancer, and their key risk factors (Vo-Nguyen and Kong 2009). A healthy diet can delay or even stop the onset of the disease progression. The most long-lasting and economical method of managing chronic diseases is prevention. In the past, research has mostly concentrated on the impact of nutrients and particular food items on human health. However, in more recent years, dietary patterns that take into consideration interactions between various foods and food components have received extensive study and have been proven to be substantially associated with health (Cena and Calder 2020). The idea of what a healthy diet is always evolving, and new knowledge about the functions that various foods, important nutrients, and other food components have on health and disease are incorporated (Tamimi et al. 2016). A substantial and rising amount of research shows that consuming particular nutrients, food groupings, or general dietary patterns improves health and helps prevent many non-communicable illnesses. Increased consistency of health-promoting foods and less consumption of poor healthy alternatives are inherent components of particular regional cuisines, such as the Mediterranean diet, or have been developed as parts of diet and lifestyle intended to lower disease risk, such as the Dietary Approaches to Stop Hypertension (DASH) or Mediterranean-DASH Intervention for Neurodegenerative Delay (MIND) diets (Bakaloudi et al. 2021). These more healthful options have fewer amounts of animal-based meals, especially fatty and processed meats, and higher amounts of plant-based foods, such as fresh fruits and vegetables, whole grains, legumes, seeds, and nuts. This chapter outlines the characteristics and supporting clinical evidence for diets that have been found to prevent disease and/or have a favorable impact on health in order to better comprehend the current concept of a “balanced diet and health benefit” (Breymeyer et al. 2016).

2.2 Nutritional Requirement

Fulfilling food and nutritional requirements of world population has been the focus of nutritional scientists and policy makers around the globe. Until recently, the focus has also shifted towards finding ways to tackle excess calorie intake and overnutrition arising due to sedentary lifestyle, stress-eating, etc. (Yau and Potenza 2013). Although, problem of nutritional deficiency exists in pockets like developing countries, nutritional scientists and health influencers are working toward defining a clear concept of optimal nutritional requirement. The optimal amount of each nutrient required for proper growth and functioning of human body is nutritional requirement, and individuals in various cultural, climatic, age groups, diseased condition or special condition like pregnancy achieve this requirement by various sources of food (Bakaloudi et al. 2021). Finding out amount of nutrients needed by individuals or groups is usually done by clinical research and population-based studies, wherein required levels of any particular nutrients are determined along with its toxicity. Various government or non-government bodies conduct clinical research and surveys to recommend levels of nutritional requirement as guidelines for policy makers and for population in general (Yau and Potenza 2013). In the United States, these recommendations are in the form of various dietary reference intakes (DRIs) which are defined set of quantitative estimates of nutritional aspects indicating the status of nutritional uptake. Dietary reference intakes (DRIs) constitute various parameters, such as

(a) *Recommended Dietary Allowance (RDA)*—It is the measure of average daily dietary intake needed to fulfill nutritional requirement of almost all healthy persons in any particular group.
(b) *Adequate Intake (AI)*—It is a value indicating realized or experimentally dictated rough estimates of daily nutrient uptake by any group. This measure is a substitute for RDA, when RDA is unavailable (Manz et al. 2002).
(c) *Tolerable Upper Intake Level (UL)*—It is the measure of maximum daily nutrient uptake that is non-toxic and poses no threat to health of individuals of any group (Turck et al. 2022).
(d) *Estimated Average Requirement (EAR)*—An estimated value of nutrient uptake that meets nutritional requirements of half of healthy individuals in any group (Szwiega et al. 2021).

In Europe, the European Food Safety Authority (EFSA) publishes nutritional parameters as Dietary Reference Values (DRVs). Indian Council of Medical Research (ICMR) and National Institute of Nutrition (NIN) conduct studies and surveys and publish their findings of nutritional requirements as Recommended Dietary Allowance (RDA) in their bi-annual reports (Nair and Augustine 2018).

2.3 Balanced Diet

In order to reflect our evolving knowledge of how different meals serve different purposes of the functions that various foods, important nutrients, and other food components play in health and disease, the concept of what constitutes a healthy diet is always emerging (Lorenzo et al. 2022). Intake of certain minerals, food groups, or general nutritional trends are all backed up by a substantial and the growing amount of research finding is a positive impact on health and helping to prevent non-communicable diseases (NCDs) (Wickramasinghe et al. 2018). A balanced diet is one that incorporates adequate micronutrients and fluids to fulfill the body's natural physiologic requirements while also ingesting sufficient macronutrients in the proper amounts to support energetic and physiologic needs without overeating (McBurney et al. 2021). Sugars, proteins, and fats, termed as macronutrients, provide the energy required for normal biological operations. For optimal growth, development, metabolism, and physiologic functioning, micronutrients (such as vitamins and minerals) must be consumed in relatively modest amounts (Savarino et al. 2021). Figure 2.1 shows the generalized representation of a healthy and balanced diet. It is justified by research that the diet we favor to eat—or not to eat effects an attribute of our life. Science is concentrating on food and its effect on health and how to design a balanced diet for each and every age group. We all need the same nutritional constituents, but the quantity we need depends on sex, age, physical activeness, and other factors. For example, women who are in their

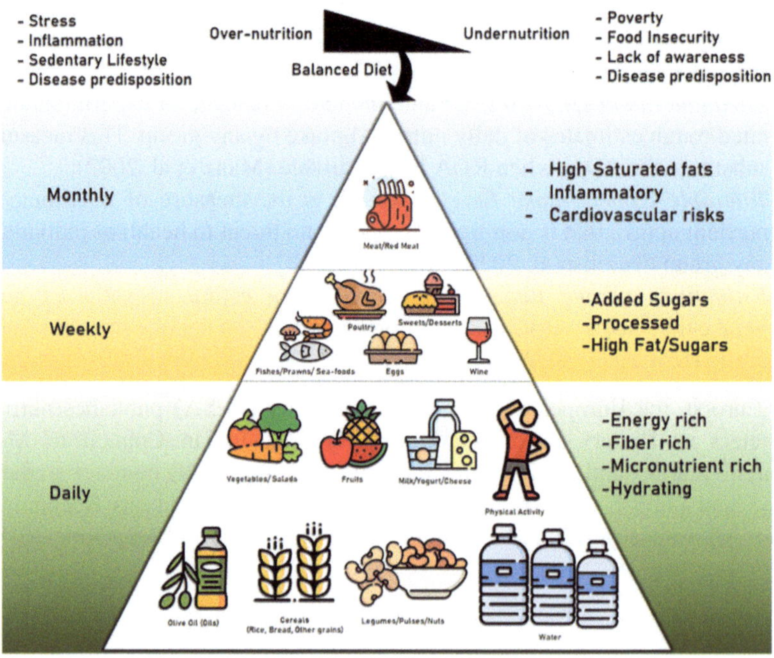

Fig. 2.1 Generalized representation of a healthy and balanced diet

pregnancy stage or breastfeeding, need more nutrients (Nutrition 2002). Dietary fibers support our gastrointestinal system in a proper way and also decrease the chances of cholesterol-related diseases. There are various non-communicable diseases such as obesity, high blood pressure, diabetes, lymphoma, and respiratory abnormalities affecting the whole world. Food choices contribute to risk for developing obesity, hypertension, and other diseases (hypercholesterolemia, diabetes) which are associated with mortality, including respiratory diseases and gastrointestinal abnormalities (Cena and Calder 2020). Balanced diet is just one approach to reducing the chances of abnormalities. Balancing caloric intake to maintain a healthy weight and shape, regular workout, and zero smoking are mandatory strategies. The data of Nurses' Health study shows that women with balanced lifestyle pattern that includes these three mandatory strategies were 80% less likely to develop cardiovascular diseases (CVD) over a 14-year period compared to all other women in the study (Errett and Willett 2010). According to the ministry of health and welfare and the Korean nutrition society, a balanced diet should contain approximately 55–60% carbohydrates, 15–20% protein, and 15–20% fat (for 3-year-old individuals). In modern times, people are highly interested in the low-carb high-fat (LCHF) diet. The LCHF diet reduces carbohydrate intake to 5–10% (Lim 2018).

2.4 Composition of a Balanced Diet and Its Health Benefit

The two main categories of nutrients that make up a balanced diet or nutrition are macronutrients and micronutrients (Cena and Calder 2020). The macronutrients, which can be broadly categorized as carbs, proteins, and lipids, are the primary building blocks of various tissues and make up the majority of caloric intake, which serves as the body's main source of energy. Similarly, micronutrients are dietary substances that, despite being required in smaller amounts, can still be considered important for health and key processes, while not contributing considerably to caloric consumption (Sanders et al. 2021). They are largely made up of water- and fat-soluble minerals and vitamins. Because shortages in both macro- and micronutrients can have a substantially detrimental effect on the physiology and overall operation of the human body, particularly on the different growth-related processes (Savarino et al. 2021). Figure 2.2 represents the composition of the daily diet.

2.4.1 Dietary Proteins

The amino acids that the body needs but cannot make on its own are included in dietary proteins, which also serve as a source of energy (i.e., essential amino acids). For the maintenance of lean body mass over the course of a lifetime, adequate dietary protein intake is essential. Protein is also important for avoiding the aging-related problem of skeletal muscle mass in elderly people. Animal sources of dietary proteins include meat, dairy, fish, and eggs, while plant sources include legumes, soy products, grains, nuts, and seeds. The former is thought to be a richer source of amino acids due to its wide range, high digestibility, and higher bioavailability

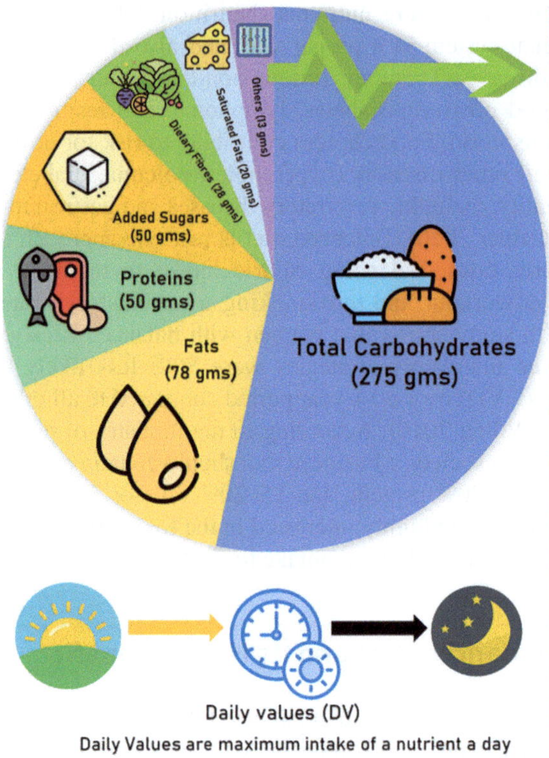

Other Nutrients	Daily Values(gm/mcg)
Potassium (K)	4700mg
Chlorine (Cl)	2300mg
Sodium (Na)	2300mg
Calcium (Ca)	1300mg
Phosphorus (P)	1250mg
Choline	550 mg
Magnesium Mg)	420mg
Cholesterol	300mg
Manganese (Mn)	2.3mg
Iron (Fe)	18mg
Zinc (Zn)	11 mg
Niacin	16 mg
Vitamin E	15 mg
Riboflavin	1.3 mg
Thiamine	1.2 mg
Copper (Cu)	0.9 mg
Vitamin A	900 mcg
Folate/Folic acid	400 mcg
Iodine	150 mcg
Vitamin K	120 mcg
Vitamin C	90 mcg
Selenium (Se)	55 mcg
Molybdenum (Mo)	45 mcg
Chromium (Cr)	35 mcg
Biotin	30 mg
Vitamin D	20 mcg
Vitamin B12	2.4 mcg
Vitamin B6	1.7 mcg

Fig. 2.2 Daily values of nutrients intake. It is the maximum amount of each nutrient recommended for consumption in a day. (Source: Food and Drug Administration 2022)

(Lonnie et al. 2018). Unfortunately, animal-based forms of protein comprise saturated fatty acids, which have been connected to heart disease, dyslipidemia, and several malignancies. Red meat, and processed meat, in particular, have been linked to an increased risk of colon cancer, while the underlying mechanisms are unknown. The dietary acid load is also increased by animal-derived proteins, shifting the body's acid–base balance in the direction of acidosis. Insulin resistance, poor glucose homeostasis, and the emergence of urinary calcium stones have all been associated with the increased metabolic acid burden (Lescinsky et al. 2022).

2.4.2 Carbohydrates

Our primary energy source comes from dietary carbs. Generally, they are divided into simple and complicated carbohydrates depending on the length of the polymer, which does not always represent their effect on health. The Institute of Medicine established a Recommended Daily Intake (RDA) for carbs for adults and children over the age of 1 year at 130 g/d. This figure was derived using the amount of sugars and starches required to feed the brain with a sufficient amount of glucose (Naude et al. 2022). For carbohydrates, the IOM determined an acceptable macronutrient distribution range (AMDR) of 45–65% of total calories. As a result, contemporary dietary advice includes eating carbohydrate-rich meals such as cereals, vegetables, fruits, legumes, nuts, seeds, and dairy products. Carbohydrate-rich foods are abundant in fiber and other nutrients (Savarino et al. 2021). Despite having similar energy efficiency and calorie content, simple sugars like fructose, glucose, and lactose have significantly different metabolic consequences that, when ingested in excess, increase the risk for a variety of chronic diseases. Recent research further shows that, in addition to the total amount of carbs taken, the dietary type or level of processing can modify the energy effectiveness and the cardiometabolic risk linked to particular carbohydrates (Martinez-Perez et al. 2021). In order to take into account both of these perspectives, the quality of carbs as well as its food type, multiple measures can be established to help identify carbohydrate-rich food sources and differentiate between those that would encourage the development of chronic diseases and those that may contribute to their prevention (Naude et al. 2022).

2.4.3 Dietary Fats

Along with protein and carbs, dietary fat is one of the three macronutrients that make up the majority of our meals. It is a nutrient with high energy density that offers necessary fatty acids (FAs) and facilitates the absorption of fat-soluble vitamins (Hooper et al. 2020). Dietary fats typically get into our diets through the consumption of animal fats or through the usage of kinds of butter and oils in a range of foods. The majority of dietary fats are triacylglycerol, which is created when fatty acids are esterified to glycerol. The amount of double bonds, where the double bonds are located in the carbon chain (e.g., n-6, n-3), and the orientation of the double bonds can all vary amongst fatty acids (cis or trans). The main sources of fat calories (energy) are SAFA (C12:0-C18:0, no double bond), MUFA (mostly cis-C18:1 oleic acid), and PUFA. Omega-6 linoleic acid (C18:2) and some n-3 alpha-linolenic acid are the major PUFA found in seed oils (C18:3, ALA) (Nettleton et al. 2018). n-3 PUFAs, which have very long chains and at least five double bonds, are present in seafood in lesser quantities (predominantly C20:5 eicosapentaenoic acid [EPA] and C22:6 docosahexaenoic acid [DHA]). Animal products tend to be high in SAFA, whereas nuts and vegetable oils are often high in PUFA (Carughi et al. 2016). Animal and vegetable sources both contain sizable levels of MUFA. Though vegetable fats like coconut and palm kernel oil are quite high in SAFA, the main sources of SAFA in western diets are meat and dairy (Imamura et al. 2017). Vegetable oils account for the majority of dietary PUFA, while some also come from meat, fish, and cereals. Dietary lipids significantly reduce the chance of heart disease (Lauber et al. 2022). There is a tonne of research that suggests replacing certain saturated fatty acids with unsaturated fatty acids lowers the risk of developing coronary heart disease and improves the blood lipid and lipoprotein profile. Fish contains very long-chain polyunsaturated n-3 or omega-3 fatty acids (n-3 VLCPUFA), which have a variety of advantageous metabolic effects and are linked to a decreased risk of catastrophic CHD and stroke when consumed regularly (Abdelhamid et al. 2018).

2.4.4 Micronutrients

Micronutrients are dietary elements that, despite having a minor impact on calorie intake, are still essential for maintaining better health and performing other essential bodily activities. They mostly consist of minerals and vitamins, both fat- and water-soluble. Micronutrients are administered in little amounts, yet they are essential for healthy growth, metabolism, and various biological process at all ages of human life, especially zinc, iron, vitamin D, folic acid, and potassium (Peña-Rosas et al. 2019). They have a number of functions, including supporting the body in the production of hormones, enzymes, and other materials required for healthy growth and development. Iron, vitamin A, and iodine deficits are the most common dietary deficiencies worldwide, particularly in children and pregnant women (Enebe et al. 2020). Micronutrient deficiencies are disproportionately frequent in low- and middle-income nations. Anyone who consumes a diet high in fruits, vegetables, and lean proteins can typically acquire all the vitamins they require from their food. However, those who consume fewer fruits and vegetables and those who have digestive issues might need to take a vitamin supplement to prevent or lessen a deficiency. By including the following foods in their diet, a person can make sure they get enough minerals:. red meat (limit their use and choose lean cuts), iodized table salt, seafood (less than 2300 milligrams), dairy products such as milk and other dairy products, nuts and seeds, fruits, vegetables, leafy greens, poultry, fortified bread and cereals, egg yolks, whole grains, beans and legumes, etc. (Field et al. 2021).

2.4.5 Water and Electrolytes

In the human body, water plays a wide range of roles. It serves as a construction material, a lubricant, a shock absorber, a solvent, a reaction medium, and a reactant. It also serves as a carrier for nutrients and waste products. Due to the fact that a loss of 1% of bodily water is often made up for in 24 h, the management of water balance is quite accurate. Water balance is attained by controlling both water intake and water retention. Young adults are able to control their body's water balance, but young new born and the elderly are more susceptible to dehydration. Dehydration can impair awareness and cause tachycardia, orthostatic hypotension, ocular hypotonia, weakness in the extremities, and speech incoherence (Setty et al. 2019). Human water demands are not established by a minimal intake because doing so may result in a water deficit due to a variety of factors that change water demand (whether, physical activeness, diet, and so on). In order to safeguard health and life, the water cycle must be properly regulated. Since water is the only liquid nutrient that is truly necessary for bodily hydration, an average inactive adult should consume 1.5 liters of water daily (Liska et al. 2019).

Electrolytes are so important for proper functioning of living cells such as maintaining electrical neutrality, generating and conducting action potential in nerves. Na, K, and Cl are significant electrolytes along with Mg, Ca, P, and $HCO3^-$ and obtained from our diet (Dermatol 2015). Cationic electrical charges must be equal to anionic charges both outside and inner side of the cell. The negatively charged ions which are present in the intracellular area are largely polyvalent and too large to penetrate the plasma membrane (Bradbury 1973). The balance of normal components and volumes of ICF and ECF in the human body is the result of basic transport and different metabolic processes operating at the cellular level. The process is in part controlled by the concentration of components determining the metabolic and transportation rates and in part by an over-riding influence from the nervous system and hormonal control system (Bradbury 1973) (Table 2.1).

Table 2.1 Essential electrolytes and their significance

Electrolytes	Source	Function	Disorders due to imbalance
Sodium (Na)	Celery, beets and milk, breads, rolls, colds, cuts, pizzas, poultry, etc.	Regulation of membrane potential and extracellular fluid volume	Confusion, irritability, coma, headache, cerebral-edema and osmotic demyelination syndrome
Potassium (K)	Dried fruits (raisins, apricots), beans, lentils, potatoes, Winter squash (acorn, butternut), spinach, broccoli	Regulation of Na-K pumps, controlling muscle contraction, regulation of digestion processes	Hyponatremia, Cushing's syndrome, Gitelman syndrome, Liddle syndrome, Bartter syndrome, Fanconi syndrome due to low potassium
Calcium (ca)	Cheese, yogurt, sardines and canned salmon, beans and lentils, almonds, leafy greens	Skeletal mineralization, muscle contraction, transmission of nerve impulse, blood clotting, secretion of hormones	Hypocalcemia (hypoparathyroidism), hypercalcemia, (hyperparathyroidism), osteoporosis
Bicarbonate (HCO3)	Fruits and vegetables, such as avocados, bananas, potatoes, and spinach	Maintaining the acid–base balance	Metabolic alkalosis (high HCO3), metabolic acidosis (low HCO3)
Magnesium (Mg)	Green leafy vegetables, whole grains, nuts, and legumes, milk, yogurt, and fortified foods	ATP metabolism, contraction and relaxation of muscle, neurological functioning, neurotransmitter secretion	Hypomagnesemia, gastrointestinal and renal losses—ventricular arrhythmias
Chloride (Cl)	Table salt, salt containing food.	Balance of body fluids (helps regulate blood pressure)	Hyperchloremia, congestive heart failure
Phosphorus (P)	Lentils, nuts, beans, meats, milk products	Growth and maintenance of cell and tissue, essential component of DNA and RNA	Cardiovascular diseases, osteoporosis

2.5 Diet Habits Across the Globe

Dietary patterns, which are characterized by the amounts, ratios, variety, or combinations of various foods and beverages, as well as the frequency with which they are routinely consumed, are also linked to either a higher or lower incidence of chronic diseases. Globally, balanced diets that support locally available food and are based on realistic, long-term, and health-promoting dietary recommendations are the norm for preventive measures (Schulze et al. 2018). To preserve natural resources for future generations while providing enough food for a growing global population, major changes in food production and consumption are required.

Since Paleolithic man first appeared on Earth, the patterns of human food, exercise, and body composition have undergone significant changes. Broad patterns of food usage and corresponding nutrition-related diseases have been identified as typical states, which have undergone a series of significant modifications in the human diet and nutritional status. In some parts of the world over the past three centuries, the rate of nutritional change appears to have increased (Popkin 2006). These modifications are mirrored in nutritional outcomes, such as modifications in average stature and body composition. Along with significant changes in health status, huge demographic shifts, and significant socioeconomic shifts, food and activity patterns also alter over time. The WHO advises making dietary modifications such as balancing energy intake, cutting back on saturated and trans fats and boosting consumption of unsaturated fats, increasing intake of fruits and vegetables, and cutting back on sugar and salt.

A good diet has a beneficial effect on one's health, and encouraging healthy eating among the populace is a concern for public health. In general, replacing lower quality, highly processed foods with a variety of whole foods such as fruits, vegetables, legumes, whole grains, nuts, seeds, and seafood will help you maintain a balanced diet (Milani et al. 2021). The Vegetarian, Mediterranean, DASH, New Nordic, and Vegan diets are the ones that better understand these patterns. Each approach incorporates the culture, identity, and traditions of a particular demographic. These are all healthy eating habits that, despite their variances, have certain key things in common because they are all based on regional foods (De Cosmi et al. 2022). These patterns share a high intake of fresh fruits and nuts, veggies, lentils (a source of dietary, polyphenols, and plant proteins), cereals, and fish, as well as a low intake of meats. For food advice and nutrition education, above-mentioned pyramids (Fig. 2.1) are clear, understandable visual aids.

2.5.1 Vegetarian Diet

A vegetarian diet constitutes food products largely based on plants, avoiding animal-derived food products like meat, fish, and eggs. However, religiously and culturally motivated vegetarians, largely belonging to eastern religions like Hinduism, Buddhism, Jainism, and Sikhism do consume dairy-based food products (Lee et al. 2016). Inclusion of dairy-based food products in vegetarian diet fulfills essential amino acid requirements and thus constitutes a balanced food choice. Vegetarian diet has higher intake of dietary fibers, lower intake of saturated fats and cholesterol along with health promoting phytochemicals such as vitamin B and C, other antioxidants, Polyphenols, Carotenoids, Magnesium, Iron, and Zinc (Ahnen et al. 2019). Although iron and zinc from plant-based food sources has limited bioavailability which should be compensated by higher intake of such plant-based food (Gibson 2007). Additionally, there are few nutrients of concern in a vegetarian diet whose intake is limited such as vitamin B12, vitamin D, iron, zinc, and calcium along with no intake of omega-3-fatty acids, which can be compensated by using fortified food products and supplements (Craig 2010). Vegetarians have a lower LDL cholesterol level, lower blood pressure, lower body mass index, and reduced risk of cancers. Vegetarian diet is also found to be associated with less risk of cardiovascular diseases, heart strokes, ischemic heart diseases, Type II diabetes, hypertension, etc. According to the American Dietetic Association, a well-balanced and planned vegetarian diet comprising a variety of plant sources and dairy products can be a viable option for leading a healthy life and preventing various diseases (Craig 2009). Quite recently, plant-based food habits like vegetarianism have gained appeal among young adults who are consciously choosing plant-based food because of various benefits like healthy lifestyle, reduced cardiovascular disease risk and obesity, climatic change concerns, etc., and have a very positive perception of vegetarian diet (Lea et al. 2006). These positive perceptions about vegetarianism and similar plant-based diet habits is a result of various studies which showed vegetarianism and plant-based food lifestyle to be less taxing to the environment and is helpful to tackle bigger threats like climate change. It is estimated that vegetarian and ovo-lactovegetarian food production produces 50% and 35% lower greenhouse gases than average omnivore food production (Fresán and Sabaté 2019). Therefore, vegetarian diet is not only beneficial for physical health of individuals but also helpful for the planet. Vegetarian diet not just contributes to better physical and environmental health but also gives the individual a sense of better moral and ethical conduct concerned with spirituality and environment, along with strong emotional sense of belonging (to a vegetarian community), which overall has balanced correlation with the Quality of life (Hargreaves et al. 2021). However, it must also be noted that irrespective of the perceived spiritual and mental health benefits, many studies investigating mental health and depression found increased risk of depression and a lower risk of anxiety among vegetarians/vegans (Iguacel et al. 2021).

2.5.2 Vegan Diet

Vegan diet is an exclusively plant-based diet which excludes all kinds of animal-based food products such as meat, fish, dairy, and even honey. Inspiration for practicing this diet habit stems from ethical and environmental reasons rather than just their physical health benefits. Comparative studies showed that vegan diets have low energy and high fiber contents when compared to a typical omnivore diet, followed by vegetarians, semi-vegetarians, and presco-vegetarians (Clarys et al. 2014).

Like all plant-based diets, vegans are also reported to have lower cholesterol, lower blood pressure, lower BMI, etc., to reduced overall risk of cardiovascular diseases, hypertension, strokes, lowered risks of various cancers, and lower risk of metabolic syndromes (Marrone et al. 2021). Vegans usually replace animal food products and essential amino acid needs by using plant-based meat and milk alternatives. Plant-based milk alternatives are usually derived from soy, a protein-rich plant product which can be used to prepare soy curd, soy cheese, and soy milk. Soy curd is also pressed to make blocks rich in soy proteins called tofu, which is a viable alternative for cheese for vegans. Extracts from legumes, nuts, seeds, and pseudo-cereals resemble milk and act as a plant-based milk alternative. Plant based-meat alternatives are derived from soy, wheat gluten, mushrooms, and mycoproteins along with recently marketed cultured meat or lab-grown meat. All these food products derived from plants are nutritionally equivalent to animal-based food products and are often chosen by vegans as an alternative food option (Alcorta et al. 2021).

2.5.3 Mediterranean Diet

Mediterranean Diet or Med Diet is the diet pattern traditionally observed by inhabitants of countries surrounding the Mediterranean Sea. These countries are Italy, Greece, Spain, Morocco, Portugal, Cyrus, and Croatia. Common food groups in Med Diet include high consumption of vegetables, fruits, nuts, legumes, high intake of extra virgin olive oil, moderate consumption of dairy products low in fat, moderate consumption of poultry, fish, wine, and low consumption of red meat, sweets, and processed food (Keys and Keys 2006). In traditional Mediterranean diet, beverages like tea made with a variety of aromatic herbs is also recommended. In 2010, the United Nations Educational, Scientific and Cultural Organization (UNESCO) has recognized this diet pattern as an "intangible cultural heritage of humanity" for being a collection of practices, traditions, skills relating to agriculture, animal husbandry, fisheries, crops, harvesting, processing, conserving and feeding generations of humans, and make a blend of culture and diet (Trichopoulou 2021).

Various studies have associated Mediterranean Diet with many health benefits and lower mortality. Adherence to Med Diet was associated to reduced total mortality which has been attributed to moderate alcohol consumption, high vegetable, fruits, and nut consumption along with low consumption of meat and meat products. Health benefits of Med Diet is also because of high legume consumption and high monounsaturated to saturated lipid ratio (Trichopoulou et al. 2009). Various studies have shown that individuals who adhere to Med Diet enjoy better quality sleep and also lead quality of life (Godos et al. 2019a, b). Observational studies have also suggested that individuals practicing adherence to Med Diet have lower risk of metabolic and cardiovascular diseases and ultimately lower risk of mortality. These health benefits of Med Diet is most likely because of well-balanced bioactive components like fibers, mono and polyunsaturated fatty acids, polyphenols, etc. (Schwingshackl et al. 2020). In large clinical studies, Med Diet is found to decrease total blood lipid levels which includes total LDL (Low-density lipids), apo-B Cholesterol, and Triglycerides (Ambring et al. 2004). Higher adherence to a Med

Diet is also associated with lower risk and incidence of Cancer cases in Mediterranean countries (Schwingshackl and Hoffmann 2016). Lower risk of cancers due to adherence to a Mediterranean diet is probably because of its protective effects on cells and DNA as it induces lowered oxidative and inflammatory processes (Mentella et al. 2019) and therefore Med Diet can be considered a powerful lifestyle choice for managing cancers and cardiovascular diseases (Portugal-Nunes et al. 2021).

2.5.4 Flexitarian Diet or Semi-Vegetarian Diet (SVD)

Flexitarian Diet as the name suggests is flexible considering their occasional consumption of meat or fish but remaining vegetarian primarily. Flexitarians or Semi-Vegetarians choose vegetarianism as their primary food habit but do not strictly adhere to it. They are sometimes referred to as "meat-reducers" who unlike "meat-eaters" do not consume meat everyday but consume it once in a while depending on their will (Derbyshire 2017). People following this diet acknowledge importance of animal food as a source of proteins, fats, and micronutrients but at the same time avoid it liberally, considering ethical arguments against animal-based food products. They also acknowledge the fact that long term and high intake of red meat and food derived from them can cause serious risk of Cardiovascular diseases and various cancers, namely of the colon (Battaglia Richi et al. 2015). Flexitarian diet has been found to be helpful in weight loss, preventing diabetes, managing metabolic and cardiovascular diseases (Derbyshire 2016) (Table 2.2).

2.5.5 DASH Diet

DASH stands for Dietary approaches to stop hypertension (DASH) was originally a dietary intervention in a study group by National Institute of Health (NIH) to understand the importance of dietary interventions in reducing hypertension. It was

Table 2.2 Diet patterns and few relevant parameters of disease and disease risk from various studies

Diet pattern	Mean BMI	Cases of diabetes	Metabolic syndrome prevalence	Iron deficiency
NVs (non-vegetarians)	~28.7 kg/m^2	2.1%	39.7%	25.5
Semi-Vegetarians (SVs)	~27.4 kg/m^2	0.92%	37.6%	38.6%
Presco-Vegetarians (PVs)	~26.1 kg/m^2	1.3%	–	–
Lacto-Ovo Vegetarians (LOV)	~26.1 kg/m^2	1.1%	25.2%	–
Strict vegetarians	~24.0 kg/m^2	0.54%	–	42.6%
Study	Rizzo et al. (2013)	Tonstad et al. (2013)	Rizzo et al. (2011)	Baines et al. (2007)

observed that dietary interventions alone can bring down blood pressure significantly without any other lifestyle modifications. Lately, it was adopted as a dietary recommendation helpful for individuals at the risk of hypertension and cardiovascular diseases (Soltani et al. 2020). DASH diet suggests more use of fruits, vegetables, dairy products, lean meat, nuts, and seeds in an individual's diet. A typical DASH diet may include 5–6 daily servings of vegetables and fruits, two daily servings of low-fat dairy products and lean meat, about seven servings of food with carbohydrate and about 2–3 weekly consumption of nuts and seeds. A DASH diet recommends moderate use of both animal- and plant-based proteins along with high intake of vegetables and fruits (Wickman et al. 2021). With lean meat, low fat dairy products, eggs, fish, legumes, nuts, and seeds, DASH diet makes a balanced combination of animal- and plant-sourced foods. Individuals following DASH diet can complete their fat requirement by using olive oil, nuts, hempseeds, flaxseeds, fish with omega-3 fatty acids, etc. Green leafy vegetables like spinach, fruits like bananas and oranges constitute a popular and healthy choice of food under this dietary approach (Sacks et al. 2001).

Many studies have found the importance of DASH diet in maintaining blood glucose, triglycerides, and LDL levels and also reduce insulin resistance. Adherence to DASH Diet is also helpful in controlling and managing type-2 diabetes (Campbell 2017). DASH diet recommends the use of less dietary sodium and replacing it with Mg2+, K+, and Ca+, thereby helps in managing the risk of heart failures and strokes (Dos Reis Padilha et al. 2018). This diet is also found useful in controlling incidence of Colorectal cancer in average-risk white populations (Jones-McLean et al. 2015). It is also helpful in controlling chronic liver diseases, celiac disease, and diverticular diseases (Tyson et al. 2012). In some studies, adhering to DASH diet has been found to be associated with bringing down all-cause mortality rates (Soltani et al. 2020).

2.5.6 MIND Diet

Stands for Mediterranean-DASH intervention for Neurodegenerative Delay, is a hybrid of Mediterranean diet and DASH diet, tailored to maintain a better brain health. This diet is rich in nutrients like folate, vitamin E, flavonoids, leutin-zeaxanthin, etc., which are pro-cognition in nature along with anti-inflammatory and anti-oxidative properties. This diet slows down the usual cognitive decline which occurs when people age and significantly reduce the risk of Alzheimer's and other neurodegenerative diseases (Morris et al. 2015a). MIND diet includes nearly 10 brain-healthy group of food which includes green leafy vegetables, beans/legumes, other vegetables, nuts, berries, olive oil, fish, poultry, wine, and whole grains. Studies which score for MIND diet in individuals considers five brain-unhealthy food groups such as red meat, fried and fast foods, pastry/sweets, butter, and cheese. Enough studies have reported the importance of MIND diet in slowing down the onset of Alzheimer's disease and reduce its overall incidence (Morris et al. 2015b). MIND diet has also been found to lower the risk of cardiovascular diseases and help maintain a healthy heart (Golzarand et al. 2022). MIND diet is also found to delay cognitive decline in post-stroke individuals (Gadgil et al. 2013).

Other Forms of Vegetarianism

Vegetarianism has many other types based on the inclusion of some specific food like fishes or eggs or milk products in their diet in addition to their primary plant-based diet. A group referred to as presco-vegetarians include individuals who are primarily vegetarians but includes fish and seafood in their diet. Some others are identified as Ovo-lactovegetarians who prefer to use eggs and milk/milk products in their diet as a matter of choice. These subgroups understand the importance of animal-based proteins in their diet and therefore include few animal-based food in their diet.

2.5.7 Nordic Diet

The Nordic Diet is mainly derived from the conventional eating habits of the Nordic regions, which include Greenland, Iceland, Denmark, Norway, Sweden, and Finland. Among the foods and cooking techniques that are largely the same across the aforementioned nations are berries (such as lingonberries), cabbage, apples, pears, root vegetables, oats, rye, and fermented milk. These traditional foods from the Nordic region have all been linked to positive health effects. The Nordic Nutrition Recommendations were jointly published as a result of decades of cooperation between the Nordic countries, and they set criteria for dietary composition and reference values for nutrient intake (NNR) (Johansson et al. 2021). According to the NNRs, fats should account for 25–40% of total energy consumption, carbohydrates for 45–60%, and protein for 10–20%. This is known as the macronutrient recommended daily energy distribution (as energy percent, E percent) (Andersen et al. 2014; Mithril et al. 2012). Although ND covers numerous nations, each Nordic nation's food-based dietary recommendations (FBDGs) differ slightly from one another. ND advises consuming more legumes because they help boost the quantity of protein in the diet while also have a positive impact on lowering the environmental pressure because the meat is the least environmentally friendly meal. Additionally, the Nordic nations have a rich marine archipelago that is a wonderful supply of fish and other seafood, which are an essential component of the diet (Mithril et al. 2013). Rapeseed, sometimes referred to as canola oil, is the most popular type of added fat found in the ND. It is obtained from the *Brassica napus* plant, a member of the *Cruciferae* family, which also produces rapeseed. Since the rapeseed plant is primarily grown in its winter form, the geographical position of the countries can probably be attributed to this. The Nordic Nutrition Recommendations (NNR) are designed to promote general well-being and lower the risk of diet-related chronic illnesses that are prevalent in Nordic populations (Kesson et al. 2013). According to a study done by Laccopidan et al., a negative correlation exists between a healthy Nordic index and the risk of T2D in both sexes. To avoid T2D, the Nordic diet's beneficial components may be helpful. Promoting local diets could be a successful and long-lasting strategy for enhancing public health (Lacoppidan et al. 2015). Low-grade inflammation (LGI) has been connected to the etiology of several chronic illnesses, including type 2 diabetes, cardiovascular disease, certain malignancies, and neurological diseases. Numerous chronic disorders, including type 2 diabetes, cancer, certain malignancies, and neurological diseases have been linked to the etiology of low-grade inflammation (LGI). Despite sharing many parallels with MD, the effects of the healthy Nordic diet (HND) on LGI are less well understood. According to various studies, ND reduces various markers of LGI and play a role in chronic disease prevention (Lankinen et al. 2019).

2.5.8 TLC Diet

The TLC diet, also known as the Therapeutic Lifestyle Changes diet, is a heart-healthy dietary strategy. It was created by the National Institutes of Health to reduce the risk of coronary diseases, stroke, and cardiovascular disease. In terms of maintaining clear arteries and improving heart health, the diet aims to reduce blood levels of total and LDL cholesterol. To prevent heart disease, it combines elements of a healthy diet, exercise, and weight management (Centre for Disease Control, NHLBI 2005). The TLC diet differs from other weight-loss plans in that it is meant to be maintained over time and is more of a lifestyle change than a quick fix. The TLC diet has been linked to various additional health advantages besides decreasing cholesterol, including improved immunological function, decreased oxidative stress, and many more (Thompson et al. 2017). The TLC diet combines dietary changes with lifestyle adjustments that have been proven to aid with heart health. It entails varying the kinds of fat you consume and boosting your consumption of nutrients that are good for you, such as soluble fiber and plant sterols that can decrease cholesterol (Bazzano 2008). To help with weight management and improve the heart muscle, it also combines dietary adjustments with increased physical activity. The primary recommendations for adhering to the TLC diet are to consume just enough calories to be within a healthy range. Daily calorie intake should be 25–35% fat, daily calorie intake should contain no more than 7% saturated fat. Less than 200 mg of dietary cholesterol should be consumed per day, daily soluble fiber intake should range between 10 and 25 grams. Consume at least 2 grams of stanols or plant sterols daily. Engage in daily moderate-intensity physical activity for at least 30 min. To increase your intake of fiber, the TLC diet often calls for eating more fruits, vegetables, whole grains, legumes, nuts, and seeds. It is also advised that you increase your daily physical activity by 30 min (NHLBI 2005; Thompson et al. 2017). This can be done by walking, running, cycling, or swimming. To maximize benefits, restrict high-fat and cholesterol-rich foods including processed foods, dairy products, egg yolks, and fatty cuts of meat to stay under the daily recommended allowance. The National Cholesterol Education Program Expert Panel recommends a therapeutic lifestyle change (TLC) diet to reduce the risk of CHD. In a 32-day randomized double-blind research, 18 subjects ate both a Western diet (38% fat) and a TLC diet (28% fat). Proinflammatory mediators such as tumor necrosis factor-, IL-6, IL-1, and prostaglandin E2 were also assessed, as were cellular immunological responses such as delayed-type hypersensitivity (DTH), in vitro lymphocyte proliferation, and interleukin (IL)-2 production. DTH reaction and lymphocyte proliferative response both increased slightly after ingesting a TLC diet (29% and 27%, respectively). When ingested by older people with high cholesterol levels, the TLC diet increases T cell-mediated immune responses. Given the loss of T cell-mediated immunological capacities with aging and the evidence of lower immune function associated to hypercholesterolemia, this might be a clinically meaningful benefit (Han et al. 2003; Khosla et al. 1997; Mirmiran et al. 2017; Singh et al. 1997).

2.5.9 Ornish Diet

The Ornish Diet is a renowned dietary pattern that promises to help reverse chronic disease as well as boost health. It entails adopting significant lifestyle modifications and adhering to plant-based, low-fat diet rich in fruits, vegetables, whole grains, and legumes. However, it also limits the number of nutritious food groups and may raise your risk of nutritional deficiencies if not planned for properly. The plan is essentially a low-fat, lacto-ovo-vegetarian diet. Dr. Dean Ornish is a medical professional, researcher, and founder of the Preventive Medicine Research Institute in Sausalito, California, who created the Ornish Diet. The researcher of the plan claims that altering your eating habits will help you lose weight and slow the advancement of chronic diseases like diabetes, heart disease, and prostate cancer (Issahaku and Alhassan 2021). It is claimed to function by turning on genes that support good health and slow down cellular aging. The Ornish Diet, in contrast to many other fad diets, is simple and simple to follow. Except for the majority of animal products, you do not have to count calories or monitor your nutritional intake, and no foods are entirely forbidden as part of the diet. Although high-fat foods like nuts, seeds, and vegetable oils are allowed, meat, fish, and chicken are not part of the diet. To follow the Ornish Diet, individuals should eat a lot of fruits, vegetables, whole grains, legumes, and soy products. In addition to being allowed, non-fat dairy products like milk and yogurt are also allowed in quantities of up to two per day. Naturally occurring fats found in complete foods like whole grains and legumes should account for roughly 10% of your daily caloric intake. You can also have three servings or less of foods like nuts and seeds each day (Issahaku and Alhassan 2021). Although the serving sizes are relatively modest, it is crucial to remember that each dish should have no more than 3 grams of fat. Additionally, limiting caffeine-containing beverages, refined carbohydrates, sugar, alcohol, and low-fat packaged meals should be part of the diet. To maximize benefits, it is advised that you modify your diet and engage in at least 30 min of moderate activity each day. There may be several health advantages to the Ornish diet. The Ornish Diet is a great option if you are trying to lose weight because it emphasizes nutrient-dense foods like fruits, vegetables, and plant-based proteins. Dansinger et al. (2005) studied 40 overweight and obese people between the ages of 22 and 72 who had known hypertension, dyslipidemia, or fasting hyperglycemia and kept them on the Ornish Diet for a year.

The average weight loss caused by the Ornish Diet was 3.5% (3.6 kg) after 6 months and 3.2% (3.3 kg) after a year in this trial. Gardner et al. (2007) randomly assigned 311 overweight and obese premenopausal women between the ages of 25 and 50 to the Ornish Diet (n = 76), the Atkins Diet (n = 77), the Zone Diet (n = 79), or the LEARN (Lifestyle, Exercise, Attitudes, Relationships, and Nutrition) Diet (n = 79) for 12 months. According to chart analysis, the Ornish Diet resulted in an average weight loss of 2.9% (2.4 kg) after 6 months and 2.6% (2.2 kg, 95% CI: 3.6 to 0.8 kg) after 12 months. According to promising research, the Ornish Diet may aid in the prevention of chronic disease. Research suggests that vegetarian diets may reduce the risk of heart disease, diabetes, and obesity. One short study with 18 participants examined the effects of three well-known diets, including the Ornish Diet, over the course of 4 weeks. The Ornish Diet reduces levels of inflammation, triglycerides, LDL (bad) cholesterol, and total cholesterol, all of which are cardiovascular disease risk factors (Harmon et al. 2016).

2.5.10 Glycemic Index Diet

The glycemic index (GI) was created by Jenkins et al. in the early 1980s and measures the impact of consuming carbohydrate-rich diets on postprandial glucose concentrations (Jenkins et al. 2002). GI is defined as the difference between the area under the glucose curve (AUC) 2 h after consuming 50 g of carbohydrates in test food and the AUC for standard food. An eating strategy focused on how foods affect blood sugar levels, also known as blood glucose levels, glycemic index (low-GI) diet (Vega-López et al. 2018). The glycemic index assigns food a score between 0 and 100. Foods that have a minimal impact on blood sugar levels are found towards the bottom end of the scale. Foods with a significant impact on blood sugar levels are found on the high end of the spectrum. The glycemic index serves as the primary tool for meal planning on a low-GI diet (Jenkins et al. 1981; Ni et al. 2022). The glycemic index is one of many methods that people can use to decide what foods and meals to eat. Foods are ranked according to how they affect postprandial blood sugar levels on the glycemic index. Diabetes, coronary heart disease, and cancer have all been linked to high energy intake, obesity, and lack of physical activity. These factors are also associated with insulin resistance and hyperinsulinemia (Blumenthal et al. 2010). There are two ways to determine the GI of a diet: one is to directly measure the GI of the diet, and the other is to calculate it using the GI of the individual components. For the latter, the amount of carbohydrates in each component is multiplied by its GI to determine its contribution, which is then added to the sum of all contributions to determine the diet's overall GI (Henry et al. 2021). Previous research has demonstrated that the dietary GI values produced using these two techniques have good validity and that both may be used to precisely predict the blood glucose response to a varied diet. Recently, carbohydrates have received a lot of attention among dietary factors as a primary culprit; nevertheless, different carbohydrates result in diverse glycemic and insulinemic reactions (Jenkins et al.

2002). Two short-term and one long-term clinical studies were published for the Glycemic Index Diet. Ebbeling et al. (2007) studied 36 obese young adults (ages 18–35 years old, BMI 30 kg/m^2) allocated to a low glycemic-index diet for 18 months and discovered that the diet resulted in an average weight loss of 4.3% (4.5 kg) after 6 months and 2.9% (3.0 kg) after 12 months (Ebbeling et al. 2007). Melanson et al. (2012) studied 59 inactive, overweight, and obese adults (aged 25–50 years and BMI = 27.0–35.0 kg/m^2) allocated to a low glycemic index diet for 3 months and discovered that the diet resulted in an average weight loss of 4.0% (3.4 kg) over this time (Melanson et al. 2012).

2.5.11 Macrobiotic Diet

A disciple of George Ohsawa's, Michio Kushi, introduced macrobiotics, a plant-based diet, to the United States around the beginning of the twentieth century. Macrobiotics is more than just a diet; it is based on a set of philosophical ideas that were thought to encourage a healthy way of life and lengthened life (Ohsawa 1965). The term macrobiotics comes from the Greek words makros, which means "long," and bios, which means "life," or makrobiotikos, which means "long-lived." According to Michio Kushi, adopting the macrobiotic philosophy would ultimately result in world peace. He saw macrobiotics as a way to achieve optimal health through eating wholesome, natural foods. A macrobiotic diet consists mainly of vegetarian foods and is low in fat, rich in fiber, and complex carbohydrates. It is connected to a way of life and a spiritual view of the world (Kushi 1977). Contrary to many diets, the composition can be changed depending on a person's health. Personalized based on a person's age, gender, amount of exercise, location, and overall health, among other factors. For instance, eating seasonal, local foods is a key component of macrobiotic philosophy. According to newly revised dietary guidelines, whole grains make up the majority of the diet, accounting for 35–50% of the daily caloric intake. Whole grains include brown rice, barley, millet, wheat, oats, rye, buckwheat, and corn. Grain products that have been processed, such as pasta and bread, are typically avoided. The daily dietary allowance for vegetables ranges from 25% to 35%, emphasizing variety, including leafy green, oblong, and root vegetables (Horowitz and Tomita 2002). Macrobiotics is among the most well-liked supplemental or alternative full-scale lifestyle approaches to cancer. The mainstay of macrobiotics is a largely vegetarian, whole-foods diet that has grown in popularity as a result of remarkable case reports of people who attribute their recovery from cancers with poor prognoses to macrobiotics and the strong evidence that the numerous dietary factors advocated by macrobiotics are linked to lowered cancer risk (Kushi et al. 2001). Women who follow macrobiotic diets had somewhat lower levels of circulating estrogen, which may indicate a reduced risk of breast cancer. The high phytoestrogen content of the macrobiotic diet may contribute to this in some way. There has been little research examining the usefulness of the macrobiotic diet in reducing pain or extending the survival of cancer, similar to most dietary elements used in cancer therapy. In conjunction with a healthy lifestyle, a carefully planned macrobiotic diet may help avoid cancer, diabetes, cardiovascular disease, and obesity. People who already have these illnesses may find it therapeutic (Lerman 2010; Soare et al. 2014).

2.6 Conclusion

Balanced or healthy diets, whether created by traditionally or designed, have many characteristics in common and typically support the WHO International Implementation Plan for the Control and Prevention of Noncommunicable Diseases. These more healthier selections feature fewer amounts of animal-based meals, notably fatty and processed meats, and greater quantities of plant-based foods, such as fresh fruits and vegetables, whole grains, legumes, seeds, and nuts. According to evidence from epidemiologic research and clinical trials, these dietary patterns appear to lower the risks of NCDs, which include everything from cancer to cardiovascular disease. In order to make healthy eating accessible, doable, and sustainable, more efforts must be made to include these beneficial food and lifestyle choices into day-to-day life in communities all over the world.

References

Abdelhamid AS, Brown TJ, Brainard JS, Biswas P, Thorpe GC, Moore HJ, Deane KH, AlAbdulghafoor FK, Summerbell CD, Worthington HV, Song F, Hooper L (2018) Omega-3 fatty acids for the primary and secondary prevention of cardiovascular disease. Cochrane Database Syst Rev 7(7):CD003177. https://doi.org/10.1002/14651858.CD003177.pub3

Ahnen RT, Jonnalagadda SS, Slavin JL (2019) Role of plant protein in nutrition, wellness, and health. Nutr Rev 77(11):735–747. https://doi.org/10.1093/nutrit/nuz028

Alcorta A, Porta A, Tárrega A, Alvarez MD, Vaquero MP (2021) Foods for plant-based diets: challenges and innovations. Foods 10(2). https://doi.org/10.3390/foods10020293

Ambring A, Friberg P, Axelsen M, Laffrenzen M, Taskinen M-R, Basu S, Johansson M (2004) Effects of a Mediterranean-inspired diet on blood lipids, vascular function and oxidative stress in healthy subjects. Clin Sci (London, England: 1979) 106(5):519–525. https://doi.org/10.1042/CS20030315

Andersen R, Biltoft-Jensen A, Christensen T, Andersen EW, Ege M, Thorsen AV, Dalskov SM, Damsgaard CT, Astrup A, Michaelsen KF, Tetens I (2014) Dietary effects of introducing school meals based on the New Nordic Diet – A randomised controlled trial in Danish children. The OPUS School Meal Study. Br J Nutr 111(11):1967–1976. https://doi.org/10.1017/S0007114514000634

Baines S, Powers J, Brown WJ (2007) How does the health and well-being of young Australian vegetarian and semi-vegetarian women compare with non-vegetarians? Public Health Nutr 10(5):436–442. https://doi.org/10.1017/S1368980007217938

Bakaloudi DR, Chrysoula L, Kotzakioulafi E, Theodoridis X, Chourdakis M (2021) Impact of the level of adherence to Mediterranean diet on the parameters of metabolic syndrome: a systematic review and meta-analysis of observational studies. Nutrients 13(5):1514. https://doi.org/10.3390/nu13051514

Battaglia Richi E, Baumer B, Conrad B, Darioli R, Schmid A, Keller U (2015) Health risks associated with meat consumption: a review of epidemiological studies. Int J Vitamin Nutr Res/

Internationale Zeitschrift Fur Vitamin- Und Ernahrungsforschung/Journal International de Vitaminologie et de Nutrition 85(1–2):70–78. https://doi.org/10.1024/0300-9831/a000224
Bazzano LA (2008) Effects of soluble dietary fiber on low-density lipoprotein cholesterol and coronary heart disease risk. Curr Atheroscler Rep 10(6):473–477. https://doi.org/10.1007/S11883-008-0074-3
Blumenthal JA, Babyak MA, Sherwood A, Craighead L, Lin PH, Johnson J, Watkins LL, Wang JT, Kuhn C, Feinglos M, Hinderliter A (2010) Effects of the dietary approaches to stop hypertension diet alone and in combination with exercise and caloric restriction on insulin sensitivity and lipids. Hypertension (Dallas, Tex: 1979) 55(5):1199–1205. https://doi.org/10.1161/HYPERTENSIONAHA.109.149153
Bradbury MWB (1973) Physiology of body fluids and electrolytes. Br J Anaesth 45(9):937–944. https://doi.org/10.1093/bja/45.9.937
Breymeyer KL, Lampe JW, McGregor BA, Neuhouser ML (2016) Subjective mood and energy levels of healthy weight and overweight/obese healthy adults on high-and low-glycemic load experimental diets. Appetite 107:253–259. https://doi.org/10.1016/j.appet.2016.08.008
Campbell AP (2017) DASH eating plan: An eating pattern for diabetes management. Diabetes Spectr 30(2):76–81. https://doi.org/10.2337/ds16-0084
Carughi A, Feeney MJ, Kris-Etherton P, Fulgoni V 3rd, Kendall CWC, Bulló M, Webb D (2016) Pairing nuts and dried fruit for cardiometabolic health. Nutr J 15:23. https://doi.org/10.1186/s12937-016-0142-4
Cena H, Calder PC (2020) Defining a healthy diet: evidence for the role of. Nutrients 12(334):1–15. https://doi.org/10.3390/nu12020334
Centre for Disease Control, NHLBI (2005) Can lifestyle modifications using theraputic lifestyle changes (TLC) reduce weight and the risk of chronic disease?
Clarys P, Deliens T, Huybrechts I, Deriemaeker P, Vanaelst B, De Keyzer W, Hebbelinck M, Mullie P (2014) Comparison of nutritional quality of the vegan, vegetarian, semi-vegetarian, pesco-vegetarian and omnivorous diet. Nutrients 6(3):1318–1332. https://doi.org/10.3390/nu6031318
Craig WJ (2009) Position of the American Dietetic Association: vegetarian diets. J Am Diet Assoc 109(7):1266–1282. https://doi.org/10.1016/j.jada.2009.05.027
Craig WJ (2010) Nutrition concerns and health effects of vegetarian diets. Nutr Clin Pract 25(6):613–620. https://doi.org/10.1177/0884533610385707
Dansinger ML, Gleason JA, Griffith JL, Selker HP, Schaefer EJ (2005) Comparison of the atkins, ornish, weight watchers, and zone diets for weight loss and heart disease risk reduction: A randomized trial. J Am Med Assoc, 293(1):43–53. https://doi.org/10.1001/jama.293.1.43
De Cosmi V, Mazzocchi A, Milani GP, Agostoni C (2022) Dietary patterns vs. dietary recommendations. Front Nutr 9. https://doi.org/10.3389/fnut.2022.883806
Derbyshire EJ (2016) Flexitarian diets and health: A review of the evidence-based literature. Front Nutr 3:55. https://doi.org/10.3389/fnut.2016.00055
Derbyshire EJ (2017) Flexitarian diets and health: A review of the evidence-based literature. Front Nutr 3:55. https://doi.org/10.3389/fnut.2016.00055
Dermatol D (2015) Full text links 12(10):8–9
Dos Reis Padilha G, Sanches Machado d'Almeida K, Ronchi Spillere S, Corrêa Souza G (2018) Dietary patterns in secondary prevention of heart failure: a systematic review. Nutrients 10(7). https://doi.org/10.3390/nu10070828
Ebbeling CB, Leidig MM, Feldman HA, Lovesky MM, Ludwig DS (2007) Effects of a low-glycemic load vs low-fat diet in obese young adults: a randomized trial. JAMA 297(19):2092–2102. https://doi.org/10.1001/JAMA.297.19.2092
Enebe JT, Dim CC, Ugwu EO, Enebe NO, Meka IA, Obioha KC, Eleje GU, Nwagha UI (2020) Serum antioxidant micronutrient levels in pre-eclamptic pregnant women in Enugu, south-East Nigeria: a comparative cross-sectional analytical study. BMC Pregnancy Childbirth 20(1):392. https://doi.org/10.1186/s12884-020-03081-w
Errett PJ, Willett WC (2010) Essentials of healthy eating: A guide. J Midwifery Womens Health 55(6):492–501. https://doi.org/10.1016/j.jmwh.2010.06.019

Field MS, Mithra P, Peña-Rosas JP (2021) Wheat flour fortification with iron and other micronutrients for reducing anaemia and improving iron status in populations. The. Cochrane Database Syst Rev 1(1):CD011302–CD011302. https://doi.org/10.1002/14651858.CD011302.pub3

Food and Drug Administration (2022) Daily value and percent daily value: changes on the new nutrition and supplement facts labels daily value vs. % Daily Value. Retrieved January 31, 2023, from www.FDA.gov/NewNutritionFactsLabel

Fresán U, Sabaté J (2019) Vegetarian diets: planetary health and its alignment with human health. Adv Nutr (Bethesda, Md.) 10(Suppl_4):S380–S388. https://doi.org/10.1093/advances/nmz019

Gadgil MD, Appel LJ, Yeung E, Anderson CAM, Sacks FM, Miller ER 3rd. (2013) The effects of carbohydrate, unsaturated fat, and protein intake on measures of insulin sensitivity: results from the OmniHeart trial. Diabetes Care 36(5):1132–1137. https://doi.org/10.2337/dc12-0869

Gardner CD, Kiazand A, Alhassan S, Kim S, Stafford RS, Balise RR, Kraemer HC, King AC (2007) Comparison of the atkins, zone, ornish, and LEARN diets for change in weight and related risk factors among overweight premenopausal women: The a TO Z weight loss study: a randomized trial. J Am Med Assoc, 297(9):969–977. https://doi.org/10.1001/jama.297.9.969

Gibson RS (2007) The role of diet- and host-related factors in nutrient bioavailability and thus in nutrient-based dietary requirement estimates. Food Nutr Bull 28(1 Suppl International):S77–S100. https://doi.org/10.1177/15648265070281S108

Godos J, Castellano S, Marranzano M (2019a) Adherence to a Mediterranean dietary pattern is associated with higher quality of life in a cohort of Italian adults. Nutrients 11(5). https://doi.org/10.3390/nu11050981

Godos J, Ferri R, Caraci F, Cosentino FII, Castellano S, Galvano F, Grosso G (2019b) Adherence to the Mediterranean diet is associated with better sleep quality in Italian adults. Nutrients 11(5). https://doi.org/10.3390/nu11050976

Golzarand M, Mirmiran P, Azizi F (2022) Adherence to the MIND diet and the risk of cardiovascular disease in adults: a cohort study. Food Funct 13(3):1651–1658. https://doi.org/10.1039/D1FO02069B

Han SN, Leka LS, Lichtenstein AH, Ausman LM, Meydani SN (2003) Effect of a therapeutic lifestyle change diet on immune functions of moderately hypercholesterolemic humans. J Lipid Res 44(12):2304–2310. https://doi.org/10.1194/JLR.M300181-JLR200

Hargreaves SM, Raposo A, Saraiva A, Zandonadi RP (2021) Vegetarian diet: an overview through the perspective of quality of life domains. Int J Environ Res Public Health 18(8). https://doi.org/10.3390/ijerph18084067

Harmon ME, Campen MJ, Miller C, Shuey C, Cajero M, Lucas S, Pacheco B, Erdei E, Ramone S, Nez T, Lewis J (2016) Associations of circulating oxidized LDL and conventional biomarkers of cardiovascular disease in a cross-sectional study of the Navajo population. PLoS One 11(3):e0143102. https://doi.org/10.1371/journal.pone.0143102

Henry CJ, Quek RYC, Kaur B, Shyam S, Singh HKG (2021) A glycaemic index compendium of non-western foods. Nutr Diabetes 11(1):1–36. https://doi.org/10.1038/s41387-020-00145-w

Hooper L, Abdelhamid AS, Jimoh OF, Bunn D, Skeaff CM (2020) Effects of total fat intake on body fatness in adults. Cochrane Database Syst Rev 6(6):CD013636. https://doi.org/10.1002/14651858.CD013636

Horowitz J, Tomita M (2002) The macrobiotic diet as treatment for cancer: review of the evidence. Perm J 6(4):34

Iguacel I, Huybrechts I, Moreno LA, Michels N (2021) Vegetarianism and veganism compared with mental health and cognitive outcomes: a systematic review and meta-analysis. Nutr Rev 79(4):361–381. https://doi.org/10.1093/nutrit/nuaa030

Imamura F, Sharp SJ, Koulman A, Schulze MB, Kröger J, Griffin JL, Huerta JM, Guevara M, Sluijs I, Agudo A, Ardanaz E, Balkau B, Boeing H, Chajes V, Dahm CC, Dow C, Fagherazzi G, Feskens EJM, Franks PW et al (2017) A combination of plasma phospholipid fatty acids and its association with incidence of type 2 diabetes: the EPIC-InterAct case-cohort study. PLoS Med 14(10):e1002409–e1002409. https://doi.org/10.1371/journal.pmed.1002409

Issahaku I, Alhassan M (2021) Nutrition knowledge, dietary practices and nutritional status of non-academic staff at the Tamale campus of University for Development Studies. Heliyon 7(4):e06635. https://doi.org/10.1016/j.heliyon.2021.e06635

Jenkins DJA, Wolever TMS, Taylor RH, Barker H, Fielden H, Baldwin JM, Bowling AC, Newman HC, Goff DV (1981) Glycemic index of foods: a physiological basis for carbohydrate exchange. Am J Clin Nutr 34(3):362–366. https://doi.org/10.1093/AJCN/34.3.362

Jenkins DJA, Kendall CWC, Augustin LSA, Franceschi S, Hamidi M, Marchie A, Jenkins AL, Axelsen M (2002) Glycemic index: overview of implications in health and disease. Am J Clin Nutr 76(1). https://doi.org/10.1093/AJCN/76/1.266S

Johansson U, Lindberg L, Öhlund I, Hernell O, Lönnerdal B, Lundén S, Sandell M, Lind T (2021) Acceptance of a Nordic, protein-reduced diet for young children during complementary feeding-A randomized controlled trial. Foods (Basel, Switzerland) 10(2):275. https://doi.org/10.3390/foods10020275

Jones-McLean E, Hu J, Greene-Finestone LS, de Groh M (2015) A DASH dietary pattern and the risk of colorectal cancer in Canadian adults. Health Promot Chronic Dis Prev Can 35(1):12–20. https://doi.org/10.24095/hpcdp.35.1.03

Kesson AA, Andersen LF, Kristjánsd6 Ttir G, Roos E, Trolle E, Voutilainen E, Wirfält E (2013) Health effects associated with foods characteristic of the Nordic diet: a systematic literature review. Food Nutr Res. https://doi.org/10.3402/fnr.v57i0.22790

Keys A, Keys M (2006) How to eat well and stay well. The Mediterranean way. FDM

Khosla P, Hajri T, Pronczuk A, Hayes KC (1997) VIIth Asian congress of Nutrition: lipid symposium proceedings replacing dietary palmitic acid with Elaidic acid (t-C18:1D9) depresses HDL and increases CETP activity in Cebus monkeys. J Nutr 127:531–536. https://academic.oup.com/jn/article/127/3/531S/4728708

Kushi M (1977) The book of macrobiotics the universal way of health and happiness. https://philpapers.org/rec/KUSTBO

Kushi LH, Cunningham JE, Hebert JR, Lerman RH, Bandera EV, Teas J (2001) The macrobiotic diet in cancer. J Nutr. https://doi.org/10.1093/jn/131.11.3056S

Lacoppidan SA, Kyrø C, Loft S, Helnaes A, Christensen J, Hansen CP, Dahm CC, Overvad K, Tjønneland A, Olsen A (2015) Adherence to a healthy Nordic food index is associated with a lower risk of type-2 diabetes-the Danish diet, Cancer and Health Cohort Study. Br J Nutr. https://doi.org/10.3390/nu7105418

Lankinen M, Uusitupa M, Schwab U (2019) Nordic diet and inflammation-A review of observational and intervention studies. Nutrients 11(6). https://doi.org/10.3390/nu11061369

Lauber C, Gerl MJ, Klose C, Ottosson F, Melander O, Simons K (2022) Lipidomic risk scores are independent of polygenic risk scores and can predict incidence of diabetes and cardiovascular disease in a large population cohort. PLoS Biol 20(3):e3001561–e3001561. https://doi.org/10.1371/journal.pbio.3001561

Lea EJ, Crawford D, Worsley A (2006) Public views of the benefits and barriers to the consumption of a plant-based diet. Eur J Clin Nutr 60(7):828–837. https://doi.org/10.1038/sj.ejcn.1602387

Lee BR, Ko YM, Cho MH, Yoon YR, Kye SH, Park YK (2016) Effects of 12-week vegetarian diet on the nutritional status, stress status and bowel habits in middle school students and teachers. Clin Nutr Res 5(2):102–111. https://doi.org/10.7762/cnr.2016.5.2.102

Lerman RH (2010) The macrobiotic diet in chronic disease. Nutr Clin Pract 25(6):621–626. https://doi.org/10.1177/0884533610385704

Lescinsky H, Afshin A, Ashbaugh C, Bisignano C, Brauer M, Ferrara G, Hay SI, He J, Iannucci V, Marczak LB, McLaughlin SA, Mullany EC, Parent MC, Serfes AL, Sorensen RJD, Aravkin AY, Zheng P, Murray CJL (2022) Health effects associated with consumption of unprocessed red meat: a Burden of Proof study. Nat Med 28(10):2075–2082. https://doi.org/10.1038/s41591-022-01968-z

Lim S (2018) Eating a balanced diet: a healthy life through a balanced diet in the age of longevity. J Obes Metab Syndr 27(1):39–45. https://doi.org/10.7570/JOMES.2018.27.1.39

Liska D, Mah E, Brisbois T, Barrios PL, Baker LB, Spriet LL (2019) Narrative review of hydration and selected health outcomes in the general population. Nutrients 11(1):70. https://doi.org/10.3390/nu11010070

Lonnie M, Hooker E, Brunstrom JM, Corfe BM, Green MA, Watson AW, Williams EA, Stevenson EJ, Penson S, Johnstone AM (2018) Nutrients protein for life: review of optimal protein intake, sustainable dietary sources and the effect on appetite in ageing adults. Nutrients. https://doi.org/10.3390/nu10030360

Lorenzo PM, Izquierdo AG, Rodriguez-Carnero G, Fernández-Pombo A, Iglesias A, Carreira MC, Tejera C, Bellido D, Martinez-Olmos MA, Leis R, Casanueva FF, Crujeiras AB (2022) Epigenetic effects of healthy foods and lifestyle habits from the Southern European Atlantic diet pattern: A narrative review. Adv Nutr (Bethesda, Md.) 13(5):1725–1747. https://doi.org/10.1093/advances/nmac038

Manz F, Wentz A, Sichert-Hellert W (2002) The most essential nutrient: defining the adequate intake of water. J Pediatr 141(4):587–592. https://doi.org/10.1067/mpd.2002.128031

Marrone G, Guerriero C, Palazzetti D, Lido P, Marolla A, Di Daniele F, Noce A (2021) Vegan diet health benefits in metabolic syndrome. Nutrients 13(3). https://doi.org/10.3390/nu13030817

Martinez-Perez C, San-Cristobal R, Guallar-Castillon P, Martínez-González MÁ, Salas-Salvadó J, Corella D, Castañer O, Martinez JA, Alonso-Gómez ÁM, Wärnberg J, Vioque J, Romaguera D, López-Miranda J, Estruch R, Tinahones FJ, Lapetra J, Serra-Majem L, Bueno-Cavanillas A, Tur JA et al (2021) Use of different food classification systems to assess the association between ultra-processed food consumption and Cardiometabolic health in an elderly population with metabolic syndrome (PREDIMED-Plus Cohort). Nutrients 13(7):2471. https://doi.org/10.3390/nu13072471

McBurney MI et al (2021) Beyond nutrient deficiency-opportunities to improve nutritional status and promote health modernizing DRIs and supplementation recommendations. Nutrients 13(6):1844. https://doi.org/10.3390/nu13061844

Melanson KJ, Summers A, Nguyen V, Brosnahan J, Lowndes J, Angelopoulos TJ, Rippe JM (2012) Body composition, dietary composition, and components of metabolic syndrome in overweight and obese adults after a 12-week trial on dietary treatments focused on portion control, energy density, or glycemic index. Nutr J 11(1). https://doi.org/10.1186/1475-2891-11-57

Mentella MC, Scaldaferri F, Ricci C, Gasbarrini A, Miggiano GAD (2019) Cancer and Mediterranean diet: a review. Nutrients 11(9). https://doi.org/10.3390/nu11092059

Milani GP, Silano M, Mazzocchi A, Bettocchi S, de Cosmi V, Agostoni C (2021) Personalized nutrition approach in pediatrics: a narrative review. Pediatr Res. https://doi.org/10.1038/s41390-020-01291-8

Mirmiran P, Hosseinpour-Niazi S, Azizi F (2017) Therapeutic lifestyle change diet enriched in legumes reduces oxidative stress in overweight type 2 diabetic patients: a crossover randomised clinical trial. Eur J Clin Nutr 72(1):174–176. https://doi.org/10.1038/ejcn.2017.113

Mithril C, Dragsted LO, Meyer C, Blauert E, Holt MK, Astrup A (2012) Guidelines for the New Nordic Diet. Public Health Nutr 15(10):1941–1947. https://doi.org/10.1017/S136898001100351X

Mithril C, Dragsted LO, Meyer C, Tetens I, Biltoft-Jensen A, Astrup A (2013) Dietary composition and nutrient content of the New Nordic Diet. Public Health Nutr 16(5):777–785. https://doi.org/10.1017/S1368980012004521

Morris MC, Tangney CC, Wang Y, Sacks FM, Barnes LL, Bennett DA, Aggarwal NT (2015a) MIND diet slows cognitive decline with aging. Alzheimers Dement 11(9):1015–1022. https://doi.org/10.1016/j.jalz.2015.04.011

Morris MC, Tangney CC, Wang Y, Sacks FM, Bennett DA, Aggarwal NT (2015b) MIND diet associated with reduced incidence of Alzheimer's disease. Alzheimers Dement 11(9):1007–1014. https://doi.org/10.1016/j.jalz.2014.11.009

Nair KPM, Augustine LF (2018) Country-specific nutrient requirements & recommended dietary allowances for Indians: current status & future directions. Indian J Med Res 148(5):522–530. https://doi.org/10.4103/ijmr.IJMR_1762_18

Naude CE, Brand A, Schoonees A, Nguyen KA, Chaplin M, Volmink J (2022) Low-carbohydrate versus balanced-carbohydrate diets for reducing weight and cardiovascular risk. Cochrane Database Syst Rev 1(1):CD013334. https://doi.org/10.1002/14651858.CD013334.pub2

Nettleton JA, Brouwer IA, Mensink RP, Diekman C, Hornstra G (2018) Fats in foods: current evidence for dietary advice. Ann Nutr Metab 72(3):248–254. https://doi.org/10.1159/000488006

Nhlbi (2005) Your guide to lowering your cholesterol with TLC

Ni C, Jia Q, Ding G, Wu X, Yang M (2022) Low-glycemic index diets as an intervention in metabolic diseases: A systematic review and meta-analysis. Nutrients 14(2). https://doi.org/10.3390/NU14020307

Nutrition H (2002) Encyclopedia of foods: a guide to healthy nutrition. Choice Rev Online 40(01):40-0025-40–0025. https://doi.org/10.5860/choice.40-0025

Ohsawa G (1965) Zen macrobiotics:the art of rejuvenation and longevity [Pocket book ed.]. Ohsawa Foundation

Peña-Rosas JP, Mithra P, Unnikrishnan B, Kumar N, De-Regil LM, Nair NS, Garcia-Casal MN, Solon JA (2019) Fortification of rice with vitamins and minerals for addressing micronutrient malnutrition. The. Cochrane Database Syst Rev 2019(10):CD009902. https://doi.org/10.1002/14651858.CD009902.pub2

Popkin BM (2006) Global nutrition dynamics: the world is shifting rapidly toward a diet linked with noncommunicable diseases. Am J Clin Nutr 84(2):289–298. https://doi.org/10.1093/ajcn/84.2.289

Portugal-Nunes C, Nunes FM, Fraga I, Saraiva C, Gonçalves C (2021) Assessment of the methodology that is used to determine the nutritional sustainability of the Mediterranean diet-A scoping review. Front Nutr 8:772133. https://doi.org/10.3389/fnut.2021.772133

Rizzo NS, Sabaté J, Jaceldo-Siegl K, Fraser GE (2011) Vegetarian dietary patterns are associated with a lower risk of metabolic syndrome: the adventist health study 2. Diabetes Care 34(5):1225–1227. https://doi.org/10.2337/dc10-1221

Rizzo NS, Jaceldo-Siegl K, Sabate J, Fraser GE (2013) Nutrient profiles of vegetarian and nonvegetarian dietary patterns. J Acad Nutr Diet 113(12):1610–1619. https://doi.org/10.1016/j.jand.2013.06.349

Sacks FM, Svetkey LP, Vollmer WM, Appel LJ, Bray GA, Harsha D, Obarzanek E, Conlin PR, Miller ER 3rd, Simons-Morton DG, Karanja N, Lin PH (2001) Effects on blood pressure of reduced dietary sodium and the Dietary Approaches to Stop Hypertension (DASH) diet. DASH-Sodium Collaborative Research Group. N Engl J Med 344(1):3–10. https://doi.org/10.1056/NEJM200101043440101

Sanders LM, Zhu Y, Wilcox ML, Koecher K, Maki KC (2021) Effects of whole grain intake, compared with refined grain, on appetite and energy intake: a systematic review and meta-analysis. Adv Nutr (Bethesda, Md.) 12(4):1177–1195. https://doi.org/10.1093/advances/nmaa178

Savarino G, Corsello A, Corsello G (2021) Macronutrient balance and micronutrient amounts through growth and development. Ital J Pediatr 47(1):109. https://doi.org/10.1186/s13052-021-01061-0

Schulze MB, Martínez-González MA, Fung TT, Lichtenstein AH, Forouhi NG (2018) Food based dietary patterns and chronic disease prevention. BMJ 361. https://doi.org/10.1136/BMJ.K2396

Schwingshackl L, Hoffmann G (2016) Does a Mediterranean-type diet reduce cancer risk? Curr Nutr Rep 5:9–17. https://doi.org/10.1007/s13668-015-0141-7

Schwingshackl L, Morze J, Hoffmann G (2020) Mediterranean diet and health status: active ingredients and pharmacological mechanisms. Br J Pharmacol 177(6):1241–1257. https://doi.org/10.1111/bph.14778

Setty K, Loret J-F, Courtois S, Hammer CC, Hartemann P, Lafforgue M, Litrico X, Manasfi T, Medema G, Shaheen M, Tesson V, Bartram J (2019) Faster and safer: research priorities in water and health. Int J Hyg Environ Health 222(4):593–606. https://doi.org/10.1016/j.ijheh.2019.03.003

Singh RB, Rastogi SS, Rao PV, Das S, Madhu SV, Das AK, Sahay BK, Fuse SM, Beegom R, Sainani GS, Shah NA (1997) Diet and lifestyle guidelines and desirable levels of risk factors for the prevention of diabetes and its vascular complications in Indians: a scientific statement of the International College of Nutrition. J Cardiovasc Risk 4(3):201–208. https://doi.org/10.1097/00043798-199706000-00007

Soare A, Khazrai YM, del Toro R, Roncella E, Fontana L, Fallucca S, Angeletti S, Formisano V, Capata F, Ruiz V, Porrata C, Skrami E, Gesuita R, Manfrini S, Fallucca F, Pianesi M, Pozzilli P (2014) The effect of the macrobiotic Ma-Pi 2 diet vs. the recommended diet in the management of type 2 diabetes: the randomized controlled MADIAB trial. Nutr Metab 11(1):39. https://doi.org/10.1186/1743-7075-11-39

Soltani S, Arablou T, Jayedi A, Salehi-Abargouei A (2020) Adherence to the dietary approaches to stop hypertension (DASH) diet in relation to all-cause and cause-specific mortality: a systematic review and dose-response meta-analysis of prospective cohort studies. Nutr J 19(1):37. https://doi.org/10.1186/s12937-020-00554-8

Szwiega S, Pencharz PB, Rafii M, Lebarron M, Chang J, Ball RO, Kong D, Xu L, Elango R, Courtney-Martin G (2021) Dietary leucine requirement of older men and women is higher than current recommendations. Am J Clin Nutr 113(2):410–419. https://doi.org/10.1093/ajcn/nqaa323

Tamimi RM, Spiegelman D, Smith-Warner SA, Wang M, Pazaris M, Willett WC, Eliassen AH, Hunter DJ (2016) Population attributable risk of modifiable and nonmodifiable breast cancer risk factors in postmenopausal breast cancer. Am J Epidemiol 184(12):884–893. https://doi.org/10.1093/aje/kww145

Thompson SV, Hannon BA, An R, Holscher HD (2017) Effects of isolated soluble fiber supplementation on body weight, glycemia, and insulinemia in adults with overweight and obesity: a systematic review and meta-analysis of randomized controlled trials. Am J Clin Nutr 106(6):1514–1528. https://doi.org/10.3945/AJCN.117.163246

Tonstad S, Stewart K, Oda K, Batech M, Herring RP, Fraser GE (2013) Vegetarian diets and incidence of diabetes in the Adventist Health Study-2. Nutr Metab Cardiovasc Dis 23(4):292–299. https://doi.org/10.1016/j.numecd.2011.07.004

Trichopoulou A (2021) Mediterranean diet as intangible heritage of humanity: 10 years on. Nutr Metab Cardiovasc Dis 31(7):1943–1948. https://doi.org/10.1016/j.numecd.2021.04.011

Trichopoulou A, Bamia C, Trichopoulos D (2009) Anatomy of health effects of Mediterranean diet: Greek EPIC prospective cohort study. BMJ 338:b2337. https://doi.org/10.1136/bmj.b2337

Turck D, Bohn T, Castenmiller J, De Henauw S, Hirsch-Ernst KI, Knutsen HK, Maciuk A, Mangelsdorf I, McArdle HJ, Peláez C, Pentieva K, Siani A, Thies F, Tsabouri S, Vinceti M, Aggett P, Crous Bou M, Cubadda F, de Sesmaisons Lecarré A et al (2022) Guidance for establishing and applying tolerable upper intake levels for vitamins and essential minerals: draft for internal testing. EFSA J 20(1):e200102. https://doi.org/10.2903/j.efsa.2022.e200102

Tyson CC, Nwankwo C, Lin P-H, Svetkey LP (2012) The Dietary Approaches to Stop Hypertension (DASH) eating pattern in special populations. Curr Hypertens Rep 14(5):388–396. https://doi.org/10.1007/s11906-012-0296-1

Vega-López S, Venn BJ, Slavin JL (2018) Relevance of the glycemic index and glycemic load for body weight, diabetes, and cardiovascular disease. Nutrients 10(10). https://doi.org/10.3390/NU10101361

Vo-Nguyen BQ, Kong HY (2009) Symbol Error Rate expression for decode-and-forward relaying using generalized selection combining over Rayleigh fading channels. IEICE Trans Commun E92-B(4):1369–1372. https://doi.org/10.1587/transcom.E92.B.1369

Wickman BE, Enkhmaa B, Ridberg R, Romero E, Cadeiras M, Meyers F, Steinberg F (2021) Dietary Management of Heart Failure: DASH diet and precision nutrition perspectives. Nutrients 13(12):4424. https://doi.org/10.3390/nu13124424

Wickramasinghe K, Wilkins E, Foster C, Fadhil I, Hammerich A, Slama S, El Berri H, Elimam M, Adib S, Al-Mudwahi M, Townsend N (2018) The development of national multisectoral action plans for the prevention and control of noncommunicable diseases: experiences of national-level stakeholders in four countries. Glob Health Action 11(1):1532632. https://doi.org/10.1080/16549716.2018.1532632

Yau YHC, Potenza MN (2013) Stress and eating behaviors. Minerva Endocrinol 38(3):255–267

Nutrition Biology: A New Paradigm for Human Health

3

Manoj Kumar Tripathi, Nidhi V. Maheshwari, Anil Kumar, Aman Kumar, Adinath Kate, Rajpal Singh Jadam, Samreen Khan, and Riya Chouhan

Abstract

The nutrition transition, characterized by a shift from traditional diets to modern dietary patterns with high-energy density and reduced nutrient diversity, is closely linked to the prevalence of acquired metabolic syndromes. The human diet comprises a complex array of both nutrient and non-nutrient components, which serve as fundamental substrates for various metabolic pathways at the cellular level. Additionally, these dietary constituents and their metabolites play a crucial role in modulating gene expression and regulating diverse cellular functions through intricate molecular mechanisms. While certain dietary components exert beneficial effects, others may have cytotoxic or adverse metabolic consequences. Recent studies highlight that metabolic activity is influenced by multiple factors, including extrinsic determinants (e.g., dietary composition, environmental exposure, xenobiotics) and intrinsic determinants (e.g., sex, age, genetic polymorphisms). Furthermore, interactions between the host and gut microbiota significantly modulate metabolic processes, impacting susceptibility to acquired metabolic disorders. Emerging evidence underscores the importance of consuming low-energy, nutrient-dense diets in promoting and maintaining optimal physiological health. In developing nations, plant-based foods constitute a predominant portion of the diet, largely due to the limited consumption of animal-derived products, which is constrained by economic factors and cultural

M. K. Tripathi (✉) · A. Kumar · A. Kate · R. S. Jadam · S. Khan · R. Chouhan
ICAR- Central Institute of Agricultural Engineering, Bhopal, Madhya Pradesh, India
e-mail: tripathimanoj007@gmail.com

N. V. Maheshwari
Somaiya Vidyavihar University, Mumbai, Maharashtra, India

A. Kumar
Rani Lakshmi Bai Central Agricultural University, Jhansi, Uttar Pradesh, India

A. Kumar et al. (eds.), *Innovations in Ayurvedic Nutrition*,
https://doi.org/10.1007/978-981-95-1213-3_3

or religious practices. However, reliance on plant-based diets is frequently associated with micronutrient deficiencies and suboptimal bioavailability of essential nutrients. Several dietary factors influence nutrient assimilation, including the food matrix composition, nutrient interactions, and the presence of anti-nutritional compounds such as polyphenols, phytates, dietary fiber, oxalates, proteins, lipids, and ascorbic acid. Additionally, food processing techniques significantly affect nutrient bioavailability. Consequently, there is an urgent need for dietary interventions and processing strategies aimed at minimizing the inhibitory effects of anti-nutrients and enhancing micronutrient bioavailability to support better health outcomes.

Keywords

Nutrition biology · Nutrigenomics · Biomolecules · Microbiome · Bioactive compounds · Human health

3.1 Introduction

Human nutrition involves the biochemical and physiological mechanisms by which cells, organelles, tissues, and organ systems assimilate and metabolize essential nutrients derived from dietary intake to sustain structural integrity and optimal physiological function. The investigation of nutrient interactions at molecular, cellular, and systemic levels, along with the extrinsic and intrinsic factors influencing these processes, necessitates an interdisciplinary approach encompassing molecular biology, genetics, biochemistry, and nutritional sciences. Recent advancements at the genetic level have elucidated the role of nutrients in modulating phenotypic expression by influencing transcription, translation, and post-translational modifications. Dietary components can directly impact gene expression, determining the synthesis of specific RNAs and proteins (Fenech 2012). For instance, glucose, a carbohydrate, stimulates transcriptional activity, enhancing the synthesis and activation of glucokinase. Iron regulates translational efficiency for ferritin synthesis, whereas vitamin K facilitates post-translational carboxylation of glutamic acid residues, essential for prothrombin activation. Nutrients thus serve as key regulators of gene expression, contributing to the synthesis of structural and functional proteins at the molecular level (Popkin et al. 2012). Additionally, nutrients act as substrates and cofactors in metabolic pathways essential for growth, development, and homeostasis. The circulatory system ensures the transport of nutrients and oxygen while concurrently facilitating the removal of metabolic waste products and toxic substances, which are excreted via the skin, kidneys, and intestines. A comprehensive, integrative approach to human nutrition is illustrated in Fig. 3.1, highlighting the dynamic interplay between nutritional status and organ system health, which collectively determine overall nutrient requirements.

Food represents a complex biochemical matrix composed of a diverse array of constituents, broadly categorized into nutrients and non-nutrient compounds. Nutrients are further classified based on their quantitative requirements into

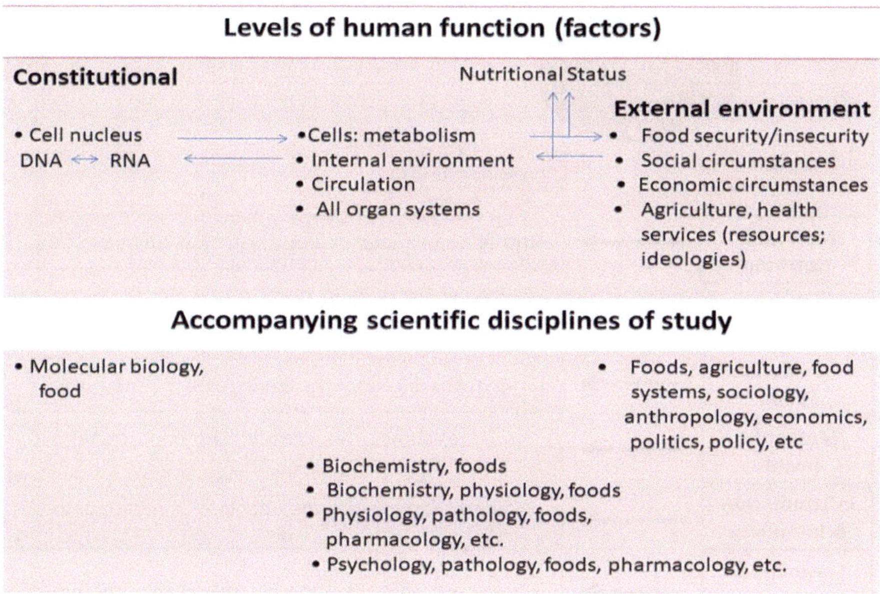

Fig. 3.1 Basic approach of human nutrition

macronutrients and micronutrients. The nutritional demands of plants and animals differ significantly, leading to the biosynthesis of distinct metabolic compounds that may not be universally present across both biological kingdoms. Micronutrients, encompassing essential vitamins and minerals, are required in minute concentrations to facilitate enzymatic catalysis and protein-mediated biochemical processes. In contrast, macronutrients which include carbohydrates, proteins, and lipids are indispensable in larger quantities, playing a crucial role as structural components of cells and serving as primary sources of metabolic energy. Certain species lack the metabolic capacity to synthesize vital compounds necessary for survival, necessitating their dietary acquisition. These vital biochemical compounds, categorized as essential nutrients, encompass distinct amino acids, essential fatty acids, micronutrients such as vitamins, and inorganic elements classified as minerals. These substances play a crucial role in maintaining physiological homeostasis, supporting metabolic functions, and facilitating biochemical pathways necessary for cellular growth, repair, and overall systemic health. Non-nutrient dietary components, which do not fall within the macronutrient or micronutrient categories, exhibit diverse physiological effects. They include beneficial compounds such as dietary fiber and polyphenols, non-beneficial additives and preservatives, and potentially harmful xenobiotics and antibiotics. Some polyphenolic compounds derived from plants may exert both beneficial and adverse effects (Suez et al. 2014). Emerging research indicates that both nutrients and non-nutrient dietary components, along with their metabolites, modulate key molecular mechanisms, including gene expression, protein functionality, and epigenetic modifications (Hardy and Tollefsbol 2011). These

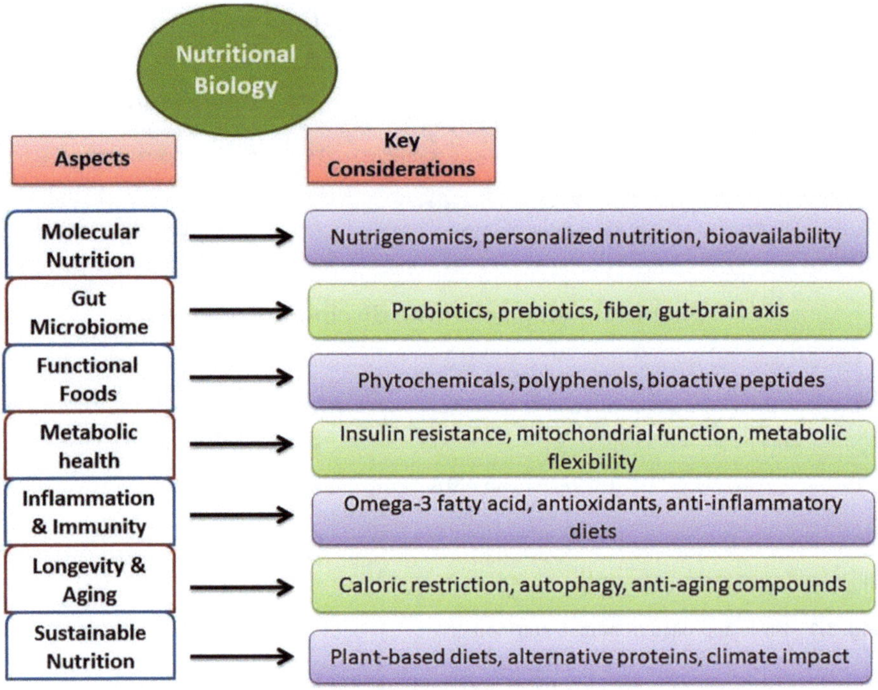

Fig. 3.2 Nutrition biology: a new paradigm for human health

findings underscore the complex and dynamic interactions between diet and human physiology, emphasizing the important role of diet in health and sickness prevention.

The field of human dietetics and nutritional science seeks to analyze the intricate interactions between sociocultural and biological determinants that shape dietary behaviors, metabolic functions, and overall health outcomes. This multidisciplinary perspective advances the thoughtfulness of the etiological aspects contributing to malnutrition while elucidating the complex interdependence between nutrient intake and physiological homeostasis (Fig. 3.2).

3.2 Nutrients

Nutrients are essential biochemical compounds derived from food during digestion. The three primary macronutrient groups—carbohydrates, proteins, and lipids—are required in varying quantities to support physiological functions (Gropper and Smith 2012). These macronutrients play a key part in cellular growth, tissue repair, maintenance, and energy production necessary for metabolic processes (Soetan et al. 2010). Additionally, dietary fiber, vitamins, and minerals contribute to various biological functions and are present in differing concentrations across food sources. Optimal nutrition necessitates a well-balanced intake of these nutrients in appropriate proportions to sustain overall health. Malnutrition, in its various forms—undernutrition, micronutrient deficiencies, and overnutrition—remains a significant global health challenge. According to the World Health Organization (2021), approximately one-third of the global population experiences malnutrition in some capacity. Deficiencies in essential nutrients have profound implications for both physiological and psychological health (Doll and Peto 1981). Over the past four decades, diet-related mortality has persisted as a major public health concern, with suboptimal dietary patterns contributing to approximately 20% of global deaths, primarily due to cardiovascular diseases and cancer (Afshin et al. 2019). Beyond physical health, increasing evidence suggests that dietary patterns significantly influence mental well-being. Large-scale observational studies and clinical interventions indicate a strong correlation between dietary quality, mental health, and overall well-being, with nutritional supplementation demonstrating beneficial effects on conditions such as depression and anxiety.

3.2.1 Essential Nutrients for Energy

1. Carbohydrates are organic compounds consisting of saccharide units and are categorized based on their structural complexity. Monosaccharides, oligosaccharides, and polysaccharides serve as primary energy sources for cellular metabolism.
2. Protein molecules have amino acid monomeric form linked with peptide bonds. Proteins play a crucial role in tissue synthesis, enzymatic reactions, and immune system. Certain amino acids, named essential amino acids, cannot be endogenously made and must be obtained through dietary intake. During digestion, proteins undergo hydrolysis into free amino acids, which are subsequently absorbed and utilized for biosynthetic processes.
3. Fat molecules contain a glycerol backbone and esterified to fatty acids. Fatty acids are classified as saturated (containing only single bonds) or unsaturated (containing one or more double bonds). Lipids are essential for cellular membrane integrity, thermoregulation, organ protection, and dermal health. Certain fatty acids, known as essential fatty acids (e.g., omega-3 and omega-6), cannot be synthesized de novo and come from dietary sources.

3.2.2 Link Between Nutrition and Health

Humans consume food rather than isolated nutrients; however, the composition and proportion of nutrients within ingested foods ultimately determine health outcomes. It is crucial to recognize that, beyond nutrition, several extrinsic factors—such as lifestyle and environmental influences—affect human health and well-being. Scientific evidence highlights the fundamental role of nutrition as a regulatory and influential factor in helping human health, preventing and managing diseases, and enhancing overall value of life (Phillips 2017). To develop a complete thoughtful of nutrition, it is important to explore various aspects of nutrients, including:

I. The biochemical structure and physicochemical properties of nutrients.
II. The dietary sources, compositional attributes, and the effect of food processing on nutrient integrity and bioavailability.
III. The mechanisms of digestion, absorption, systemic circulation, and cellular uptake of nutrients.
IV. Nutrient metabolism, physiological functions, storage mechanisms, and routes of excretion.
V. Nutrient requirements for maintaining health, managing disease states, and supporting specific physiological conditions (e.g., pregnancy, lactation, athletic performance), accounting for individual variability.
VI. Nutrient interactions with other nutrients, bioactive compounds, anti-nutrients, and pharmacological agents.
VII. The consequences of nutrient deficiencies and toxicities due to inadequate or excessive intake.
VIII. The therapeutic applications of nutrients in disease management and clinical nutrition.

Food and nutritional security, alongside food safety, are critical components of public health and well-being. The human diet comprises over 50 essential nutrients, in addition to a wide array of bioactive compounds, which play an essential role in modulating physiological functions and influencing complete health outcomes (Gibson et al. 2006).

3.2.3 Role of Nutrition in Chronic Disease

Dietary patterns, influenced by cultural diversity, play a key role in human health, growth, and development. Lifestyle factors, including tobacco consumption and physical inactivity, significantly affect health outcomes, either positively or negatively. In the absence of a health-supportive environment, the escalating prevalence of chronic diseases presents a critical global public health challenge. Currently, 79% of mortality associated with chronic diseases occurs in developing nations, predominantly affecting middle-aged men (WHO 2003). Emerging evidence suggests that the predisposition to chronic diseases originates during fetal development and persists throughout the aging process (Kim and Giovannucci 2022). The manifestation of chronic illnesses in adulthood is a consequence of cumulative lifetime exposure to adverse physical and social determinants (Fig. 3.3). Chronic diseases, characterized as conditions persisting for at least 1 year and necessitating ongoing medical intervention, encompass cardiovascular disorders, malignancies, diabetes mellitus, and neurodegenerative conditions such as Alzheimer's disease. According to the Centers for Disease Control and Prevention (CDC), an estimated 60% of adults in the United States have been clinically diagnosed with at least one chronic disease, whereas approximately 40% present with comorbid chronic conditions. Chronic diseases, which include ailments such as cardiovascular disorders, diabetes mellitus, and chronic respiratory conditions, contribute significantly to morbidity

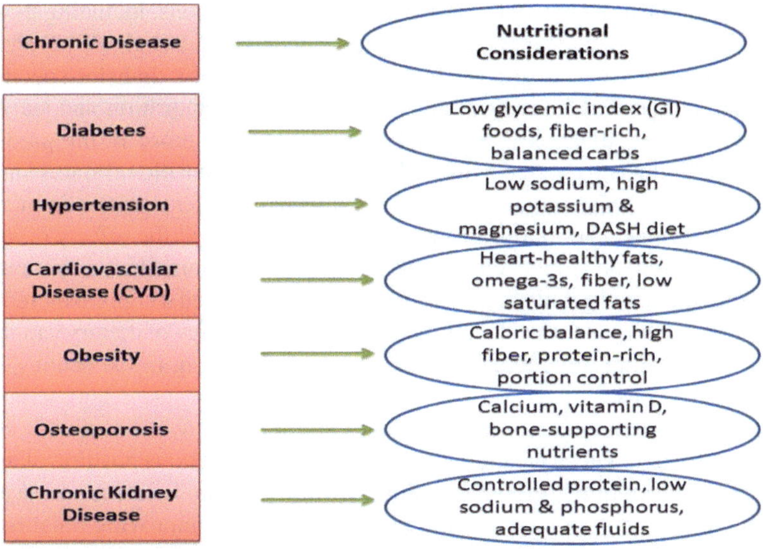

Fig. 3.3 Nutritional consideration in chronic diseases

and healthcare burden. These conditions often result from a complex interplay of genetic predisposition, environmental influences, and lifestyle factors, necessitating long-term medical intervention and management. These diseases constitute a leading cause of mortality worldwide, accounting for approximately 70% of global deaths (Kimokoti and Millen 2016; Pesudovs et al. 2015; Correction Naghavi et al. 2015).

Diet, acknowledged as a fundamental determinant of overall health and well-being, exerts a profound influence on the pathophysiology of multiple chronic diseases. These include cardiovascular disorders, obesity, essential hypertension, type 2 diabetes mellitus, cerebrovascular accidents (stroke), metabolic syndrome, and malignancies affecting various organ systems. Furthermore, emerging evidence suggests a potential association between dietary patterns and certain neurodegenerative conditions. Additionally, the coexistence of one pathological condition may potentiate the susceptibility to others through interrelated physiological mechanisms, thereby compounding the overall disease burden. For instance, obesity and excess body weight are key risk reasons for type 2 diabetic condition, hypertension, metabolic syndrome, and specific cancers (Ding et al. 2022).

For decades, diet has been acknowledged as a key determinant of chronic disease risk (Willett and Skerrett 2005). Since the mid-twentieth century, substantial dietary transitions have been observed globally, particularly in developing nations. Traditional plant-derived foods have increasingly been substituted by energy-dense and fat-rich foods with a high proportion of animal-derived diets. Although diet is a crucial factor in disease prevention, it represents only one of many risk determinants. Physical inactivity, now widely regarded as a primary contributor to health deterioration, also plays a critical role in chronic disease pathogenesis.

In disease management and treatment, dietary interventions, including the use of nutritional supplements, have shown promise. López-Gómez et al. (2022) showed a comprehensive study to assess the therapeutic potential of a diabetes-specific oral nutritional supplement in mitigating the incidence of malnutrition and sarcopenia among individuals diagnosed with diabetes mellitus and those in the prediabetic stage. Their findings indicated a marked improvement in nutritional status and muscle preservation, suggesting a pivotal role of targeted supplementation in metabolic health management. Similarly, Basiri et al. (2022) explored the effects of specialized nutritional involvements on systemic inflammatory biomarkers in patients suffering from diabetic foot ulcers. Their research demonstrated a significant reduction in pro-inflammatory cytokine levels, highlighting the efficacy of dietary supplementation in modulating inflammatory responses and promoting tissue healing in diabetic complications.

Food and nutrient interactions are complex and show a crucial function in chronic disease prevention. Dietary patterns reflect the overall nutritious position of an individual at any given time. Adopting health-promoting dietary habits has been associated with alleviating multiple chronic conditions, such as improving renal function and reducing serum uric acid levels (Yokose et al. 2021). Obesity, a persistent metabolic disorder linked to various pathophysiological abnormalities, can be mitigated through evidence-based nutritional forms, with the Mediterranean diet, the dietary approaches to stop hypertension (DASH) food, and other regionally adapted nutritional regimens (Zhu and Zhang 2024). Among these, the Mediterranean and DASH diets are globally recognized for their efficacy in managing multiple chronic diseases (Zhu and Zhang 2024).

3.3 Functional Foods: A New Development

Functional foods represent a novel category of food products specifically intended to confer healthiness beyond basic nutrition. These foods are developed through targeted formulation and fortification to address specific physiological needs. Phytosterol-fortified lipid emulsions have demonstrated efficacy in lowering circulating low-density lipoprotein (LDL) cholesterol concentrations, consequently diminishing the predisposition to coronary artery disease. Likewise, the integration of resistant starch into carbohydrate-rich food matrices has been associated with attenuated postprandial glycemic responses, contributing to improved glycemic regulation and a reduced incidence of type 2 diabetes mellitus. The research, development, and evaluation of functional foods constitute a rapidly expanding domain within food science and human nutrition. These foods play a pivotal role in enhancing dietary quality and addressing nutritional deficiencies. Functional foods have gained significant attention due to their potential in the prevention and management of chronic diseases such as cardiovascular disorders, cancer, osteoporosis, diabetes, and hypertension. The presence of bioactive nutraceutical compounds in these products confers both nutritional and therapeutic benefits (Rani et al. 2021). Furthermore, the interplay between functional ingredients' technological and physiological properties has facilitated improvements in food quality, including enhanced sensory attributes, oxidative stability, and emulsification properties. These advancements contribute to the development of innovative functional food products that align with contemporary manufacturing trends and evolving consumer preferences.

The increasing global interest in functional foods is primarily attributed to the rising consumer inclination toward natural, health-enhancing dietary products (Baker et al. 2022). As public awareness of health and nutrition expands, there is a growing demand for food items rich in bioactive compounds that contribute to overall well-being, optimize physiological functions, and mitigate the risk of chronic diseases. However, despite their potential health benefits, the large-scale commercialization of functional foods remains a complex endeavor. This transition from research and development (R&D) to market availability is impeded by several critical factors, including the physicochemical stability and bioavailability of bioactive constituents, intricate regulatory frameworks governing health claims and food safety, as well as consumer perception, acceptance, and trust in these novel products. Nevertheless, functional foods exhibit significant potential, particularly in the realm of personalized nutrition, by delivering essential bioactive compounds (e.g., polyphenolic antioxidants) and beneficial microorganisms (e.g., probiotics) (Ahluwalia 2021).

3.3.1 Bioactive Compounds/Phytochemicals

Bioactive compounds and phytochemicals are naturally occurring constituents in plants, widely recognized for their health-promoting properties. These bioactive molecules, including polyphenols, flavonoids, carotenoids, and alkaloids, play a significant part in the prevention and management of numerous chronic diseases. They exhibit diverse pharmacological actions such as anti-inflammatory, antioxidant, antiatherogenic, antimicrobial, antithrombotic, cardioprotective, and vasodilatory effects (Kumar et al. 2023; Mohamed 2015). Antioxidants, a prominent class of bioactive compounds, are crucial in neutralizing free radicals, which contribute to oxidative stress and the pathogenesis of multiple diseases. These compounds are abundant in a wide range of dietary sources, predominantly fruits, vegetables, herbs, spices, cereals, legumes, chocolate, and beverages such as tea, coffee, and wine (Mohamed 2015). Additionally, bioactive compounds in plants exist in bioactive proteins form and phytochemical forms and each contributing to essential physiological functions. They are extensively worked for therapeutic purpose in conditions such as cardiovascular diseases, cancer, and diabetes.

Beyond plant-derived compounds, bioactive molecules are also sourced from animals and microorganisms. For instance, omega-3 fatty acids, primarily obtained from fish, have demonstrated potent anti-inflammatory and cardioprotective effects. Similarly, probiotics—beneficial microorganisms—are associated with enhanced gut microbiota balance, improved immune function, and overall gastrointestinal health.

3.3.2 Challenges Facing Functional Food Development

The functional food industry faces several challenges that must be addressed to achieve the full utilization of plant and microbial resources in food production. The primary obstacles is the high cost associated with large-scale microbial cultivation. This is primarily due to the significant capital and operational expenses required for constructing and maintaining photo-bioreactors (Assunção and Malcata 2020). To keep the integrity of bioactive functional components, advanced preservation techniques such as cold-chain logistics, microencapsulation, and freeze-drying are employed, further driving up technological and transportation costs. Moreover, the purity requirements for natural bioactive ingredients in functional foods exceed those for animal feed, necessitating enhanced processing methodologies. Regulatory constraints also present a significant hurdle, as the commercialization of microbiological food products is subject to stringent safety approval procedures that are often lengthy and complex.

Many plants and microorganisms, while rich in bioactive compounds, also contain toxic or antinutritional constituents that pose potential health risks. Examples include cyanogenic glycosides in cassava leaves, solanine in potato tubers, and β-ODAP in leguminous seeds. These hazardous compounds must be effectively removed or reduced to safe consumption thresholds during food processing. Another major challenge in the functional food sector is preserving the bioactivity and efficacy of functional ingredients throughout processing and storage (Nazir et al. 2019). Certain natural bioactive components may interact with other food constituents, leading to issues such as reduced solubility, oxidation, and degradation. Moreover, functional ingredients may influence digestion and metabolism, affecting their bioavailability post-ingestion. For instance, dairy consumption has been shown to negatively impact the metabolism of flavonoid compounds, thereby limiting their concurrent use in functional formulations. Comprehensive scientific research is essential to ensure food safety and optimize the production of high-quality, health-promoting functional foods (Gohara-Beirigo et al. 2022).

Despite the rapid growth of the functional food sector, regulatory frameworks governing functional claims and product efficacy remain insufficient. The digestion, absorption, and metabolism of bioactive compounds involve multiple stages within the human gastrointestinal tract, including mastication in the oral cavity, enzymatic hydrolysis in the stomach, and microbial fermentation in the intestine. The acidic gastric environment and interactions with gut microbiota can contribute to the degradation or inactivation of functional components, ultimately impacting their effectiveness.

Consumer awareness concerning health and nutrition has been progressively increasing, thereby fostering a heightened requirement for functional diets known as natural and efficacious substitutes to synthetic additives (Topolska et al. 2021). Functional food products fortified with bioactive constituents, including antioxidants, polyphenols, and essential micronutrients, are extensively acknowledged for their potential to confer health-promoting effects and mitigate the risk of chronic diseases. Contemporary consumers exhibit greater scrutiny regarding the nutritional composition of food products and their corresponding physiological benefits (Baker et al. 2022). This paradigm shift is evident in the growing preference for functional phytochemical compounds, for example phenolic acids, flavonoids, dietary fibers, essential micronutrients, omega-3 polyunsaturated fatty acids, prebiotic and probiotic microorganisms, which collectively contribute to improved metabolic and immunological functions. While increased consumer awareness is a key driver of market expansion, misleading health claims can contribute to misconceptions about dietary benefits, potentially resulting in suboptimal nutritional choices (Williams and Ghosh 2008).

3.4 Human Body Composition

The human body composition can be analyzed at multiple levels, including atomic, molecular, cellular, tissue, and whole-body scales. Various chemical elements are integral to human physiology, with six major elements, carbon, oxygen, hydrogen, nitrogen, calcium, and phosphorus, constituting over 98% of total body mass (Table 3.1).

The human body comprises various chemical elements in molecular form, primarily categorized into water, lipids, proteins, minerals, and carbohydrates. Water constitutes approximately 60–70% of total body mass (Wang et al. 1999). Total water in body is distributed in cell compartments, and the ratio between these compartments serves as a critical physiological marker influencing the onset of numerous health conditions. Lipids within the human body manifest in various forms, with fundamental structural lipids including phospholipids, which constitute a crucial component of cellular membranes, and sphingomyelin, an essential element of the nervous system containing a relatively small proportion of the total lipid reservoir. The predominant lipid class comprises nonessential triglycerides, which serve as the primary energy reserve. In a healthy adult with normal body weight, adipose tissue accounts for approximately 10–25% of total body mass in males and 15–35% in females. Proteins constitute 10–15% of body composition, with a higher proportion observed in males due to greater skeletal muscle mass. The mineral content of the human body ranges between 3% and 5%, largely influenced by fat percentage. Calcium and phosphorus are the predominant minerals, primarily localized in

Table 3.1 A 70 kg man body composition (atomic level)

Atoms	Quantity (kg)	Total (body weight %)
Carbon	16	23
Oxygen	43	61
Nitrogen	1.8	2.6
Hydrogen	7	10
Calcium	1.0	1.4
Phosphorus	0.6	0.8
Total	69.4	98.8

Table 3.2 A 70 kg man body composition at the molecular level (Wang et al. 1999)

Component	Amount (kg)	Amount (body weight %)
Water component		
Extracellular	18	26
Intracellular	24	34
Protein	10.1	14.4
Lipid component		
Essential	1.5	2.1
Nonessential	12	17
Mineral	3.7	5.3
Total	69.8	99.4

osseous tissue. Carbohydrates are primarily stored as glucose in circulation and as glycogen—a polysaccharide stored in hepatic and skeletal muscle tissues—serving as a critical short-term energy reservoir (Table 3.2).

3.5 Energy Balance and Human Nutrition

The regulation of energy homeostasis is fundamental to human nutrition, playing an important function in body weight management and health. An imbalance in energy dynamics where caloric intake surpasses expenditure leads to weight gain and obesity, whereas an energy deficit results in weight reduction. Maintaining equilibrium in energy metabolism is essential for devising effective dietary and lifestyle interventions to promote health and prevent metabolic disorders. Energy balance is governed by three primary components: energy consumption, energy expenditure, and energy storage (Hill et al. 2003). Disruptions in body weight occur when energy intake does not match energy expenditure over a given timeframe. The human diet provides energy through macronutrients: proteins, carbohydrates, and lipids, with a minor contribution from ethanol. Energy expenditure transpires via three principal pathways: resting metabolic rate (RMR), the thermic effect of food (TEF), and physical activity energy expenditure (PAEE). RMR predominantly correlates with body composition, particularly fat-free mass, whereas TEF is contingent on the total caloric consumption and the macronutrient composition of the diet. The caloric contributions of macronutrients are as follows: carbohydrates (16.8 kJ/g), proteins (16.8 kJ/g), fats (37.8 kJ/g), and alcohol (29.4 kJ/g). Energy obtained from food can be stored within the body as adipose tissue, glycogen, or, to a lesser extent, protein, which is typically not utilized for energy production except under extreme metabolic stress. Stored energy plays a key function in sustaining essential functional processes, including metabolic, cellular, and biomechanical functions such as respiration, myocardial activity, and skeletal muscle contractions. Energy assessment adheres to thermodynamic principles, wherein 4.2 kJ of energy is necessary to increase the temperature of 1 liter of water by 1 °C. The caloric value of food is commonly determined using bomb calorimetry, a technique that involves the complete combustion of a specified food sample within a sealed chamber, enabling the measurement of heat released during oxidative degradation. Current research suggests that energy homeostasis is regulated through an intricate physiological control system comprising afferent signals from peripheral tissues that convey energy status and efferent signals that modulate energy intake and expenditure (Sandoval et al. 2008). Furthermore, interactions among the components of energy balance can result in either a positive or negative energy state (Stubbs et al. 2014), both of which are critical in maintaining metabolic equilibrium and preventing energy imbalances that contribute to metabolic diseases.

3.6 Protein and Nutrition

Proteins are the primary nitrogen-containing macronutrients essential for physiological functions and cellular integrity. As fundamental biomolecules, they serve as the structural and functional components of all cells. The molecular composition of proteins consists of many amino acids linked through peptide bonds. Dietary protein is crucial for cellular repair, tissue regeneration, and biosynthesis of enzymes and hormones. Furthermore, adequate protein intake is essential for growth and development, particularly in children, adolescents, and pregnant women. During digestion, dietary proteins undergo enzymatic hydrolysis, and hydrolyzed in to amino acids, which are subsequently absorbed and utilized for metabolic processes. The human body needs a diverse range of amino acids to sustain homeostasis and overall health.

Amino acids are broadly categorized into essential and nonessential. Essential amino acids are not endogenously synthesized and must be attained from dietary sources and nonessential amino acids are synthesized de novo by metabolic pathways utilizing essential amino acids or through protein turnover. Animal-derived protein sources provide a complete amino acid profile, while plant-based sources, including soy, legumes, nuts, and specific grains like quinoa and wheat germ, contribute significantly to dietary protein intake.

3.6.1 Achieving Nitrogen Balance

Adequate quantities of amino acids must be supplied through dietary intake, either in their preformed state or as appropriate precursors that facilitate the synthesis of a balanced amino acid profile. This ensures sufficient availability for protein biosynthesis and various metabolic pathways. The body's nitrogen and essential amino acid requirements, crucial for protein metabolism, can only be fulfilled through dietary sources. The dynamic flux of amino acids within the system is commonly illustrated using a standardized model, as represented in Fig. 3.4.

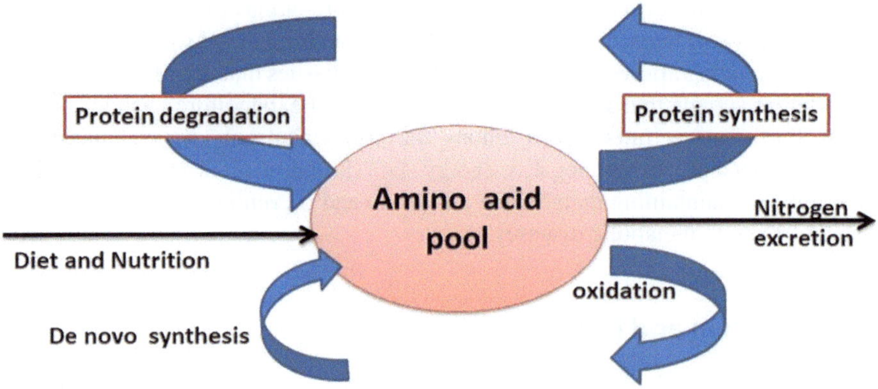

Fig. 3.4 Amino acid interchanges in human body system

3.6.2 Protein Quality

The efficiency of nitrogen balance maintenance in the human body for a given amount of absorbed dietary nitrogen is quantitatively expressed as biological value (BV). BV is determined by the composition of essential amino acids in relation to physiological demand, facilitating the classification of dietary proteins. Deficiencies in one protein source can be compensated by an excess in another, ensuring a balanced amino acid profile. It is important to recognize that BV is significantly influenced by the ratio of essential to nonessential amino acids, along with the presence of other nitrogenous compounds (Millward and Rivers 1988; Jackson 1995). The culmination of the Human Genome Project in the year 2000 elucidated that the human genome consists of approximately 30,000 protein-coding genes. However, the diversity of human traits and physiological processes is primarily governed by the vast array of proteins they encode. This has led to the emergence of *nutrigenomics*, a discipline that investigates the intricate interactions between nutrition and the genome, with implications for human health and disease prevention. Within the human body, proteins and amino acids play diverse and essential roles, as outlined in Table 3.3.

3.6.3 Biology of Amino Acid and Protein Requirements

A fundamental and quantifiable function of dietary α-amino acid nitrogen and indispensable amino acids is their role as precursors for intracellular protein biosynthesis, thereby sustaining optimal cellular and organ protein homeostasis (Elango et al. 2009). As a result, total body protein mass serves as a key determinant of daily protein requirements. Even among individuals with similar age, body composition, sex, and physiological state, variations in body size contribute to distinct demands for nitrogen and essential amino acids.

Table 3.3 Some major functions of amino acid and proteins

Biomolecule (Biological functions)	Major examples
Proteins	
Enzymatic catalysis	Branched chain ketoacid dehydrogenase
Messengers/signals	Growth hormone; IGF-1, Insulin
Movement	Myosin, kinesin
Storage	Ferritin
Immunity	Cytokine, antibodies, chemokines
Growth	Peptide growth factors
Gene expression	Transcription factors

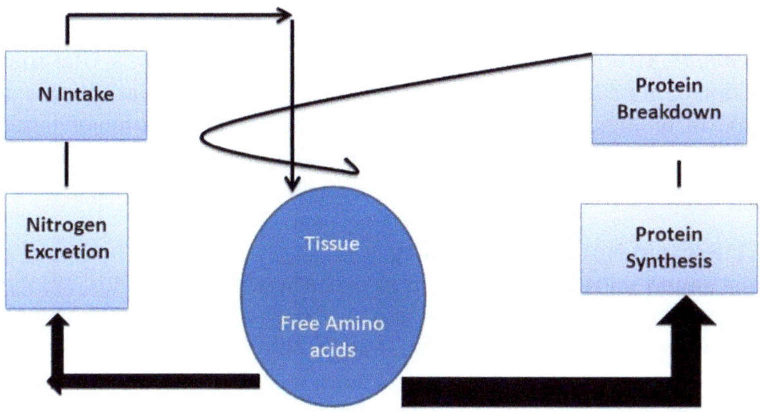

Fig. 3.5 The major systems/process in amino acid uptake, utilization, and catabolism

At present, direct in vivo quantification of total body protein remains impractical; however, a range of indirect methodologies enables the estimation of nitrogen (protein) content across different developmental stages. Research findings suggest that nitrogen accrual occurs at an accelerated rate from infancy through childhood and early adulthood, reaching a peak around the third decade of life. Thereafter, nitrogen levels exhibit a gradual decline with advancing age, with this reduction occurring more prominently in males than in females (Wolfe et al. 2018).

In adults, protein requirements are primarily defined by the minimal dietary intake necessary to maintain nitrogen homeostasis, typically assessed via short-term experimental methodologies. In contrast, infants, growing children, and pregnant individuals require additional protein intake to support tissue anabolism. Proteins undergo continuous synthesis and degradation through a highly regulated dynamic process known as protein turnover. The principal metabolic pathways governing protein and amino acid equilibrium are depicted in Fig. 3.5. These regulatory mechanisms ensure the preservation of physiological protein balance and overall metabolic stability.

3.6.4 Amino Acids and Synthesis of Important Nitrogen Compounds

Amino acids serve as fundamental building blocks in the biosynthesis of essential nitrogen-containing compounds, which are crucial for cellular, organ, and systemic functions. These biomolecules contribute to various physiological processes and facilitate the production of vital substances within the body, including:

1. *Arginine*: Arginine, a conditionally essential amino acid, functions as a critical precursor in the endogenous synthesis of nitric oxide (NO). The total NO produced and metabolized within a 24-h period represents less than 1% of the overall arginine turnover in the human body and contributes to less than 1% of the daily dietary arginine consumption.
2. *Glutamate, Glycine, and Cysteine*: These amino acids play a vital role in the creation of glutathione, a key intracellular thiol and significant antioxidant compound in biological system. Glutathione is described as a major intracellular antioxidant molecule that plays a crucial defense system against many reactive oxygen species in body.

3.6.4.1 Protein Nutritional Quality

Essential amino acids, also referred to as indispensable amino acids, are those that cannot be endogenously synthesized at a sufficient rate to meet the physiological demands of an organism and must therefore be obtained through dietary intake. In contrast, nonessential amino acids, also known as dispensable amino acids, can be endogenously synthesized in adequate amounts to fulfill metabolic requirements. The ability of dietary proteins to satisfy physiological nitrogen requirements and provide indispensable amino acids varies significantly. The bioavailability and concentration of essential amino acids are critical factors influencing the nutritional quality of dietary proteins. The composition and relative abundance of these amino acids vary between plant-based and animal-derived protein sources. For example, lysine is present in significantly lower concentrations in most predominant plant-based protein sources compared to animal proteins, often making it the primary limiting amino acid in plant-based diets (Wu 2009). The nutritional implications of these disparities can be evaluated using various methodologies. A widely adopted approach is amino acid scoring, which compares the amino acid composition of a given protein against a reference pattern that represents human amino acid requirements. The most robust and internationally recommended method for this evaluation is the Protein Digestibility-Corrected Amino Acid Score (PDCAAS) (Henley and Kuster 1994). This method integrates amino acid composition with protein digestibility to provide an accurate assessment of protein quality. The PDCAAS scoring system utilizes the amino acid requirement patterns for the children aged 2–5 years as a reference, given their relatively higher protein needs. This scoring method also facilitates the optimization of protein intake through complementary food blending, thereby enhancing nitrogen utilization and ensuring adequate amino acid supply.

The PDCAAS is calculated using the formula: **PDCAAS** = Concentration of most limiting, digestibility-corrected amino acid in a test protein/Concentration of that amino acid.

By applying this approach, researchers and nutritionists can effectively evaluate protein quality and optimize dietary formulations to meet essential amino acid requirements.

3.6.4.2 Primary Dietary Sources of Protein

Proteins are macronutrients essential for numerous physiological functions and are abundant in various food sources of both animal and plant origin. They are extensively promoted within the sports supplement industry due to their critical role in muscle synthesis and recovery. Major dietary protein sources include whey, casein, and soy, derived from both animal and plant-based origins. The efficacy is determined by assessing its protein biochemical quality and digestibility. Protein quality is characterized by the availability of essential amino acids necessary for physiological processes, whereas digestibility refers to the extent to which the body efficiently absorbs and utilizes the protein. Plant-based proteins are often considered incomplete due to deficiencies in some essential amino acids. Protein digestibility indices, such as the Protein Digestibility-Corrected Amino Acid Score (PDCAAS), biological value (BV), net protein utilization (NPU), and protein efficiency ratio (PER), are commonly used to evaluate the bioavailability and utilization efficiency of protein sources. Typically, animal proteins exhibit superior scores in these indices compared to plant proteins.

The dietary proportion of animal versus plant-based protein sources varies globally due to geographical, economic, and cultural factors. In developed nations, animal protein consumption accounts for approximately 60–70% of the total protein consumption, whereas in developing regions, plant proteins, particularly cereals, constitute around 60–80% of total protein consumption. Given the variations in amino acid composition among different protein sources, disparities in indispensable amino acid intake are observed across diverse populations (FAO/WHO 2013). Nutrient requirements are not uniform across individuals of the same age, sex, or body composition due to genetic variability. Additionally, environmental, physiological, psychological, and pathological factors contribute to the heterogeneity in protein and overall nutrient needs.

Recent emphasis on protein consumption has extended beyond athletic populations to the general public, particularly for weight management (Johnston et al. 2004). The rationale behind these diets is based on the increased satiety effects of protein, which may lead to reduced voluntary caloric intake (Araya et al. 2000). Empirical evidence suggests that the Atkins diet induces greater weight loss at three and 6 months compared to conventional low-fat, high-carbohydrate diets aligned with U.S. dietary guidelines (Foster et al. 2003). However, concerns regarding the long-term safety of high-protein diets have been raised. The American Heart Association issued a statement in 2001 highlighting potential risks associated with excessive protein intake, including metabolic, cardiovascular, renal, skeletal, and hepatic complications (St Jeor et al. 2001). Consequently, balanced dietary approaches that incorporate adequate protein intake while ensuring overall nutritional adequacy remain essential for optimal health and well-being.

3.7 Carbohydrate and Nutrition

Carbohydrate is the common macronutrient without any recognized minimum requirement. Although various persons depend upon carbohydrates as their main energy source and some people continued with very low or without carbohydrate intake for long periods (Håglin 1991). The great brain of current society humans has energy requirement and needed considerably more portion of dietary energy than other primates (Hardy et al. 2015). The greater nutritional with energy density of animal-based food helped in the development of a smaller digestive tract efficiently pay compensation for the brain's higher energy necessities (Leonard et al. 2007).

Carbohydrates are important classes of biomolecules playing a significant part in the metabolism process and ultimately in life. The key parts of carbohydrates are mentioned below:

I. *Primary Sources of Metabolic Fuels and Energy Reserves*
Metabolic fuels primarily originate from carbohydrates, lipids, and proteins, serving as essential energy substrates. Carbohydrates, in the form of monosaccharides, disaccharides, and polysaccharides, contribute to immediate and stored energy. Lipids, mainly triglycerides, function as long-term energy reservoirs, while proteins can be catabolized to provide energy under specific metabolic conditions.

II. *Structural Components of Deoxyribonucleic acid (DNA) and Ribonucleic acid (RNA)*
Nucleotides, the structural building blocks of DNA and RNA, comprise of a pentose sugar in deoxyribose in DNA and ribose sugar in RNA covalently linked via N-glycosidic bonds to nitrogenous bases. These nucleotides polymerize to form the genetic material essential for cellular function, replication, and protein synthesis.

III. *Role in Protein and Lipid Structures: Cell Recognition and Molecular Targeting*
Carbohydrates are integral components of glycoproteins and glycolipids, contributing to structural stability and functionality in cellular membranes. These biomolecules play a crucial role in cell–cell interactions, immune responses, and molecular signaling pathways. Their recognition properties are essential in physiological processes, including receptor–ligand binding, and cellular adhesion mechanisms.

A comprehensive overview of dietary carbohydrate sources and their metabolic breakdown pathways is presented in Table 3.4.

Table 3.4 Carbohydrates present in food their possible fates in digestive system

Carbohydrates	Examples	Primary place in digestive system	List of absorbed metabolites
Monosaccharides	Glucose, fructose	Small intestine	Glucose, fructose
Disaccharides	Sucrose, lactose	Small intestine	From sucrose: Glucose, fructose From lactose: Glucose, galactose
Oligosaccharides	Raffinose, inulin	Large intestine	Short-chain fatty acids (SCFAs)
Polysaccharides	Starches	Predominantly small intestine	Glucose
Non-starch polysaccharides	Dietary fiber (e.g., cellulose, hemicellulose)	Large intestine	Short-chain fatty acids (SCFAs)

3.7.1 Dietary Management of Blood Glucose Concentration

Dietary management is a very important approach for the prevention of blood glucose diabetes mellitus, particularly type-2 diabetes. Suitable foods play an important part in controlling the levels of blood sugar to improve insulin sensitivity and reduce the risk of problems linked with blood glucose level.

Carbohydrate molecules considerably affect glucose levels in blood since they hydrolyzed into glucose during digestion. Management of type and quantity of carbohydrates utilized during food intake is vital for blood sugar regulation and control.

- *Low Glycemic Index (GI) Foods*: Diets with a low glycemic index are absorbed in blood slowly, producing a slow rise in blood glucose level. The low glycemic index foods comprise whole grains, legumes, non-starchy vegetables, and fruits, e.g. apples and berries.
- *Glycemic Load (GL)*: Glycemic load reflects both the GI and the quantity of carbohydrate during consumption of food. Foods with a low glycemic load are better as they have a minimal impact on blood sugar levels.
- *Carbohydrate Counting*: Observing the total carbohydrate consumption with each and every meal prevents unnecessary spikes in blood glucose, and useful in diabetes management.

3.7.2 Glycemic Index

The glycemic index (GI) was introduced by as a dietary tool for managing blood glucose levels in individuals with diabetes. The GI quantifies postprandial blood glucose responses to equivalent amounts of digestible carbohydrates from various food sources. When categorized based on their glycemic index (GI) values, carbohydrate-rich foods demonstrate a strong linear correlation with their rapidly digestible glucose (RDG) content, as quantified through in vitro analysis. This in vitro technique serves as an efficient and cost-effective alternative to traditional in vivo glycemic index measurements. Carbohydrates that resist absorption in the small intestine transit to the large intestine, where they undergo partial or complete fermentation by colonic microbiota. Carbohydrates also classified into "available" and "unavailable" categories, distinguishing those that are readily digestible and absorbed from those that contribute to colonic fermentation.

3.7.3 Dietary Fiber

The importance of dietary fiber emerged as a focal point of scientific inquiry in the early 1970s, following the hypothesis proposed by Burkitt and Trowell (1975). They suggested that the high incidence of chronic diseases among Western populations was associated with insufficient dietary fiber consumption. Despite ongoing debates regarding its precise definition, dietary fiber remains a widely accepted term within scientific, consumer, and regulatory domains. The necessity of an accurate characterization and quantification method for dietary fiber is critical for both scientific research and food labeling regulations. Burkitt and Trowell (1975) initially defined dietary fiber as a complex matrix of structural polysaccharides that form the primary constituents of plant cell walls and exhibit resistance to enzymatic degradation within the human small intestine. Over time, this definition was expanded to encompass non-digestible storage polysaccharides that are sequestered within plant cellular compartments, further emphasizing their physiological significance in human nutrition and digestive processes. Various analytical techniques have been developed to quantify dietary fiber, yet they often measure distinct components. The standard methodology begins with drying and grinding the food sample, followed by lipid extraction using an organic solvent. Traditional methods involved treating the residue with strong acids, which hydrolyzed starch and a subset of polysaccharides into their monosaccharide constituents. The insoluble fraction obtained post-filtration was termed "crude fiber" and was conventionally used in food composition databases. Acid hydrolysis facilitates the breakdown of specific carbohydrates that exhibit resistance to enzymatic digestion within the small intestine. However, this process may result in an underestimation of total dietary fiber content due to the degradation of structural polysaccharides. Contemporary analytical techniques employ enzymatic hydrolysis using α-amylase to selectively depolymerize starch into soluble monosaccharides and oligosaccharides. These hydrolyzed products are then effectively separated from the fiber matrix through advanced filtration or centrifugation methods, ensuring a more accurate assessment of dietary fiber composition. The residual fraction primarily comprises dietary fiber, along with proteins and inorganic compounds. These advancements in methodology ensure a more precise estimation of dietary fiber, facilitating improved nutritional labeling and dietary assessment.

3.8 Lipids in Nutrition

Dietary fat encompasses all lipid types resulting from plant-based and animal-based sources in consumable forms. The predominant classes of fats and oils belong to the glycerolipid category, primarily composed of triglycerides. Fatty acids, essential components of dietary lipids, play a crucial role in energy metabolism, biochemical pathways, and structural functions within the human body. Based on saturation, dietary fatty acids are categorized into three primary groups: a). saturated fatty acids (SFA), comprise single bonds only; b). monounsaturated fatty acids (MUFA), characterized by a single double bond; c) polyunsaturated fatty acids (PUFA), which have two or more double bonds. These fatty acids typically exhibit an even number of carbon atoms and maintain a linear, unbranched structure (Sundram et al. 2003). Naturally unsaturated fatty acids predominantly found in cis configuration.

Lipids, similar to other organic biomolecules, consist of a carbon backbone substituted with hydrogen and oxygen atoms, while certain lipid molecules also incorporate nitrogen, sulfur, and phosphorus. Certain lipid categories, such as short-chain to medium-chain fatty acids, saponified lipids, and specific complex lipid molecules, demonstrate aqueous solubility (Katan and Deslypere 1993). Lipids are systematically classified into four principal categories: simple lipids, complex (compound) lipids, derived lipids, and miscellaneous lipids (Table 3.5). Simple lipids consist of fatty acid esters conjugated with alcohols, including glycerol or cholesterol molecules, encompassing triacylglycerols, waxes, cholesteryl esters, and esterified derivatives of lipophilic vitamins such as vitamins A and D. Compound lipids consist of fatty acid esters conjugated with both alcohols and additional functional groups, encompassing phospholipids, glycolipids, cerebrosides, sulfolipids, lipoproteins, and lipopolysaccharides. Derived lipids result from the hydrolytic breakdown of simple or complex lipids, generating molecules such as free fatty acids, monoacylglycerols, diacylglycerols, sterols, steroids, and straight-chain or cyclic alcohols (Sundram et al. 2003). Miscellaneous lipids include diverse lipid compounds such as wax esters, carotenoids, squalene, and fat-soluble vitamins E and K.

Table 3.5 Classification of lipids

Lipids	Significant examples
Simple lipids	
Fatty acids esterified with alcohols	Fats, Waxes
Complex lipids Fatty acids esterified with alcohols and other groups	Phospholipids
	Glycolipids
	Sulfolipids (with sulfur containing functional group)
	Lipoproteins (Attach with plasma or other proteins) Lipopolysaccharides (with polysaccharides)
Derived lipids Obtained by hydrolysis of simple or complex lipids	Fatty acids (saturated, monounsaturated, or polyunsaturated) Monoacylglycerols and diacylglycerols alcohols (include sterols, steroids, vitamin D, vitamin A)

3.8.1 Lipids as Components of the Diet

Cholesterol is exclusively derived from animal lipids, whereas plants contain a diverse range of phytosterols. Dietary phospholipids are abundant in soybean seeds, leafy plants, and lean animal tissues. Triacylglycerols (TAGs) are predominantly found in animal fats and plant oils extracted from seeds or nuts. In higher plants, both foliar and fruit tissues contain phospholipids and sterols, whereas seeds primarily accumulate lipids in the form of triacylglycerols. Notably, edible green leaves generally exhibit elevated levels of α-linolenic acid compared to seeds, with exceptions such as flaxseed (*Linum usitatissimum*), which possesses a significant α-linolenic acid content. Seed-derived lipids are typically enriched with either linoleic acid or oleic acid, depending on species-specific lipid metabolism. The predominant phytosterols in plant tissues include β-sitosterol, β-sitostanol, and campesterol. Functional food products fortified with plant sterol esters are widely employed to attenuate plasma cholesterol levels by impeding intestinal cholesterol absorption (Kris-Etherton and Harris 2003).

Phospholipids and cholesterol constitute fundamental lipid components in various biological tissues, including the gastrointestinal epithelium, renal structures, and neural tissues, and are also present in numerous species of edible macroalgae. In general, tropical fish species tend to accumulate higher concentrations of arachidonic acid compared to their cold-water counterparts. Industrial food processing frequently employs partial hydrogenation to manipulate the degree of fatty acid unsaturation, thereby modifying lipid functionality in processed food systems (St-Onge and Heymsfield 2003). While complete hydrogenation results in highly saturated and rigid fats, it is less economically viable than partial hydrogenation. The selection of hydrogenation methodology depends on the specific physicochemical attributes required for the end-product and the initial composition of the lipid substrate. From a manufacturing perspective, partial hydrogenation remains a cost-effective strategy for modulating lipid characteristics in food production. Additionally, diacylglycerols and monoacylglycerols function as emulsifying agents in food formulations, promoting the stabilization of biphasic systems such as oil-in-water emulsions found in ice cream and mayonnaise.

3.9 Vitamins in Nutrition

Table 3.6 presents an overview of vitamins along with their biological functions. Extensive research has demonstrated that the vitamin B complex comprises multiple compounds with distinct biochemical activities within the human body. These compounds are systematically designated as vitamin B1 (thiamine), vitamin B2 (riboflavin), and so forth. However, numerical discontinuities exist within the B-vitamin classification due to historical revisions and subsequent scientific discoveries. For instance, when a compound that could have been labeled as vitamin B3 was identified, it was recognized as nicotinic acid (niacin), a previously known substance, and thus was not assigned a new numerical designation. Compounds that

Table 3.6 Vitamins and their biological functions

Name	Vitamins	Biological functions
Retinol, β-Carotene	**A**	Essential for phototransduction in visual pigments, facilitates cellular differentiation; β-Carotene functions as an antioxidant
Tocopherols	**E**	Actions as an antioxidant, protective for cell membranes from free radicals.
Phylloquinone	**K**	Serves as a coenzyme in γ-carboxylation of glutamate residues, essential for blood coagulation and bone matrix formation
Thiamine	**B1**	Functions as a coenzyme in biological reaction
Riboflavin	**B2**	Integral component of flavoproteins, participating in redox reactions as a coenzyme in electron transport and metabolism
Cobalamin	B12	Facilitates the transfer of one-carbon units, playing a crucial role in folate metabolism and DNA synthesis
Ascorbic acid	C	As cofactor during collagen synthesis, serves as an antioxidant, and enhances iron absorption

were initially misidentified as vitamins, such as B4 and B5, were subsequently recognized as either nonessential for human physiology or reclassified under established biochemical designations. The naming conventions for vitamins C, D, and E corresponded to the chronological order of their discovery (Hemila 2017). The term "vitamin F" historically denoted essential fatty acids, while "vitamin G" was an early designation for riboflavin (vitamin B2). Biotin is occasionally still referred to as "vitamin H" due to its historical classification (Traber and Atkinson 2007). Vitamin K was identified by Henrik Dam in relation to its crucial role in blood coagulation and was named accordingly, derived from the Danish word "koagulation" (Holick 2007).

Certain bioactive compounds are integral to various metabolic pathways but are not classified as vitamins due to their ability to be endogenously synthesized in sufficient quantities to meet physiological demands. These biomolecules include carnitine, choline, inositol, taurine, and ubiquinone, each of which contributes to distinct biochemical functions such as lipid metabolism, neurotransmission, and cellular energy production.

However, vitamin D and niacin are categorized as essential vitamins despite their intrinsic biosynthetic potential. Vitamin D is synthesized in the epidermal layers of the skin from 7-dehydrocholesterol through a photochemical reaction triggered by ultraviolet (UV) radiation. This process leads to the formation of cholecalciferol (vitamin D3), which undergoes subsequent hydroxylation steps in the liver and kidneys to produce its biologically active form, calcitriol.

3.9.1 Roles of Vitamins in Nutrition

- *Antioxidant*: Some important vitamins (e.g., vitamin C and E) play a major role in the biological defense system as antioxidants, defend the body from several types of oxidative stress in body, which can damage cells and lead to chronic diseases.

- *Immune Function*: Several vitamins (e.g., vitamin C, vitamin D, and vitamin A) play a major role in keeping a healthy immune system.
- *Bone Health*: Vitamins D, K, and A are mainly significant for bone health, serving to prevent bone fractures and osteoporosis.
- *Energy Metabolism*: Vitamins B are very vital in converting food into energy and keeping cellular function.
- *Cognitive Health*: Some important vitamins, such as B12 and folate, play an important role for cognitive function.

Vitamins are vital nutrients that contribute to several roles in the body as immune defense, energy metabolism, cognitive health, and bone integrity. A balanced food, including fruits, vegetables, dairy, and protein sources, naturally delivers all the vitamins as body needs to keep optimal health.

3.10 Minerals and Trace Elements in Nutrition

Micronutrients, with minerals and vitamins, play an essential role in keeping human health and improving immunity of the body system. These important nutrients, needed in small quantities but essential for many physiological activities and functions, comprising growth, development, and disease prevention (Al-Khalidy and Al-Hamdani 2021). In spite of their much importance, a deficiency in micronutrient is widespread and causes serious global health problem, affecting particularly peoples in developing countries (Kretchmer et al. 1996).

Some important minerals like zinc, iron, and selenium are very vital for immune health. Zinc is important for the activation of immune cells, including T-immune cells. Iron shows a vital function in the development of immune cells and worked against generation of reactive oxygen species to support against infections. Selenium, an important micronutrient, plays an essential part of several antioxidant enzymes, helps against oxidative stress, and improves the body's capacity to fight infections and inflammation (Isaacs and Oates 2008).

Food is the major way to confirm suitable micronutrient consumption. Vitamins and minerals-rich foods such as fruits, vegetables, whole grains, nuts, and lean proteins must be taken with daily meals for fulfilling the daily requirement of body for their biological functions. Some major sources such as citrus fruits, bell peppers, and spinach are exceptional sources of vitamin, although fatty fish, eggs, and several fortified dairy foods are rich source of vitamin D. Several plant sources such as legumes, seeds, and seafood are rich in zinc, iron, and selenium (Süttmann et al. 1996).

Essential minerals play a vital role in human nutrition and are primarily obtained through dietary intake. Macrominerals are required in gram quantities per day, whereas trace elements are needed in milligram to microgram amounts daily. While all elements have the potential to exhibit toxic effects at excessive levels, deficiencies in certain essential elements can lead to physiological disorders. Notably, deficiencies in four key inorganic elements have been identified in human populations.

Among these, iodine and iron deficiencies are widely recognized and prevalent, contributing to well-documented health conditions. In contrast, zinc and selenium deficiencies are more restricted and typically observed in specific populations under distinct physiological or environmental conditions.

3.10.1 Calcium

Calcium, a very crucial nutrient, found over 3% of the Earth's crust is also rich in bones, milk, dairy, and several plant-based foods. It plays a crucial role in bone health and also works as the body's major calcium pool. Dairy-based products are the chief dietary source, although plant-based food items contribute lesser but it is very significant. Currently, development and available calcium-fortified foods and supplements enrich intake options for calcium. Unlike other nutrients, calcium supplies focus on keeping ideal reserves rather than only metabolic functions. Suitable calcium consumption cares bone growth, development, and maintenance which make it important for complete health (Mertz and Tredwell 2020).

3.10.2 Magnesium

Magnesium (Mg) is an alkaline earth metal with chemical properties analogous to calcium and is the eighth most abundant element in the Earth's lithosphere. It predominantly exists in nature in the form of mineral deposits such as magnesite ($MgCO_3$) and dolomite ($CaMg(CO_3)_2$), among other magnesium-bearing compounds. This element serves as a critical material in various industrial sectors, including pyrotechnics, high-intensity flash illumination, and distress signaling devices. Due to its lower density relative to aluminum, magnesium is a key constituent in the development of lightweight structural alloys utilized in aerospace engineering, particularly in the fabrication of aircraft and missile components.

From a nutritional perspective, magnesium is primarily obtained through dietary sources such as whole grains, legumes, dark green leafy vegetables, and soy-based products like tofu. Moderate quantities of this essential mineral are present in meat, fruits, and dairy products, whereas highly refined and processed foods tend to have minimal magnesium content. The bioavailability of magnesium is subject to modulation by dietary interactions; excessive consumption of calcium, phosphate, and fiber-rich food sources can impede its absorption in the gastrointestinal tract (Lönnerdal 2019).

3.10.3 Phosphorus

Phosphorus predominantly exists in combination with other minerals. Phosphate rock, primarily composed of apatite, contains phosphorus in the form of impure tricalcium phosphate and serves as a principal source of this element. In nature,

Table 3.7 Essential trace elements

Element	Specific role	Bioavailability	Deficit
Copper (Cu)	In oxidation–reduction reactions Component of several enzymes	Active transport and by passive diffusion	Menkes disease or Menkes kinky (steely) hair syndrome
Zinc (Zn)	In cell proliferation, differentiation, metabolic activity Genetic expression	Zn absorption Inhibited in the presence of phytates	Genetic disorder—Acrodermatitis enteropathica
Selenium (Se)	Regulation of immunity, thyroid function, and reproductive system	Majority absorbed and some affected by diet composition, toxic elements (mercury and arsenic)	Tissue diseases

phosphorus is predominantly present in its pentavalent oxidation state, commonly forming phosphate through its interaction with oxygen. It is an essential component of protoplasm in both plant and animal tissues and plays a crucial role in biological structures and functions. Phosphorus is a fundamental constituent of cellular membranes, nucleotides, and nucleic acids, contributing to genetic material synthesis and cellular communication. Additionally, it plays a vital role in acid–base homeostasis by acting as a buffer to regulate pH levels. Furthermore, phosphorus is integral to energy metabolism, facilitating short-term energy storage and transfer through molecules such as adenosine triphosphate (ATP).

3.10.4 Trace Elements

Trace elements are present in biological tissues in minute concentrations. Some of these elements are classified as nutritionally essential, while others are considered nonessential. Primarily, trace elements function as cofactors in enzymatic reactions, facilitating catalytic activities in various biochemical pathways (Table 3.7). Certain trace elements, such as iron and copper, play a crucial role in redox reactions, particularly in cellular energy metabolism. Iron, as an integral component of hemoglobin and myoglobin, is essential for oxygen transport and storage. However, excessive intake of trace elements over prolonged periods can exert toxic effects on physiological functions.

3.11 Conclusions

Nutrients are traditionally regarded as essential substrates for cellular growth, proliferation, and metabolic energy production. However, beyond these fundamental roles, nutrients and their metabolites actively mediate, regulate, and integrate numerous cellular processes essential for maintaining homeostasis. The efficiency of cellular function is contingent upon various factors, including sex, age, and the optimal availability of critical nutrients. The widespread consumption of processed foods, characteristic of Western dietary patterns, is a significant contributor to the escalating prevalence of acquired metabolic syndromes in industrialized societies. These foods are typically characterized by high energy density and low micronutrient diversity, leading to nutrient insufficiencies and an excessive supply of metabolic substrates. This imbalance is hypothesized to disrupt cellular nutrient and energy homeostasis, predisposing cells to chronic metabolic stress. Initially, cellular adaptations to such stressors may serve as compensatory mechanisms; however, prolonged exposure fosters persistent metabolic alterations that ultimately drives systemic metabolic dysfunction.

Recent advancements in high-throughput omics technologies, the development of transgenic and knockout animal models for metabolic disorders, and sophisticated bioinformatics tools have enhanced our capacity to formulate precise nutritional interventions. While ongoing research continues to refine dietary recommendations, current evidence suggests that prioritizing nutrient-dense, low-energy foods may mitigate cellular stress, thereby promoting metabolic equilibrium and overall physiological health.

References

Afshin A, Sur PJ, Fay KA, Cornaby L, Ferrara G, Salama JS, Mullany EC, Abate KH, Abbafati C, Abebe Z, Afarideh M (2019) Health effects of dietary risks in 195 countries, 1990–2017: a systematic analysis for the Global Burden of Disease Study 2017. Lancet 393(10184):1958–1972

Ahluwalia MK (2021) Nutrigenetics and nutrigenomics—a personalized approach to nutrition. Adv Genet 108:277–340

Al-Khalidy MRAK, Al-Hamdani ZM (2021) Role of trace elements in human health and nutrition. J Food Sci Nutr 8(1):1–15. https://doi.org/10.1007/jfsn.2021.11345

Araya H, Hills J, Alvina M, Vera G (2000) Short-term satiety in preschool children: a comparison between high protein meal and a high complex carbohydrate meal. Int J Food Sci Nutr 51(2):119–124

Assunção J, Malcata FX (2020) Enclosed "non-conventional" photobioreactors for microalga production: a review. Algal Res 52:102–107

Baker MT, Lu P, Parrella JA, Leggette HR (2022) Consumer acceptance toward functional foods: a scoping review. Int J Environ Res Public Health 19(3):1217

Basiri R, Spicer M, Levenson C, Ledermann T, Akhavan N, Arjmandi B (2022) Improving dietary intake of essential nutrients can ameliorate inflammation in patients with diabetic foot ulcers. Nutrients 14(12):2393

Correction Naghavi M, Wang H, Lozano R, Davis A, Liang X, Zhou M, Vollset SE, Ozgoren AA, Abdalla S, Abd Allah F, Aziz MIA (2015) Global, regional, and national age-sex specific all-cause and cause-specific mortality for 240 causes of death, 1990-2013: a systematic analysis for the Global Burden of Disease Study 2013. Lancet 385(9963):117–171

Ding Y, Xu X, Tian T, Yu C, Ge X, Gao J, Lu J, Ge Z, Jiang T, Jiang Y, Ma H (2022) Weight change across adulthood in relation to non-alcoholic fatty liver disease among non-obese individuals. Nutrients 14(10):2140

Doll R, Peto R (1981) The causes of cancer: quantitative estimates of avoidable risks of cancer in the United States today. JNCI J Natl Cancer Inst 66(6):1192–1308

Elango R, Humayun MA, Ball RO, Pencharz PB (2009) Evidence that protein requirements have been significantly underestimated. J Nutr 139(4):784–789

FAO/WHO (2013) Dietary protein quality evaluation in human nutrition, Report 92. Food and Agriculture Organization of the United Nations

Fenech M (2012) Nutrigenomics and personalized nutrition: science and concept. Mutat Res Fundam Mol Mech Mutagen 733(1–2):50–55

Foster GD, Wyatt HR, Hill JO, McGuckin BG, Brill C, Mohammed BS, Szapary PO, Rader DJ, Edman JS, Klein S (2003) A randomized trial of a low-carbohydrate diet for obesity. N Engl J Med 348(21):2082–2090

Gibson RS, Perlas L, Hotz C (2006) Improving the bioavailability of nutrients in plant foods at the household level. Proc Nutr Soc 65(2):160–168

Gohara-Beirigo AK, Matsudo MC, Cezare-Gomes EA, de Carvalho JCM, Danesi EDG (2022) Microalgae trends toward functional staple food incorporation: sustainable alternative for human health improvement. Trends Food Sci Technol 125:185–199

Gropper SS, Smith JL (2012) Copper, iron, and selenium: nutritional and functional significance. Adv Nutr 3(6):749–750. https://doi.org/10.3945/an.112.003392

Håglin L (1991) Nutrient intake among Saami people today compared with an old, traditional Saami diet. Arctic Med Res:741–746

Hardy TM, Tollefsbol TO (2011) Epigenetic diet: impact on the epigenome and cancer. Epigenomics 3(4):503–518

Hardy K, Brand-Miller J, Brown KD, Thomas MG, Copeland L (2015) The importance of dietary carbohydrate in human evolution. Q Rev Biol 90(3):251–268

Hemila H (2017) Vitamin C and acute respiratory infections. J Am Coll Nutr 36(2):105–108

Henley EC, Kuster JM (1994) Protein quality evaluation by the protein digestibility–corrected amino acid score method. Food Technol 48(4):74–77

Hill JO, Levine JS, Saris WHM (2003) Energy expenditure and physical activity. In: Bray G, Bouchard C (eds) Handbook of obesity, 2nd edn. Marcel Dekker, Inc, New York, pp 631–654

Holick MF (2007) Vitamin D deficiency. N Engl J Med 357(3):266–281

Isaacs E, Oates J (2008) Nutrition and cognition: assessing cognitive abilities in children and young people. Eur J Nutr 47(3):4–24

Jackson AA (1995) Salvage of urea-nitrogen and protein requirements. Proc Nutr Soc 54(2):535–547

Johnston CS, Tjonn SL, Swan PD (2004) Highprotein, low-fat diets are effective for weight loss and favorably alter biomarkers in healthy adults. J Nutr 134(3):586–591

Katan MB, Deslypere JP (1993) Dietary fats and coronary heart disease: a review of recent evidence. J Am Coll Nutr 12(3):324–335

Kim H, Giovannucci E (2022) The role of nutrition in chronic disease. Nutrients 14(3):500

Kimokoti RW, Millen BE (2016) Nutrition for the prevention of chronic diseases. Med Clin 100(6):1185–1198

Kretchmer N, Beard JL, Carlson S (1996) The role of nutrition in the development of normal cognition. Am J Clin Nutr 63(6):997S–1001S

Kris-Etherton PM, Harris WS (2003) Omega-3 fatty acids and cardiovascular disease: new developments and implications for policy. Circulation 107(2):266–269

Kumar S, Gautam V, Singh BP, Kumar D (2023) Investigating the impact of bioactive metabolites and extracts in human health and disease authors. Front Mol Biosci 10:1244316

Leonard WR, Snodgrass JJ, Robertson ML (2007) Effects of brain evolution on human nutrition and metabolism. Annu Rev Nutr 27:311–327

Lönnerdal LA (2019) Dietary minerals and their bioavailability in the human body. Nutr Rev 77(3):223–232. https://doi.org/10.1093/nutrit/nuy085

López-Gómez JJ, Gutiérrez-Lora C, Izaola-Jauregui O, Primo-Martín D, Gómez-Hoyos E, Jiménez-Sahagún R, De Luis-Román DA (2022) Real world practice study of the effect of a specific Oral nutritional supplement for diabetes mellitus on the Morphofunctional assessment and protein energy requirements. Nutrients 14(22):4802

Mertz BM, Tredwell HE (2020) Minerals and trace elements in the human diet. Adv Nutr 11(4):528–539. https://doi.org/10.1093/advances/nmaa089

Millward DJ, Rivers JP (1988) The nutritional role of indispensable amino acids and the metabolic basis for their requirements. Eur J Clin Nutr 42(5):367–393

Mohamed S (2015) Antioxidants as functional foods in health and diseases, Austin. J Nutr Food Sci 3(3)

Nazir M, Arif S, Khan RS, Nazir W, Khalid N, Maqsood S (2019) Opportunities and challenges for functional and medicinal beverages: current and future trends. Trends Food Sci Technol 88:513–526
Pesudovs K, Melaku YA, Global Burden of Disease Study 2013 Collaborators (2015) Global, regional, and national incidence, prevalence, and years lived with disability for 301 acute and chronic diseases and injuries in 188 countries, 1990–2013 diseases and injuries in 188 countries, 1990-2013: a systematic analysis for the Global Burden of Disease Study 2013. Lancet 386(9995):743–800
Phillips SM (2017) Current concepts and unresolved questions in dietary protein requirements and supplements in adults. Front Nutr 4:13
Popkin BM, Adair LS, Ng SW (2012) Global nutrition transition and the pandemic of obesity in developing countries. Nutr Rev 70(1):3–21
Rani A, Saini KC, Bast F, Mehariya S, Bhatia SK, Lavecchia R, Zuorro A (2021) Microorganisms: a potential source of bioactive molecules for antioxidant applications. Molecules 26(4):1142
Sandoval D, Cota D, Seeley RJ (2008) The integrative role of CNS fuel-sensing mechanisms in energy balance and glucose regulation. Annu Rev Physiol 70(1):513–535
Soetan KO, Olaiya CO, Oyewole OE (2010) The importance of mineral elements for humans, domestic animals, and plants: a review. Afr J Food Sci 4(5):200–222
St Jeor ST, Howard BV, Prewitt E, Bovee V, Bazzarre T, Eckel RH (2001) A statement for health-care professionals from the nutrition committee of the council on nutrition, physical activity, and metabolism of the American Heart Association. Circulation 104:1869–1874
St-Onge MP, Heymsfield SB (2003) The role of fats in body weight regulation. Curr Opin Clin Nutr Metab Care 6(6):671–675
Stubbs RJ, Hughes DA, Johnstone AM, Horgan GW, King N, Blundell JE (2014) A decrease in physical activity affects appetite, energy, and nutrient balance in lean men feeding ad libitum. Am J Clin Nutr 79:62–69
Suez J, Korem T, Zeevi D, Zilberman-Schapira G, Thaiss CA, Maza O, Elinav E (2014) Artificial sweeteners induce glucose intolerance by altering the gut microbiota. Nature 514(7521):181–186
Sundram K, Tan YA, West CS (2003) The influence of dietary fats on the fatty acid composition of phospholipids and lipoproteins. Eur J Clin Nutr 57(4):531–537
Süttmann U, Ockenga J, Schneider H, Selberg O, Schlesinger A, Gallati H, Wolfram G, Deicher H, Müller MJ (1996) Weight gain and increased concentrations of receptor proteins for tumor necrosis factor after patients with symptomatic HIV infection received fortified nutrition support. J Am Diet Assoc 96(6):565–569
Topolska K, Florkiewicz A, Filipiak-Florkiewicz A (2021) Functional food—consumer motivations and expectations. Int J Environ Res Public Health 18(10):5327
Traber MG, Atkinson J (2007) Vitamin E: its role in oxidative stress and health. J Clin Nutr 87(6):1640S–1647S
Wang Z, Wang ZM, Heymsfield SB (1999) History of the study of human body composition: a brief review. Am J Hum Biol 11(2):157–165
Willett WC, Skerrett PJ (2005) Optimal dietary patterns for prevention of chronic disease. Am J Clin Nutr 81(2):587S–591S
Williams P, Ghosh D (2008) Health claims and functional foods. Nutr Diet 65:S89–S93
Wolfe RR, Baum JI, Starck C, Moughan PJ (2018) Factors contributing to the selection of dietary protein food sources. Amino Acids 50(6):1207–1219
World Health Organization (2003) Diet, nutrition, and the prevention of chronic diseases: report of a joint WHO/FAO expert consultation, vol 916. World Health Organization
World Health Organization (2021) Fact sheet: malnutrition. WHO, Geneva
Wu G (2009) Amino acids: metabolism, functions, and nutrition. Amino Acids 37(1):1–17
Wu G (2016) Dietary protein intake and human health. Food Funct 7(3):1251–1265
Yokose C, McCormick N, Choi HK (2021) Dietary and lifestyle-centered approach in gout care and prevention. Curr Rheumatol Rep 23:1–15
Zhu Y, Zhang D (2024) Dietary patterns and multiple chronic diseases in older adults. Nutr Metab 21(1):8

Impact of Nutrigenomics on Human Nutrition

4

Nikitha Susan Varghese, Vigneshwaran Subramani, A. Nisha, Vidisha Tomer, Ghan Shyam Abrol, Anil Kumar, and Ashwani Kumar

Abstract

Nutrigenomics focuses on comprehending the intricate relationship between genomics and nutrition, with a specific emphasis on tailoring dietary strategies to prevent diet-related diseases. Macro and micro-nutrients play a crucial role in maintaining body equilibrium, and any alterations in their intake can disrupt gene regulation, potentially leading to conditions like diabetes. Genes like LIPC, APOA, PPAR, and MTHR significantly influence the development of cardiovascular disease, with their impact being shaped by both diet and environmental factors. Poor nutrition, including factors like saturated fats and moderate meat consumption, contributes to a substantial portion of cancer cases, while certain phytochemicals in food can epigenetically reduce cancer susceptibility. Moreover, dietary components assist in the detoxification of toxins and induce cancer cells to undergo apoptosis. Food intolerances can arise from either the food itself or the host's physiological response, underscoring the importance of understanding individual reactions to different nutrients. Patients with Non-Alcoholic Fatty Liver Disease (NAFLD) often consume suboptimal nutrients, potentially exacerbating their condition. Insufficient micronutrients can pose risks to the genome, leading to birth defects or increased cancer susceptibility, particularly in developing children or fetuses. The chapter highlights the need for a personalized approach to nutrition, considering individual genetic factors and

N. S. Varghese · V. Subramani · A. Nisha · V. Tomer (✉)
VIT School of Agricultural Innovations and Advanced Learning (VAIAL), Vellore Institute of Technology, Vellore, Tamil Nadu, India
e-mail: vidisha.tomer@vit.ac.in

G. S. Abrol · A. Kumar
Rani Lakshmi Bai Central Agricultural University, Jhansi, Uttar Pradesh, India

A. Kumar (✉)
Institute of Food Technology, Bundelkhand University, Jhansi, Uttar Pradesh, India

A. Kumar et al. (eds.), *Innovations in Ayurvedic Nutrition*,
https://doi.org/10.1007/978-981-95-1213-3_4

physiological responses to specific dietary components. Overall, the intricate interplay between genetics, nutrition, and environmental factors has a substantial impact on health benefits, emphasizing the importance of tailored dietary strategies in disease prevention.

Keywords

Nutrigenomics · Nutraceuticals · Nutrition · Genes · Diseases

4.1 Introduction

Food is the major source of energy and nutrients. Food choices along with genetics determine the health and well-being of a person. A balanced diet that contains all the nutrients in adequate amounts is essential for a healthy life. Nutrients can modulate the function of genes through epigenetic control mechanisms like microRNAs, DNA methylation, and modifications of histamine can be a critical predisposing factor for the onset of many diseases. The understanding of functions of genes and how they associate with a person and the environment is essential to know the health challenges a person could face. It is well researched that diet has the ability to not only change the expression, structure of gene but even the human genome. The commencement of a disease, its extent, and progression is also dependent on the interaction of genes and dietary factors (Elsamanoudy et al. 2016). A customized diet as per the genetic makeup of a person can reduce/increase the chances of several hereditary diseases. Poor nutrition, including factors like high consumption of saturated fats and moderate red meat consumption, contributes to a substantial portion of cancer cases, while certain phytochemicals in food can epigenetically reduce cancer susceptibility. Moreover, dietary components assist in the detoxification of toxins and induce cancer cells to undergo apoptosis. Food intolerances can arise from either the food itself or through the host's physiological response, emphasizing the importance of understanding individual reactions to different nutrients. Patients with Non-Alcoholic Fatty Liver Disease (NAFLD) are found to often consume suboptimal nutrients, potentially exacerbating their condition. Insufficient micronutrients can pose risks to the genome, leading to birth defects or increased cancer susceptibility, particularly in developing children or fetus.

The study of the interaction of nutrients with genes and vice versa has emerged as a new field known as "nutrigenomics." Nutrigenomics focuses on comprehending the intricate relationship between genomics and nutrition, with a specific emphasis on tailoring dietary strategies to prevent diet-related diseases. Macro and micro-nutrients play a crucial role in maintaining bodily equilibrium, and any alterations in their intake can disrupt gene regulation, potentially leading to conditions like diabetes. Genes like LIPC, APOA, PPAR, and MTHR significantly influence the development of cardiovascular disease, with their impact being shaped by both diet and environmental factors. Gene expression is known to be altered by single nucleotide polymorphism (SNPs), a type of genetic variation closely associated with nutrition (Elsamanoudy et al. 2016).

In nutrigenomics, the aim is to discover how nutrition impacts metabolic pathways, particularly in the early phases of diet-related disease, and to determine whether genetic variance plays a role. Ultimately, it holds potential for evidence-based dietary interventions to restore health and prevent diet-related illnesses (Afman and Müller 2006). This chapter highlights the need for a personalized approach to nutrition, considering individual genetic factors and physiological responses to specific dietary components. Overall, the intricate interplay between genetics, nutrition, and environmental factors has a significant impact on health benefits, emphasizing the importance of tailored dietary strategies in disease prevention.

4.2 Nutrigenomics

In this study, the transcriptome, proteome, and metabolome of cells, tissues, or organisms are examined widely based on their genome to determine the influence of herbal drugs or nutrition or dietary components.

High-throughput genomic tools have recently found applicability in nutrition research with an aim to understand the molecular mechanisms through which specific regular components or the entire diet affects metabolism and/or health in people. This strategy investigates the changes in gene and protein expression that occur in response to an individual's genotype (Fig. 4.1). From the study, it is clear that nutritional science is expected to become an increasingly important area over the next decade. The interactions between nutrients and genes play a critical role in maintaining health and also prevent or delay the onset of diseases. The lack of balanced diet results in the risk of chronic conditions such as obesity, diabetes, and cardiovascular diseases. These imbalances as well probably will lead to earlier development and stronger forms of numerous common age-related diseases.

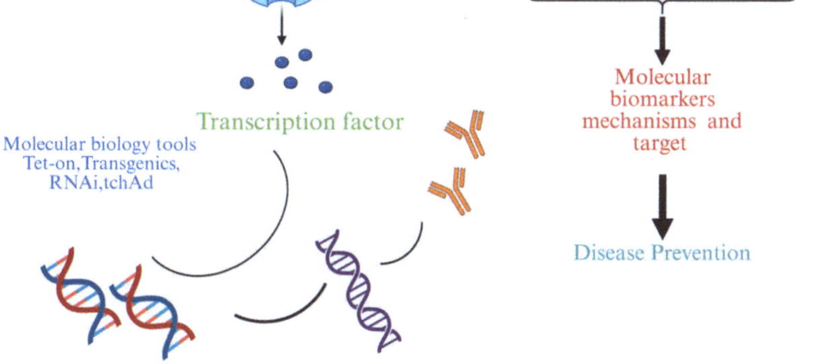

Fig. 4.1 Relationship between nutrition and disease prevention at genomic level

4.3 Role of Nutrients in Health: Nutrient–Gene Interaction

Homeostasis is a self-acting process regulated by dietary intake and the transcription factor of genes associated with various anabolic processes (Mas-Bargues et al. 2023). Diet along with environment has significant role in gene expression as shown in Fig. 4.2. Multiple genes interact with various nutrients and influence the expression of genes resulting in nutrition-dependent disorders (Elsamanoudy et al. 2016). Dietary nutrients interact with genes and influence the expression of genes either by binding or receptors or at the level of substrates (Irimie et al. 2019). These affect DNA methylation pathways through change of substrates and regulating enzyme activity (Kadayifci et al. 2018). Nutritional exposure in early life influences the metabolic and physiological changes which affect the epigenetic profile and in turn susceptible to a number of diseases. Similar influence is imparted by maternal nutrient intake and the impact continues later in life (Hjort et al. 2018; Martin et al. 2019).

Nutrients like carbohydrates, protein, fat, vitamins, and minerals play a vital role in diet. Carbohydrates contribute to 45–65% of energy value in the human diet. Different forms of carbohydrates regulate the energy balance and other metabolic processes (Ibáñez and De Molina 2019). Perception of sweetness is regulated by the taste receptors like Taste 1 receptor member 2/Taste 1 receptor member 3. Variant Ile191Val has been found to reduce sugar intake by approximately 18 percent. Val191Val variation has been correlated with enhanced carbohydrate intake and hypertriglyceridemia (Ramos-Lopez et al. 2016). The gut microbiota is influenced by prebiotics such as oligosaccharides which promote calcium and magnesium absorption (Abrams et al. 2005). High carbohydrate:fat ratio enhances histidine acetylation on sucrose-isomaltose gene in mice small intestine (Honma et al. 2007). Glycolysis, lipid metabolism, and functions of insulin are influenced by various

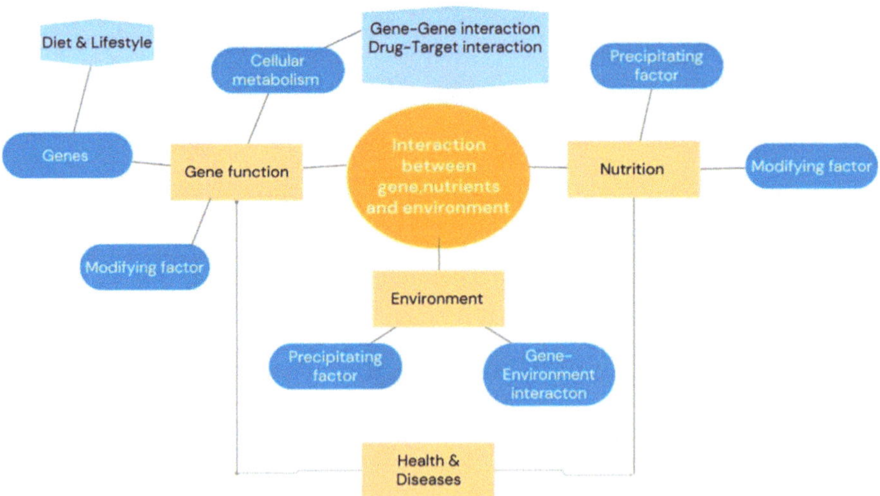

Fig. 4.2 Interaction of gene, nutrient, and environment

genes like Socs3, Irs2, Foxo1, Acadsb, Slc2a1, Pfkl, Pygf, and Ldha (Tain et al. 2016). Dosage of sugar, i.e., glucose or fructose influences metabolic functions. For example, sucrase-isomaltase gene contributes to the breakdown of sugar and a high dosage of glucose improves the activity of sucrase-isomaltase (Belmont et al. 2002; Le 2010). The transportation of carbohydrates is facilitated by GLUT and SGLT proteins. Genetic variation in GLUT2 (Thr110Ile) is associated with 30% increase in carbohydrates irrespective of the intake of other macronutrients. In vitro studies indicate high glucose consumption downregulated sucrase-isomaltase, SLC2A2, SLC2A5, SLC5A1 and ketohexokinase expression (Le 2010). Glucose consumption also influences the gene expression established in liver and pancreatic cells. It has been found that high glucose intake in the presence of insulin has exhibited overexpression of genes encoding for pyruvate kinase, fatty acid synthase promoting glucose storage, and downregulates genes responsible for gluconeogenetic pathway (Rui 2014). The intake of high glucose activates genes such as Sterol Regulatory Element Binding Protein-1 (SREBP1) and glucokinase, also enhances cellular glucose uptake. Even fructose has a similar impact. High intake of fructose during pregnancy is associated with transcriptome modification having consequences in later life (Tain et al. 2016). In vivo animal studies reported that animals provided with fructose diets have a decreased expression of glutathione peroxidase, copper-zinc superoxide dismutase, and catalase genes.

Starch is a well-known polysaccharide found in cer eals and plant-based foods frequently consumed by humans and have a potential role in the salivary amylase gene AMγ-1 (Perry et al. 2007). Resistant starch resists digestion and acts as a substrate for good bacteria in the colon. The study carried on Pig with resistant starch had higher short-chain fatty acids in their colons (Haenen et al. 2013). The intake of highly resistant starch improves the monocarboxylate transporter 1 (MCT 1) and glucagon in swine intestine (Ibáñez and De Molina 2019).

Proteins are important dietary components and integral to major body functions. Alsulami et al. (2020) reported significant interaction of genetic risk score with protein intake was observed in Southeast Asian women with respect to waist circumference and triglyceride concentrations. The women carriers of six or more alleles and having low protein intake, i.e., 13.51% of the total energy intake, were found to have lower waist circumference and levels of triglycerols compared to the carriers of five or less risk genes. The digestibility and amino acid composition of proteins also serve an essential factor in determining the gut microbiota. The intake of high as well as undigested proteins encourage pathogens and protein fermenting bacteria in gut, affects gastrointestinal tract, reduces immune system, and raises the chance of ailments (Ma et al. 2017). Beaumont et al. (2017) reported the implications of dietary protein quality and quantity on rectal mucosa gene expression in overweight humans. Researchers conducted a 3-week isocaloric supplementation study with casein and soy protein, concluded that high protein diets significantly alter gene expression in rectal mucus. Another important highlight was that animal and plant proteins exhibited distinct effects. Consumption of very high protein diets associated with disturbed normal gene expression in rectal mucosa. Impact on protein intake (protein enriched milk—20 g/day) causes changes in gene expression patterns in the mononuclear cells of old home-dwellers. Subsequently a 12-week period of treatment, 758 gene transcripts were regulated, out of which 25 genes were upregulated and 2 genes were downregulated influencing immune function and IGF signaling (Gjevestad et al. 2019).

A diet rich in fats can also have profound effects on gene expression, depending on the quantity, chemistry, and type of fat consumed (Jump and Clarke 1999). Diet-rich fat enhances the risk of colorectal cancer by modulating gut microbiota and metabolites (Ocvirk and O'Keefe 2021). High intake of saturated fatty acid leads to enhancement in phosphorylation of Mitogen-Activated Protein Kinases (MAPK), increase the regulation of gene expressions and elevation of irritant gene expression (Zhou et al. 2020). Consumption of polyunsaturated fatty acids (PUFAs), particularly omega-3 fatty acids, is associated with lowering of plasma lipid levels, increase insulin signaling and enhancing the immune response. Its consumption is also associated with the prevention of chronic diseases like rheumatoid arthritis, long diseases, coronary heart diseases, and inflammatory bowel diseases. PUFAs are believed to alter the gene expression by interacting with Liver X receptors (LxRs), Peroxisome Proliferators-Activated Receptors, and Hepatocyte Nuclear Factor (HNF) by balancing the genes of Sterol Regulatory Element Binding Proteins (SREBPs) 1 and 2 (Sampath and Ntambi 2004). Influence of Omega-3 polyunsaturated fatty acids (EPA, DHA—100 μM) function of differentiation and inflammatory activation was studied in human adipocytes which led to lower the post lipo-polysaccharides, mRNA expression and level of protein in interleukin-6, C-C motif Chemokine Ligand 2 (CCL2), and C-X3-C motif Chemokine Ligand 1 (CX3CL1) (Ferguson et al. 2019). Carbohydrate–lipid metabolism is influenced by omega-3 fatty acids and interacts with sterol regulatory element binding proteins (SREBPs), peroxisome proliferator activated receptor (PPAR), Nuclear Factor kappa light chain enhancer activated B-Cells (NF-κB), and Carbohydrate Response Element Binding Protein (ChREBP) (Rodríguez-Cruz and Serna 2017). Omega-6 fatty acids interact with the fatty acid desaturase gene (FAD) (cluster and haplotype) and apolipoprotein E gene (Bordoni et al. 2021). Research studies shows that the consumption of foods rich in omega-3,6 fatty acids (oil like fish and flaxseed) enhances the activity of Low-Density Lipoprotein Receptor (LDLR) and Peroxisome Proliferator Activated Receptor Gamma (PPAR-γ) influencing the metabolism of lipid (Bordoni et al. 2021).

Major micronutrients like minerals and vitamins essential at the micro level for metabolic processes like nutrient utilization and absorption of nutrients utilized for biological processes (Ames 2001). Table 4.1 describes the various vitamins, their target gene, and associated functions. Vitamins, especially the B vitamins, play an important role as co-factors, methyl acceptors/donors. Choline-deficient diet resulted in hypomethylation of (calcium binding protein) Calbindin-1, CDK3 (Cyclin-Dependent Kinase 3), VEGF-C (vascular endothelial growth factor-C), and Ang-2 (Angiopoietin) genes (Niculescu et al. 2006; Mehedint et al. 2010; Mahmoud and Ali 2019). Folic acid supplementation is related to *MTHFR* gene and folic acid deficiency indicators (Grimaldi 2014).

Table 4.1 Effect of micronutrients on the functioning of various genes

S. No.	Nutrient	Gene	Function of the gene	References
1	Vitamin A	RAR (Retinoic Acid Receptor)	Nuclear receptor Neural function Neuroblastoma therapy	Kawasaki and Taira (2003), Duester (2008)
2	Vitamin E	L-α-Tocopherol	Lipid metabolism Inflammation Regulation of gene and transcription factor	Woodson et al. (1999) Beckett et al. (2014)
3	Vitamin D	VDR (vitamin D Receptor) cell	Cell cycle regulation and differentiation Cancer chemo preventive	Lamprecht and Lipkin (2003)
4	Vitamin K	Gamma carboxyglutamyl carboxylase	Promotes calcium binding capacity Carboxylation	Shearer and Newman (2014)
5	Vitamin C	miRNA profiles	Collagen synthesis Neurotransmitter synthesis Hormonal function Cellular differentiation	Hung et al. (2010) Beckett et al. (2014)
6	Vitamin B3	PARP	Acts as substrate Repairment of DNA	Ames (2001)
7	Vitamin B2,B6,B9,B12	dTMP	Methylation of DNA Regulation of folate receptors	
8	Iron	DGCR8	Heme binding protein Modulation of miRNA process	Pogue et al. (2011)
9	Magnesium	RISC (miRNA processing)	Linking of specific miRNA Equalization of argonaute protein	Barr et al. (2012)
10	Zinc	TCFα	Cofactor in signaling pathways Stimulation of transcriptional factors	Prasad (2012)
11	Selenium	Se-Cys	Pro apoptotic Restoration of DNA	Lynnette and Karunasinghe (2011)

Clinical studies indicate that foods abundant in anthocyanins, notably from sources like pears, blueberries, and apples decrease the development of diabetes (DM). The food rich in plant-based origin which are abundant source of flavonoids shows that flavonoids had a positive impact on glucose regulation and control of carbohydrate digestion by influencing insulin signaling pathways (Rana et al. 2016). Certain bioactive compounds like genistein and resveratrol directly impact gene expression as ligands for transcription factors. Meanwhile, substances like choline affect gene expression indirectly by modifying signal transduction pathways and chromatin structure (Mead 2007).

4.4 Non-communicable Diseases and Nutrient–Gene Interaction

4.4.1 Diabetes Mellitus

Diabetes Mellitus (DM) is a prevalent metabolic disease known as hyperglycemia caused by the failure of insulin secretion or the reduced or impaired activity of the insulin produced (Dimple et al. 2018). It is distinguished into type-1 and type-2, where type-1 DM results from the immune disorder leads to elimination of pancreatic beta cells, decreases the insulin production, and type-2 DM causes deficiency in insulin secretion as well as insulin resistance associated with multiple organ impairment of blood vessels, heart, and kidney disorders (Georgoulis et al. 2014). Diabetes Mellitus is common among peoples of age group 40–60 years influenced by diet and other environmental factors (Federation 2019).

Exact genes regulating diabetes are not known but different studies have tried to find out associated genes. In such a study, the genes associated with Type-2 DM were found to be Transcription Factor7-Like 2 (TCF7L-2), Calpain-10 (CAPN-10) (Ali 2013). The gene, CAPN-10, belongs to the calpain family codes for cysteine protease and also serves as a mediator in post-receptor signaling and remodeling in intracellular process (Ali 2013). Research study proved that the variants of CAPN-10 are significantly linked with type-2 DM (Song et al. 2004). TCF7L-2 has been found to be active in beta cells as part of the Wnt (Wingless/Integrated) signaling pathway. Intron 3 of TCF7L-2, a risk allele, increased the level of TCF7L-2 protein in beta cells, decreases the secretion of insulin, incretin effects, and elevated level of hepatic glucose production (Lyssenko et al. 2007).

A gene SLC30A8 acts as a zinc transporter which contains protein associated with regulation of insulin production and it is stored in islets of Langerhans (Lefebvre et al. 2012). The cyclin-dependent kinase inhibitor CDKN2A/B found on chromosome 9p21 produces several transcript variants associated with type 2 diabetes (Li et al. 2013). The gene Insulin-like Growth Factor 2- mRNA binding protein-2 (IGF2BP2) generates a protein that binds with 5'UTR of Insulin Growth Factor-2 (IGF-2) and also regulates IGF-2 studies that conclude the mechanism of the above genes in causing type-2 dm remains unknown (Le et al. 2012). Risk alleles of Melatonin Receptor-1B (MTNR-1B), Solute Carrier Family 30 (SLC30A8), Transcription factor 7-Like 2 (TCF7L2), Potassium Voltage-Gated channel, Q-member (KCNQ1), and Cyclic-Dependent Kinase (subunit protein-1) (CDKAL-1) were associated with decreased beta cell function. In addition to this, the other genes like Peroxisome Proliferator Activated Receptor Gamma (PPARG), Fat mass and Obesity Gene (FTO), and Kruppel Like Factor-14 (KLF14) associated with reduced level of insulin sensitivity (Voight et al. 2010).

Nutrients can link with epigenome in distinctive ways and alters the expression of gene by causing activation or inhibition. Dietary nutrients like carbohydrates, proteins, fat, vitamins, and minerals were utilized by pancreatic β cells for secreting the insulin (Berná et al. 2014). Protein regulates the level of mammalian Target of Rapamycin (mToR), calcineurin, and Pancreatic and Duodenal home box 1(PDX1) regulates the level of insulin secretion, insulin absorption, cell proliferation, and growth. Lipids stimulate the Oxidative Phosphorylation (OXPHOS) gene, a metabolic link necessary for insulin exocytosis. The gene like PDX1 and PDX2 plays a major role in pancreatic function and development affected by long-term exposure of fat metabolites which lowers the insulin synthesis, nutrition-induced insulin release, cell survival, maintenance, and β-cell integrity (Ardestani et al. 2012; Berná et al. 2014). Hence, a strong association of nutrigenomics and diabetes can be conferred.

4.4.2 Obesity

Obesity is a multi-dimensional disease, i.e., interrelated with diabetes, cardiovascular risk, and chronic liver diseases. Obesity is a major precursor for all life-style-related diseases. Genes are also related to weight loss in accordance with diet and physical activity. It has been identified that obesity is the result of an imbalance between consumed calories and expended calories (Lin and Li 2021). The mechanism of obesity is associated with hunger pangs in obese individuals that are stimulated by gut hormone. Alterations in gut microbiota influence the secretion of fatty acids (short-chain) and enzymes which regulate the metabolism of glucose and insulin the major cause for developing obesity (Singer-Englar et al. 2019). The risk of obesity along with complications and metabolism regulations were influenced by genetic, epigenetic, and environmental factors (Dubern 2019). Genetic causes of obesity are identified as monogenic, polygenic, and syndrome obesity (Fig. 4.3) (Thaker 2017). Nucleotide Polymorphisms in FTO rs9939609 *AA* genotype have more susceptibility than non-carrier of A allele. Even the susceptibility to this allele can be modified by diet and life style changes (Hetheington 2009). Proven nutrigenetic relations exist between fat and *APOA2 2265T* > *C* variant and BMI (Table 4.2).

4.4.3 Cardiovascular Diseases

World Health Organization defines cardiovascular disease (CVD) as the inflammation of heart as well as blood vessels which in turn causes cerebrovascular accident and coronary artery disease (Mozaffarian et al. 2016). Genetics holds a major part in CVD by altering the gene expressions by interacting with selective dietary intake and environment (Peña-Romero et al. 2018).

Gene responsible for causing CVD were found to be Methylene Tetrahydrofolate Reductase (MTHR), Peroxisome Proliferator Activated Receptor (PPAR), Apo Lipoprotein (APO-A), and Hepatic Lipase (LIPC) (Peña-Romero et al. 2018).

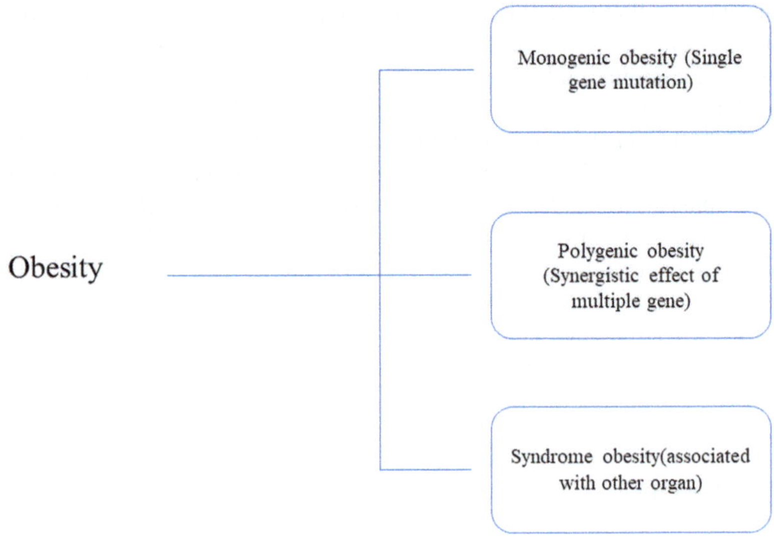

Fig. 4.3 Genetic causes of obesity identified as monogenic, polygenic and syndrome obesity (Thaker 2017)

Table 4.2 Gene associated with obesity along with their role and deficiency disorders

Monogenic obesity			
Gene	Role	Lack of expression	References
LEP (Leptin)	Satiety signal in hypothalamus	I. Hyperphagia II. Lethal bacterial infection [decreased t-cell immunity] III. Hypogonadotropic hypogonadism IV. Hyperinsulinemia V. Liver steatosis VI. Dyslipidemia	Zhang et al. (1997) Zhang et al. (1994) Funcke et al. (2014) Farooqi et al. (2002) Montague et al. (1997) Wabitsch et al. (2015)
POMC (Pro-opiomelanocortin)	Appetite regulation and pigmentation	I. Deficiency of ACTH II. Presentation of red hair due to pigmentation III. Severe obesity	Thaker (2017)
MC4R (Melanocortin receptor)	Appetite regulation	I. Hyperphagia II. High blood pressure III. Advanced bone age IV. Dysmorphic	Farooqi et al. (2000) Mountjoy and Wong (1997)

(continued)

Table 4.2 (continued)

Monogenic obesity			
Gene	Role	Lack of expression	References
PC1/3, PC 2 (Proprotein convertase)	Neuroendocrine convert endoproteases that process large precursor protein into mature bioactive products	I. Lack of adrenal, gonadotrophic, somatotrophic, and thyrotropic hormones II. Post-prandial hypoglycemic malaise III. Malabsorptive neonatal diarrhea IV. Central diabetes insipidus	Frank et al. (2013) Jackson et al. (1997) Jackson et al. (2003) Farooqi et al. (2007) O'Rahilly et al. (1995) Jansen et al. (1995)
SIM-1 (Single-minded homolog of drosophila)	Regulator of appetite	I. Hyperphagia II. Food impulsivity III. Neuro behavioral disorder	Michaud et al. (1998) Ramachandrappa et al. (2013) Michaud et al. (1998)
NTRK (Neuro trophin receptor kinase)	Regulation of food intake and body weight	I. Early onset of obesity	Han et al. (2008)
SH2B1 (Src homology 2 B adapter protein)	Regulator of leptin sensitivity	I. Hyperphagic II. Hyperinsulinemia III. Delayed speech and language	Pearce et al. (2014) Thaker (2017)
Polygenic obesity			
FTO (Fat mass and obesity)	Development of central nervous system and cardiovascular system	I. Neonatal hypotonia II. Hyperphagia III. Hypogonadism IV. Hypothyroidism V. Ghrelin abnormalities	Boissel et al. (2009) Miller et al. (2011)
Syndrome obesity			
BBS1–BBS21 (Bardet–Biedel syndrome)	Regulation of cilia composition and intra flagellar trafficking	I. Retinal dystrophy II. Obesity III. Post axial poly dactyly IV. Renal disinfection V. Hypogonadism	Nachury et al. (2007) Stoetzel et al. (2006) Forsythe and Beales (2013)
PWCR (Prader–Willi syndrome)	Development of neuron system	I. Hypotonia II. Hypogonadism III. Sleep disturbance IV. Lack of growth hormone	Cassidy et al. (2012) Zahova and Anthony (2018)

Hepatic lipase synthesized by liver cells and released into blood stream which converts fat transport molecules into low-density lipoproteins (Kobayashi et al. 2015). The study by Verdier et al. (2013) on (genotyping rs1800588) LIPC promoter shows that LIPC polymorphism and triglycerides increases the chance for cardiovascular disease (Verdier et al. 2013). The variants of APO lipoprotein A (APOA) play a vital role in causing CVD, APOA-1, high-density lipoprotein favors displacement of cholesterol and phospholipids from inside to outside of cell membrane. Another variant of Apolipoprotein was APOA5 regulating factor of plasma triglycerides also responsible for causing hypertriglyceridemia and hyperlipoproteinemia (Aouizerat et al. 2003).

PPAR ligand-regulated transcription factors regulate the expression of gene by interaction with specific response elements within promoters which are important regulators in glucose lipid interaction, inflammatory response, and adipocyte differentiation (Peña-Romero et al. 2018). Peroxisome Proliferator Activated receptor-γ2 (PPAR-γ2) promotes Pro 12Ala substitution which acts as carriers in cardio metabolic risk caused by polymorphism (García-Calzón et al. 2015). Methylene Tetra Hydro folate Reductase (MTHR), a major enzyme in homocysteine metabolism, polymorphism of MTHR by defective replacement of cytosine by thymine results in valine being replaced for alanine. Polymorphism of MTHR (rs1801133, rs1801131) in homocysteine pathway closely associates with CVD (Chen et al. 2016).

4.4.4 Cancer

Cancer can occur due to various predispositions, one among which is genetics. The alteration of a single DNA followed by the development of tumor cells is the major process occurring in carcinogenesis (Csar 2013). During this process, DNA undergoes multiple oncogenic mutations which may not be always in a single pathway (Ardekani and Jabbari 2019). According to numerous research, nutrition influences approximately 30–40% of cancer (Ardekani and Jabbari 2019; Csar 2013; Marcum 2020; Sellami and Bragazzi 2020). Women who consume more saturated fat are more likely to get breast cancer. Similarly, in a meta-analysis study conducted to check the relation of meat consumption with breast cancer, the RR was 1.11 (95% CI 1.05, 1.16) for a daily increased uptake of 120 g of red meat, and 1.09 (95% CI 1.03, 1.16) for a daily increased consumption of 50 g of processed meat. This study showed a positive correlation between red meat consumption and increased risk of breast cancer (Sellami and Bragazzi 2020). Nutrigenomics has a significant influence on modulating dietary components for human benefit, notably in cancer preventive treatment.

Phytochemicals including quercetin, kaempferol, genistein, daidzein, etc., are found to reduce the risk of cancer by epigenetic regulation (Braicu et al. 2017). There are certain ways through which carcinogenesis can be inhibited by the nutritional factors: (a) Activation of enzymes which metabolizes phase 2 drug that aids in the detoxification of carcinogenic intermediates, (b) Constraining enzymes that are dependent on Cytochrome P450, (c) targeted death of cancer cells, (d)

Disruptions in development of new cancer cells, and (e) reduction on spreading of cancer cells through blood stream (Srivastava et al. 2022). Furthermore, the absence of specific essential nutritional elements in the diet also promotes carcinogenesis. As an instance, folic acid-deficit diet may be associated with carcinogenesis, particularly in the case of colon and pancreatic cancers. Folic acid effectively preserves the integrity of DNA by repairing the strands, so low amounts of the nutrient will result in imbalance of genes through epigenetic processes (Marcum 2020). In a study conducted among 88,756 female nurses in the United States, it has been found that there is a threefold reduction in colorectal cancer in women on using nutritional supplements containing folic acid more than 400 microgram per day.

Research on nutrigenomics has shown that both micronutrients and macronutrients, such as dietary fiber, minerals, vitamins, have a key role in cancer treatment along with its prevention. This is particularly relevant when considering the hallmarks of cancer, which encompass various tumor cell characteristics, including limitless replicative potential and metastasis (Marcum 2020). Flax seeds have shown to aid in the treatment of breast cancer. The component lignan present in it binds with the estrogen receptors. This mechanism slows down the growth of cancer cells (Franklyn and Jane 2019).

Another study found that the cell surface glucose-regulated protein 78 (csGRP78), which is irregularly positioned on colorectal cancer cells (CRC), have a direct and positive correlation with the anti-CRC effects of Foxtail Millet Bran Powder (FMBP). This indicates that csGRP78 may be a potential target for FMBP's anti-CRC activity. This study, titled "Peroxidase from a secretory peroxidase of class III derived from foxtail millet bran (FMBP)," was published in *Acta Pharmaceutica* (Shan et al. 2022).

Free radicals can be bound by antioxidant phytochemicals, changing antioxidant defenses, DNA damage and repair, and tumor formation. By changing phase I and phase II enzyme activity, phytochemicals, such as cytochrome P450 and antioxidant enzymes, have been discovered to affect the bioactivation or detoxification of carcinogens (Srivastava et al. 2022).

4.5 Food Allergy and Similar Other Genetic Predispositions

The expert panel of National Institute of Allergy and Infectious Diseases have described "Food Allergy" as "an adverse health effect resulting from a specific immune response that consistently occurs upon exposure to a particular food." This definition includes all factors that trigger immune-related reactions (Valenta et al. 2015). The history of food allergy has been reported from twentieth century itself (Zukiewicz-Sobczak et al. 2023).

Hippocrates (460–377 BC) claimed that IgE antibodies have a role in allergic reactions to food, referring to them as "hostile humors" in people who experience sensitive reactions in body after consuming cheese. In 1921,Praustnizt and Kutsnerthe scientifically explained immunologically the reason of food allergy exactly a century ago for the first time (Ali et al. 2021). Food intolerances may be brought on by aspects of the food itself, such as toxic contaminants or pharmacologic properties (such as tyramine in aged cheeses), or they may be brought on by aspects of the host, such as lactase deficiency or idiosyncratic reactions (Sampson 2003). Food allergies can be classified into two, IgE-mediated and non-IgE-mediated. IgE-mediated responses often have an immediate effect, with clinical symptoms starting somewhere from a few minutes to many hours after intake. Non-IgE-mediated diseases can often be chronic and may be more challenging to treat with dietary avoidance alone than IgE-mediated diseases. IgE-mediated food allergy illness, particularly with peanut, tree nuts, and shellfish, is linked to fatal anaphylaxis (Anvari et al. 2019). The activation of genes leading to changes in signaling proteins, which in turn promote the downstream stimulation of the T cell helper (Th2) phenotype, that has been emphasized in most of the research relating to food allergies. One of the key factors in the activation of allergic responses is T cell helper (Th2), which facilitates the recruitment of IgE to further create B-cells, mast cells, and eosinophils (Ali et al. 2021).

Allergens are basically two types, based on its tolerance to heat, heat-resistant and non-heat resistant. The resistance to heat is related to the structural arrangement of amino acids; this contains heat-resistant substances that continue to function long after the product has been cooked, such as cod, milk lactoglobulin, egg white ovalbumin, and peanut allergens, and the heat sensitivity is due to the spatial structure of protein. These components which are very sensitive to heat are commonly found in fruits, vegetables, or meat, but remain active in raw fruits and vegetables. Protein gets denatured due to high heat and thereby causes inactivation of certain allergens like avidin in egg. This occurs due to the influence of high temperature on alterations in the three-dimensional structure of the protein (Zukiewicz-Sobczak et al. 2023). The rising prevalence of allergies in the population cannot only be linked to principle of mendelian inheritance. Transgenerational epigenetic inheritance provides an explanation to the transfer of environmental exposure information from parents to offsprings as well.

Phenylalanine hydroxylase (the enzyme required to convert phenylalanine to tyrosine) might exhibit genetic variations that result in decreased activity, which can cause Phenylketonuria (PKU). Without adhering to the suggested low-phenylalanine diet, people with PKU risk developing neurological impairment (severe mental retardation and convulsions). Another example is lactose intolerance, specific maldigestion of lactose carried on by a deficiency in the lactase enzyme is the cause of the classic gastrointestinal symptoms of LI. Due to the inheritance of an autosomal recessive trait, the physiological drop-in lactase activity that occurs throughout early infancy causes the lactase non-persistence (LNP) phenotype, which manifests as LI in adulthood (Porzi et al. 2021).

Allergies to fish and shellfish may co-exist but because the primary allergens are different, it is unlikely that fish and shellfish would react with each other. Parvalbumin is the primary allergen in fish, whereas tropomyosin is the primary allergy in shellfish (Berni and Di Costanzo 2013).

4.6 Liver Disease: Non-alcoholic Fatty Liver

Non-alcoholic fatty liver disease (NAFLD) is a major disorder marked by an excess of liver fat, which can vary from simple steatosis to steatohepatitis, cirrhosis, and hepatocellular carcinoma (HCC) when there is no excessive alcohol consumption (Amarapurkar et al. 2007). The condition at the clinically benign end of the spectrum is fatty liver disease, also known as hepatic steatosis. In this disorder, hepatocytes accumulate large (macro-) and small (micro-) fat droplets, primarily triglycerides, without significantly inducing hepatic inflammation, cell death, or fibrosis (Clark et al. 2002). Patients with obesity (60–95%), type2 diabetes mellitus (28–55%), and hyperlipidemia (20–92%) have a higher risk of NAFLD (Alba and Lindor 2003). In addition to the potential of treating NAFLD with calorie restriction (low in fats or carbs), several dietary components, specifically macronutrients, might directly affect the development of NAFLD (Fan and Cao 2013). Patients with NAFLD typically have a dietary pattern that includes high intakes of nutrients like Saturated fatty acids (SFA), cholesterol, and fructose but low intakes of vital nutrients like PUFAs and antioxidant vitamins (Dongiovanni and Valenti 2017). DNL, which is hepatic de novo lipogenesis, is brought on by diets high in saturated fatty acids. The peroxisome proliferator-activated receptor (PPAR)-coactivator-1 beta (PGC-1) influences how SFAs act on hepatic lipid metabolism (Lottenberg et al. 2012).

Carbohydrates also have a major part in the production of substrate that facilitates DNL in the liver and adipose tissues. The visceral adipose volume, DNL, and insulin sensitivity of overweight/obese patients are all increased by mostly fructose-containing beverages. Increased dietary fructose consumption promotes intestinal permeability and bacterial proliferation in the small intestine. It contributes to the disease progression of NAFLD by raising endotoxin levels in the portal vein (Dongiovanni and Valenti 2017).

Antioxidants like Vitamin E and betaine are proven to improve fatty liver disease in some patients and animal models. Vitamin E is a particularly appealing prospective therapy for this widespread and slowly progressing illness since it is also widely tolerated and affordable (Clark et al. 2002).

4.7 Kidney Diseases: Nephrolithiasis

Renel calculi which also called as Kidney stone is developing a condition called nephrolithiasis which happens due to crystalline formations that typically develop in the kidneys. Ideally, these stones form in the kidneys and exit the body through the urethra without causing pain. However, larger stones can be painful and may necessitate surgical intervention (Nojaba and Guzman 2023). The risk of development of nephrolithiasis is largely influenced through nutrition that is high in fat and animal protein but containing low amounts of fiber. Reduced excretion of citrate and magnesium, increased excretion of calcium, oxalate, and salt, and an acidic urine pH are all associated with this connection (D'Ambrosio et al. 2022). The consumption of 200 mL of fluids per day has been associated to a 13% decreased risk of stone development. However, not all drinks provide the same level of safety. Because

Table 4.3 Association of diet with nephrolithiasis

		Association	
Sl. No	Factors	Men	Women
1	Increased calcium intake	Decrease	Decrease
2.	Increased animal protein intake	Increase	Increase
3.	Increased fluid intake	Decrease	Decrease
4.	Vitamin D	Either way	Either way
5.	Sugar sweetened soda	Increase	Increase
6.	Fresh fruit intake	Decrease	Decrease
7.	Coffee and tea	Decrease	Decrease

Adapted from Ziemba Matlaga (2017)

soda contains sugar and fructose, it raises the excretion of calcium, oxalate, and uric acid, which increases the risk of kidney stones. In contrast to caffeinated coffee, sugar-sweetened non-cola, cola, and punch are associated to an increased risk of developing stones because caffeine increases potassium and calcium excretion and raises urine volume (Ferraro et al. 2020).

Table 4.3 shows that an increased calcium, fluid intake, coffee and tea intake reduced the risk of kidney stone both in men and women. Despite the limited evidence, there appears to be no additional risk associated with vitamin D supplementation when the objective is to restore vitamin D levels to normal. Increased intake of animal protein and sugar sweetened soda directly involved in the risk of kidney stone.

4.8 Deficiency Disorders

"Nutritional inadequacy" indicates insufficient nutrient intake below the average requirement, while "nutritional deficiency" involves critically low nutrient levels, impairing bodily functions and increases the chances of cardiac diseases, cancer, and diabetes (Kiani et al. 2022). Genetic polymorphism, a variation in genes responsible for nutrient requirements, has been discovered to alter the likelihood of organ dysfunction in individuals with low-choline diets. A notable instance of this is observed in the interaction of a specific SNP in mothers following a low-choline diet. The SNP MFTHD1-G1958A elevates the chances of neural tube defects in children of those mothers by four times more than with the ones who have higher choline consumption (Neeha and Kinth 2013).

Micronutrient deficiency can cause genomic damage, which may result in birth abnormalities or an positive impact of cancer in infants or fetuses. Specifically, low vitamin C intake has been related to increased sperm DNA oxidation and worsened birth abnormalities brought on by diabetes. When pregnant women do not take folic acid supplements, folate deficiency is linked to neural tube abnormalities in babies and an increased risk of juvenile leukemia. Zinc deficiency, which impedes repair and results in oxidative DNA damage, is teratogenic in and of itself. Furthermore, increasing genome damage in spermatogonia brought on by environmental genotoxins or nutritional deficiencies may be linked to the rising incidence of male infertility and testicular cancer (Fenech 2005). A deficiency in vitamin K could potentially exacerbate both cytokine storms (immune responses) and T helper 2 cells responses. This is due to the possibility that it will lead to an increase in the production of cytokines that promote inflammation, such as IL-6, which are involved in strengthening the inflammatory response and have both cellular and humoral (connected to body fluids) components. Additionally, vitamin K insufficiency may be a factor in the vascular calcification processes that result in problems like thrombosis and disseminated intravascular coagulation, which are indicative of the microvascular damage seen in COVID-19 patients (Rajagopal et al. 2022). Table 4.4 represents the potential deficiency diseases that can be developed from single nucleotide polymorphism due to the deficiency of the nutrients.

Table 4.4 Nutrients and its deficiency due to SNP

Nutrients	Function of the nutrient in the body	Type of gene alteration due to deficiency	Deficient disease potential
Folic acid (Vitamin B9)	Helps in amino acid metabolism and it also helps in single-carbon transfer in nucleic acid metabolism	Chromosome break and restricts the repairing of DNA	Cancer, heart disease, brain dysfunction, male infertility, leukemia
Vitamin B12 (Cobalamin)	Co-enzyme for crucial methyl transfer reaction. It has a major role in Kreb's cycle	Chromosome break and hampers DNA repair/ methylation	Same as folic acid, memory loss
Vitamin B6 (Pyridoxine)	It acts as co-enzyme for amino acid, glycogen and spingoid base metabolism	Same as folic acid	Same as folic acid
Niacin (Vitamin B3)	Main component of NAD and NADP. It also acts as a co-enzyme to dehydrogenase enzyme	Hampers DNA repair	Nerve problems, memory loss
Vitamin E (Tocopherols)	Plays key role in cell signaling, platelet aggregation	Mimics radiation damage	Colon cancer, heart disease, immune dysfunction
Vitamin D (Calciferol)	Have essential role in calcium metabolism, cell growth and development.	Prevent gene variation	Colon, breast, prostate cancer
Zinc	Essential in protein structure. Acts as a catalyst for different enzymes	Chromosome breaks	Brain and immune dysfunction
Flavonoids	Rich in antioxidants, improve immunity of the body	Alters gene expression	Cancer
Vitamin A (Retinol)	Plays important role in gene expression, reproduction, bone development, etc.	Repression of phosphoenolpyruvate carboxykinase PEPCK gene	Termination of pregnancy and fetal death
Protein	Muscle development, provide energy, regulate body processes	Alters	Gene expression kwashiorkor, marasmus
Fatty acids	Protect internal organs, plays an important role in energy storage	Alters gene expression	Obesity, CVD, diabetes

Source: Neeha and Kinth (2013), Morris and Mohiuddin (2020)

4.9 From Nutrigenomics to Nutraceutical Development

After having a clear understanding on the role of nutrigenomics, it is imperative to design strategies for delivery of nutrients in human dietary. Nutraceuticals are of significance in such scenarios. Nutraceuticals are nutritional constituents or dietary factors affecting health & diseases and having potential to act as pharmaceuticals or drugs for curing various ailments or disorders. They are a blend of nutrition and pharmaceutical components that have bio-active property and have the capacity to balance proper health of the consumers (Fig. 4.4). They gained much attention recently and paves a greater vision on the development of health through food (Puri et al. 2022). Foundation for Innovation in Medicine (New York, USA), termed "nutraceutical" in the year 1989. De Felice explained that a nutraceutical can be considered as any subject, a food or part of a food, and provides medical or health benefits including the prevention and treatment of disease.

As per the investor report of Ministry of Food Processing Industries (accessed on second June 2024), India holds at least 3.5% of global market of nutraceuticals. After the pandemic, there is a growing demand in nutraceutical exports. As per the current scenario, India imports (2.7 USD billion) more, than we export (1.5 USD billion). Looking through a global status, 90% of the market is possessed by the United States, Japan, and Europe. According to their predictions, the global market should reach USD 336 billion by 2023 from USD 247 billion in 2019 at a compound annual growth rate (CAGR) of 8%.

Nutraceuticals can be in any form like isolated nutrients, dietary supplements, and diets to genetically engineered "designer" foods, herbal products, and processed products such as cereals, soups, and beverages (Andlauer and Fürst 2002). Bioresources are the center of bioeconomy which basically include renewable sources and sustainable products from nature. They can also be used to produce high-value products (Ingle et al. 2020). Nutraceuticals can be made from bioresources, it either can be in nutrient-enriched form or in genetically modified form. Non-traditional nutraceuticals include those that are artificially prepared for the benefit of human health, which contain nutrients or bio-active components that protect from diseases (Rajasekaran 2017).

Nutrient components like dietary fiber, essential amino acids, protein isolates, fatty acids, namely Mono-Unsaturated Fatty Acids (MUFA) and Poly-Unsaturated Fatty Acids (PUFA), vitamins, and minerals can be added as enrichment agents in nutraceuticals (Da Costa 2017). Bioactive components like phenolic compounds, flavonoids, and carotenoids are present in fruit and vegetable peels which possess antioxidant capacity can also be considered as nutraceuticals. The extraction of these components using innovative and feasible methods and incorporation of these components in foods can help in reduction of many diseases. Foods that are fortified with these components are called fortified nutraceuticals (Rajasekaran 2017).

One of the main and iconic nutrient-enriched nutraceutical foods is Golden Rice that has been enriched with Vitamin A to eradicate the deficiency. Golden Rice is rich in β-carotene, precursor of vitamin A, developed through genetic engineering (Tang et al. 2009). The germplasm of the rice can form carotenoids within the

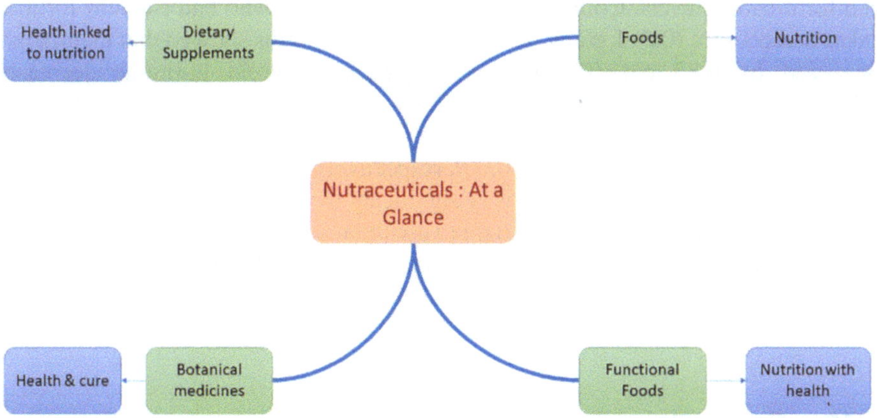

Fig. 4.4 Overview of nutraceuticals

endosperm. Golden Rice is created by inserting two genes into rice plants. The first gene comes from *Erwinia uredovora*, a soil bacterium, which encodes for *crtI* (carotene desaturase) enzyme. The second gene is sourced from the daffodil (*Narcissus pseudonarcissus*), encoding the *psy*. These genes work together to help the rice produce β-carotene. Now instead of the *Narcissus*, gene from maize is used (Amna et al. 2020). After further developments in golden rice lines, β-carotene level of Golden Rice 2 (GR2) has reached 37 μg of carotene (mainly β-carotene) was found 23 times superior to that of the initial trials (Zhao et al. 2020). Golden Rice is in the third stage of development and there is a huge potential of the rice to eradicate Vitamin A deficiency in developing countries through it (Shahbaz et al. 2020).

Vitamin D fortification can also be considered as an enriched nutraceutical. In a clinical trial, demonstrated to evaluate the effectiveness of Vitamin D fortification in edible oil (sunflower oil), showed that the method is highly effective for mass fortification to combat Vitamin D deficiency. The single blind trials, with the two sets of participants where one set have lunch made from D-fortified sunflower oil and the other control group used normal sunflower oil for a period of 12 weeks and it has been observed that Serum 25(OH)D showed a relative increase in people used fortified oils and a decrease in those who did not use fortified oils (8.8 ± 9.3–7.4 ± 6.4 ng/mL, $p < 0.001$) (Nikooyeh et al. 2020).

Wheat flour is mandated to be fortified with Calcium in the United Kingdom (except for whole meal and self-rising flour) and that is added in the form of Calcium sulfate/calcium stearoyl-2-lactylate; calcium peroxide. Commonly used other fortifications of calcium include dairy products like yogurt, cheese, and fruit juices, namely orange juice and tangerine (Palacios et al. 2021). In the research conducted to check the effect of calcium fortification on health outcomes, it has been shown that it improved the overall bone health and height of the trial children who consumed those foods. The study collected a systematic review and done meta-analysis using Revman 5.4 and performed sub-group analysis based on design, age group and fortification levels. Compared with control children who had calcium-fortified cakes and cookies (0.5–1 g/day) for a period of 8.5 months showed that their height increased by 0.83 cm. The rate of plasma parathyroid hormone decreased −1.51 pmol/L (−2.37; −0.65), urine: calcium creatinine ratio decreased −0.05, (−0.07; −0.03), femoral neck and hip bone mineral density increased 0.02 g/cm^2 (0.01; 0.04) and 0.03 g/cm^2 (0.00; 0.06), respectively (Cormick et al. 2021).

Even though nutraceuticals are very significant in maintaining a healthy lifestyle in current social systems, it is important to use them wisely. Today, market is flooded with unscientific combination ratios of nutraceuticals which needed to be controlled by the higher authorities. Nutri vigilance should be done strictly and systematically (Malve and Bhalerao 2023).

4.10 Conclusions

Nutrigenomics helps in the identification of the interaction of nutrition with genes that involve various metabolic pathways. Nutrition like carbohydrates, proteins, lipids, vitamins, and minerals which are acquired by the consumption of food interacts with genes by altering the gene expression and single nucleotide polymorphism. Environmental factors cause several non-communicable diseases. Distinct non-communicable diseases like obesity, cardiovascular disease, diabetes mellitus, kidney diseases, liver diseases, and several food allergies are closely associated with diet. Nutrigenomics helps to identify the pathogenesis of disease and helps to restore by assimilation of a balanced diet. Macronutrients like carbohydrates, proteins, and lipids are collaboratively responsible for gene functions while vitamins and minerals are micronutrients that favor the absorption of certain nutrients for the functioning of cells at the molecular level. Cardiovascular disease, diabetes mellitus, and obesity relate to lipid metabolism. Patients with NAFLD often consume large amounts of SFAs, cholesterol, and sugar while consuming relatively essential nutrients including PUFAs and antioxidant vitamins. Studies from researchers help to identify the importance of nutrigenomics as disease-causing agent and its corrective measures to be adopted.

References

Abrams SA, Griffin IJ, Hawthorne KM, Liang L, Gunn SK, Darlington G, Ellis KJ (2005) A combination of prebiotic short-and long-chain inulin-type fructans enhances calcium absorption and bone mineralization in young adolescents. Am J Clin Nutr 82(2):471–476

Afman L, Müller M (2006) Nutrigenomics: from molecular nutrition to prevention of disease. J Am Diet Assoc 106(4):569–576

Alba LM, Lindor K (2003) Non-alcoholic fatty liver disease. Alimentary pharmacology and therapeutics, 17(8):977–986

Ali O (2013) Genetics of type 2 diabetes. World J Diabetes 4(4):114

Ali A, Hamzaid NH, Ismail NAS (2021) The interplay of nutriepigenomics, personalized nutrition and clinical practice in managing food allergy. Life 11(11):1275

Alsulami S, Aji AS, Ariyasra U, Sari SR, Tasrif N, Yani FF, Lovegrove JA, Sudji IR, Lipoeto NI, Vimaleswaran KS (2020) Interaction between the genetic risk score and dietary protein intake on cardiometabolic traits in Southeast Asian. Genes Nutr 15:1–10

Amarapurkar D, Kamani P, Patel N, Gupte P, Kumar P, Agal S, Baijal R, Lala S, Chaudhary D, Deshpande A (2007) Prevalence of non-alcoholic fatty liver disease: population based study. Ann Hepatol 6(3):161

Ames BN (2001) DNA damage from micronutrient deficiencies is likely to be a major cause of cancer. Mutat Res Fundam Mol Mech Mutagen 475(1–2):7–20

Amna, Qamar S, Tantray AY, Bashir SS, Zaid A, Wani SH (2020) Golden rice: genetic engineering, promises, present status and future prospects. In: Rice research for quality improvement: genomics and genetic engineering, Volume 2: nutrient biofortification and herbicide and biotic stress resistance in rice, pp 581–604

Andlauer W, Fürst P (2002) Nutraceuticals: a piece of history, present status and outlook. Food Res Int 35(2–3):171–176

Anvari S, Miller J, Yeh CY, Davis CM (2019) IgE-mediated food allergy. Clin Rev Allergy Immunol 57(2):244–260

Aouizerat BE, Kulkarni M, Heilbron D, Drown D, Raskin S, Pullinger CR, Malloy MJ, Kane JP (2003) Genetic analysis of a polymorphism in the human apoA-V gene: effect on plasma lipids. J Lipid Res 44(6):1167–1173

Ardekani AM, Jabbari S (2019) Nutrigenomics and cancer. Avicenna J Med Biotechnol 1(1):9–17

Ardestani A, Shu L, Maedler K (2012) Targeting the metabolic syndrome and type 2 diabetes by preventing inflammation. In: Nutritional and therapeutic interventions for diabetes and metabolic syndrome, vol 5, p 233

Barr I, Smith AT, Chen Y, Senturia R, Burstyn JN, Feng G (2012) Ferric, not ferrous, heme activates RNA-binding protein DGCR8 for primary microRNA processing. Proc Natl Acad Sci 109(6):1919–1924

Beaumont M, Portune KJ, Steuer N, Lan A, Cerrudo V, Audebert M, Blachier F (2017) Quantity and source of dietary protein influence metabolite production by gut microbiota and rectal mucosa gene expression: a randomized, parallel, double-blind trial in overweight humans. Am J Clin Nutr 106(4):1005–1019

Beckett EL, Yates Z, Veysey M, Duesing K, Lucock M (2014) The role of vitamins and minerals in modulating the expression of microRNA. Nutr Res Rev 27(1):94–106

Belmont JW, Reid B, Taylor W, Baker SS, Moore WH, Morriss MC, Schwartz ID (2002) Congenital sucrase-isomaltase deficiency presenting with failure to thrive, hypercalcemia, and nephrocalcinosis. BMC Pediatr 2:1–7

Berná G, Oliveras-López MJ, Jurado-Ruíz E, Tejedo J, Bedoya F, Soria B, Martín F (2014) Nutrigenetics and nutrigenomics insights into diabetes etiopathogenesis. Nutrients 6(11):5338–5369

Berni CR, Di Costanzo M (2013) Gut microbiota as potential therapeutic target for the treatment of cow's milk allergy. Nutrients 5(3):651–662

Boissel S, Reish O, Proulx K, Takaki HK, Sedgwick B, Yeo GS, Meyre D, Golzio C, Molinari F, Kadhom N, Etchevers HC, Saudek V, Farooqi IS, Froguel P, Lindahl T, O'Rahilly S, Munnich A, Colleaux L (2009) Loss-of-function mutation in the dioxygenase-encoding FTO gene causes severe growth retardation and multiple malformations. Am J Hum Genet 85(1):106–111

Bordoni L, Petracci I, Zhao F, Min W, Pierella E, Assmann TS, Martinez JA, Gabbianelli R (2021) Nutrigenomics of dietary lipids. Antioxidants 10(7):994

Braicu C, Mehterov N, Vladimirov B, Sarafian V, Nabavi SM, Atanasov AG, Neagoe BI (2017) Nutrigenomics in cancer: revisiting the effects of natural compounds. Semin Cancer Biol 46:84–106

Cassidy SB, Schwartz S, Miller JL, Driscoll DJ (2012) Prader-willi syndrome. Genet Med 14(1):10–26

Chen YY, Wang BN, Yu XP (2016) Correlation between the 677C> T polymorphism in the methylene tetrahydrofolate reductase gene and serum homocysteine levels in coronary heart disease. Genet Mol Res 15(1):104238

Clark JM, Brancati FL, Diehl AM (2002) Non-alcoholic fatty liver disease. Gastroenterology 122:1649

Cormick G, Betran AP, Romero IB, Cormick MS, Belizán JM, Bardach A, Ciapponi A (2021) Effect of calcium fortified foods on health outcomes: a systematic review and meta-analysis. Nutrients 13(2):316

Csar J (2013) Nutrigenomics and cancer prevention. In: Cancer treatment – conventional and innovative approaches. InTech

D'Ambrosio V, Ferraro PM, Lombardi G, Friso S, Gambaro G (2022) Unravelling the complex relationship between diet and nephrolithiasis: the role of nutrigenomics and Nutrigenetics. Nutrients 14(23):4961

Da Costa JP (2017) A current look at nutraceuticals–key concepts and future prospects. Trends Food Sci Technol 62:68–78

Dimple, Kumar A, Kumar V, Tomer, V (2018) Traditional medicinal systems for treatment of diabetes mellitus: a review. Int J Pharm Pharm Sci, 10(5):7–17

Donati B, Dongiovanni P, Romeo S, Meroni M, McCain M, Miele L, Valenti L (2017) MBOAT7 rs641738 variant and hepatocellular carcinoma in non-cirrhotic individuals. Scientific reports, 7(1):4492

Dubern, Béatrice (2019) Genetics and epigenetics of obesity: keys to understand. La Revue du Praticien, 69(9):1016–1019

Duester G (2008) Retinoic acid synthesis and signaling during early organogenesis. Cell 134(6):921–931

Elsamanoudy AZ, Neamat-Allah MA, Mohamed M, Hisham F Azzahra', Hassanien M, Nada HA (2016) The role of nutrition related genes and nutrigenetics in understanding the pathogenesis of cancer. J Microsc Ultrastruct 4(3):115–122

Fan JG, Cao HX (2013) Role of diet and nutritional management in non-alcoholic fatty liver disease. J of gastroenterology and hepatology, 28:81–87

Farooqi IS, Yeo GS, Keogh JM, Aminian S, Jebb SA, Butler G, Cheetham T, O'Rahilly S (2000) Dominant and recessive inheritance of morbid obesity associated with melanocortin 4 receptor deficiency. J Clin Invest 106(2):271–279

Farooqi IS, Matarese G, Lord GM, Keogh JM, Lawrence E, Agwu C, Sanna V, Jebb SA, Perna F, Fontana S, Lechler RI, DePaoli AM, O'Rahilly S (2002) Beneficial effects of leptin on obesity, T cell hypo-responsiveness, and neuroendocrine/metabolic dysfunction of human congenital leptin deficiency. J Clin Invest 110(8):1093–1103

Farooqi IS, Volders K, Stanhope R, Heuschkel R, White A, Lank E, Keogh J, O'Rahilly S, Creemers JW (2007) Hyperphagia and early-onset obesity due to a novel homozygous missense mutation in prohormone convertase 1/3. J Clin Endocrinol Metab 92(9):3369–3373

Federation, International Diabetes (2019) Idf diabetes atlas. 2013. International Diabetes Federation

Fenech M (2005) The genome health clinic and genome health nutrigenomics concepts: diagnosis and nutritional treatment of genome and epigenome damage on an individual basis. Mutagenesis 20(4):255–269

Ferguson JF, Lee RK, Borcea C, Smith HM, Midgette Y, Shah R (2019) Omega-3 polyunsaturated fatty acids attenuate inflammatory activation and alter differentiation in human adipocytes. J Nutr Biochem 64:45–49

Ferraro PM, Bargagli M, Trinchieri A, Gambaro G (2020) Risk of kidney stones: influence of dietary factors, dietary patterns, and vegetarian–vegan diets. Nutrients 12(3):779

Forsythe E, Beales PL (2013) Bardet–biedl syndrome. Eur J Hum Genet 21(1):8–13

Frank GR, Fox J, Candela N, Jovanovic Z, Bochukova E, Levine J, Papenhausen PR, O'Rahilly S, Farooqi IS (2013) Severe obesity and diabetes insipidus in a patient with PCSK1 deficiency. Mol Genet Metab 110(1–2):191–194

Franklyn DSF, Jane A (2019) Flaxseed Lignans as important dietary polyphenols for cancer prevention and treatment: chemistry, pharmacokinetics, and molecular targets. Pharmaceuticals (Basel, Switzerland) 12(2)

Funcke JB, von Schnurbein J, Lennerz B, Lahr G, Debatin KM, Fischer-Posovszky P, Wabitsch M (2014) Monogenic forms of childhood obesity due to mutations in the leptin gene. Mol Cell Pediatr 1(1):3
García-Calzón S, Martínez-González MA, Razquin C, Corella D, Salas-Salvadó J, Martínez JA, Zalba G, Marti A (2015) Pro12Ala polymorphism of the PPARγ2 gene interacts with a mediterranean diet to prevent telomere shortening in the PREDIMED-NAVARRA randomized trial. Circ Cardiovasc Genet 8(1):91–99
Georgoulis M, Kontogianni MD, Yiannakouris N (2014) Mediterranean diet and diabetes: prevention and treatment. Nutrients 6(4):1406–1423
Gjevestad GO, Holven KB, Rundblad A, Flatberg A, Myhrstad M, Karlsen K, Mutt SJ, Herzig KH, Ottestad I, Ulven SM (2019) Increased protein intake affects pro-opiomelanocortin (POMC) processing, immune function and IGF signaling in peripheral blood mononuclear cells of home-dwelling old subjects using a genome-wide gene expression approach. Genes Nutr 14:32
Haenen D, Zhang J, da Souza SC, Bosch G, van der Meer IM, van Arkel J, van den Borne JJ, Perez Gutierrez O, Smidt H, Kemp B, Muller M, Hooiveld GJ (2013) A diet high in resistant starch modulates microbiota composition, SCFA concentrations, and gene expression in pig intestine. J Nutr 143:274e283
Han JC, Liu QR, Jones M, Levinn RL, Menzie CM, Jefferson-George KS, Adler-Wailes DC, Sanford EL, Lacbawan FL, Uhl GR, Rennert OM, Yanovski JA (2008) Brain-derived neurotrophic factor and obesity in the WAGR syndrome. N Engl J Med 359(9):918–927
Hetherington MM, Cecil JE (2009) Gene-Environment Interactions in Obesity. Forum Nutr, 63:195–203
Hjort L, Martino D, Grunnet LG, Naeem H, Maksimovic J, Olsson AH, Zhang C, Ling C, Olsen SF, Saffery R et al (2018) Gestational diabetes and maternal obesity are associated with epigenome-wide methylation changes in children. JCI. Insight 3:122572
Honma K, Mochizuki K, Goda T (2007) Carbohydrate/fat ratio in the diet alters histone acetylation on the sucraseeisomaltase gene and its expression in mouse small intestine. Biochem Biophys Res Commun 357:1124e1129
Hung PS, Chen FC, Kuang SH, Kao SY, Lin SC, Chang KW (2010) miR-146a induces differentiation of periodontal ligament cells. J Dent Res 89(3):252–257
Ibáñez C, De Molina AR (2019) Carbohydrates and nutrigenetics. In: Principles of Nutrigenetics and nutrigenomics: fundamentals of individualized nutrition. Elsevier, pp 203–209. https://doi.org/10.1016/B978-0-12-804572-5.00026-4
Ingle AP, Philippini RR, Martiniano S, Marcelino PRF, Gupta I, Prasad S, da Silva SS (2020) Bioresources and their significance: prospects and obstacles. In: Current developments in biotechnology and bioengineering. Elsevier, pp 3–40. https://doi.org/10.1016/B978-0-444-64309-4.00001-5
Irimie AI, Braicu C, Pasca S, Magdo L, Gulei D, Cojocneanu R, Ciocan C, Olariu A, Coza O, Berindan-Neagoe I (2019) Role of key micronutrients from Nutrigenetic and nutrigenomic perspectives in cancer prevention. Medicina (Kaunas) 55(6):283
Jackson RS, Creemers JW, Ohagi S, Raffin-Sanson ML, Sanders L, Montague CT, Hutton JC, O'Rahilly S (1997) Obesity and impaired prohormone processing associated with mutations in the human prohormone convertase 1 gene. Nat Genet 16(3):303–306
Jackson RS, Creemers JW, Farooqi IS, Raffin-Sanson ML, Varro A, Dockray GJ, Holst JJ, Brubaker PL, Corvol P, Polonsky KS, Ostrega D, Becker KL, Bertagna X, Hutton JC, White A, Dattani MT, Hussain K, Middleton SJ, Nicole TM, Milla PJ, Lindley KJ, O'Rahilly S (2003) Small-intestinal dysfunction accompanies the complex endocrinopathy of human proprotein convertase 1 deficiency. J Clin Invest 112(10):1550–1560
Jansen E, Ayoubi, Torik AY, Meulemans, Sandra MP, De Ven V, Wim JM (1995) Neuroendocrine-specific expression of the human prohormone convertase 1 gene: hormonal regulation of transcription through distinct camp response elements (∗). J Biol Chem 270(25):15391–15397
Jump DB, Clarke SD (1999) Regulation of gene expression by dietary fat. Annual review of nutrition, 19(1):63–90

Kadayifci FZ, Zheng S, Pan YX (2018) Molecular mechanisms underlying the link between diet and DNA methylation. Int J Mol Sci 19(12):4055

Kawasaki H, Taira K (2003) Functional analysis of micrornas during the retinoic acid-induced neuronal differentiation of human NT2 cells. Paper Presented at The Nucleic Acids Symposium Series.

Kiani AK, Dhuli K, Donato K, Aquilanti B, Velluti V, Matera G, Iaconelli A, Connelly ST, Bellinato F, Gisondi P, Bertelli M (2022) Main nutritional deficiencies. J Prev Med Hyg 63(2 Suppl 3):E93–E101

Kobayashi J, Miyashita K, Nakajima K, Mabuchi H (2015) Hepatic lipase: a comprehensive view of its role on plasma lipid and lipoprotein metabolism. J Atheroscler Thromb 22(10):1001–1011

Lamprecht SA, Lipkin M (2003) Chemoprevention of colon cancer by calcium, vitamin D and folate: molecular mechanisms. Nat Rev Cancer 3(8):601–614

Le MT (2010) Factors impacting fructose bioavailability and its adverse metabolic effects. University of Florida

Le HTT, Sorrell AM, Siddle K (2012) Two isoforms of the mRNA binding protein IGF2BP2 are generated by alternative translational initiation. PLoS One 7(3):e33140

Lefebvre, Bruno, Vandewalle, Brigitte, Balavoine, Anne-Sophie, Queniat, Gurvan, Moerman, Ericka, Vantyghem, Marie-Christine, Kerr-Conte, Julie (2012) Regulation and functional effects of ZNT8 in human pancreatic islets. J of endocrinology, 214(2):225

Li H, Tang X, Liu Q, Wang Y (2013) Association between type 2 diabetes and rs10811661 polymorphism upstream of CDKN2A/B: a meta-analysis. Actadiabetologica 50:657–662

Lin X, Li H (2021) Obesity: epidemiology, pathophysiology, and therapeutics. Front Endocrinol 12:706978

Lottenberg AM, da Silva Afonso M, Lavrador MSF, Machado RM, Nakandakare ER (2012) The role of dietary fatty acids in the pathology of metabolic syndrome. The J of nutritional biochemistry, 23(9):1027–1040

Lynnette FR, Karunasinghe N (2011) Nutrigenetics, nutrigenomics, and selenium. Front Genet 2:15

Lyssenko V, Lupi R, Marchetti P, Del Guerra S, Orho-Melander M, Almgren P, Sjögren M, Ling C, Eriksson KF, Lethagen AL, Mancarella R, Berglund G, Tuomi T, Nilsson P, Del Prato S, Groop L (2007) Mechanisms by which common variants in the TCF7L2 gene increase risk of type 2 diabetes. J Clin Invest 117(8):2155–2163

Ma N, Tian Y, Wu Y, Ma X (2017) Contributions of the Interaction Between Dietary Protein and Gut Microbiota to Intestinal Health. Current protein and peptide science, 18(8):795–808

Mahmoud AM, Ali MM (2019) Methyl donor micronutrients that modify DNA methylation and cancer outcome. Nutrients 11(3):608

Malve H, Bhalerao P (2023) Past, present, and likely future of nutraceuticals in India: evolving role of pharmaceutical physicians. J Pharm Bio Sci 15(2):68–74

Marcum JA (2020) Nutrigenetics/nutrigenomics, personalized nutrition, and precision healthcare. Curr Nutr Rep 9(4):338–345. https://doi.org/10.1007/s13668-020-00327-z. Springer

Martin C, Jima D, Sharp GC, McCullough LE, Park SS, Gowdy KM, Skaar D, Cowley M, Maguire RL, Fuemmeler B et al (2019) Maternal pre-pregnancy obesity, offspring cord blood DNA methylation, and offspring cardiometabolic health in early childhood: an epigenome-wide association study. Epigenetics 14:325–340

Mas-Bargues C, Román-Domínguez A, Borrás C, Viña J (2023) Geroscience: a unifying view on aging as a risk factor. Aging:587–600

Mead MN (2007) Nutrigenomics: the genome–food interface. Environ Health Perspect 115(12):A582

Mehedint MG, Craciunescu CN, Zeisel SH (2010) Maternal dietary choline deficiency alters angiogenesis in fetal mouse hippocampus. Proc Natl Acad Sci USA 107:12834–12839

Michaud JL, Rosenquist T, May NR, Fan C-M (1998) Development of neuroendocrine lineages requires the bHLH–PAS transcription factor SIM1. Genes Dev 12(20):3264–3275

Miller JL, Lynn CH, Driscoll DC, Goldstone AP, Gold JA, Kimonis V, Dykens E, Butler MG, Shuster JJ, Driscoll DJ (2011) Nutritional phases in Prader-Willi syndrome. Am J Med Genet A 155A(5):1040–1049

Montague CT, Farooqi IS, Whitehead JP, Soos MA, Rau H, Wareham NJ, Sewter CP, Digby JE, Mohammed SN, Hurst JA, Cheetham CH, Earley AR, Barnett AH, Prins JB, O'Rahilly S (1997) Congenital leptin deficiency is associated with severe early-onset obesity in humans. Nature 387(6636):903–908

Morris AL, Mohiuddin SS (2020) Biochemistry, nutrients

Mountjoy, Kathleen G, Wong, Jencia (1997) Obesity, diabetes and functions for proopiomelanocortin-derived peptides. Molecular and cellular endocrinology, 128(1-2):171–177

Mozaffarian D, Benjamin EJ, Go AS, Arnett DK, Blaha MJ, Cushman M, Das SR, de Ferranti S, Després JP, Fullerton HJ, Howard VJ, Huffman MD, Isasi CR, Jiménez MC, Judd SE, Kissela BM, Lichtman JH, Lisabeth LD, Liu S, Mackey RH, Magid DJ, McGuire DK, Mohler ER 3rd, Moy CS, Muntner P, Mussolino ME, Nasir K, Neumar RW, Nichol G, Palaniappan L, Pandey DK, Reeves MJ, Rodriguez CJ, Rosamond W, Sorlie PD, Stein J, Towfighi A, Turan TN, Virani SS, Woo D, Yeh RW, Turner MB, American Heart Association Statistics Committee; Stroke Statistics Subcommittee (2016) Heart disease and stroke statistics-2016 update: a report from the American Heart Association. Circulation 133(4):e38-360

Nachury MV, Loktev AV, Zhang Q, Westlake CJ, Peränen J, Merdes A, Slusarski DC, Scheller RH, Bazan JF, Sheffield VC, Jackson PK (2007) A core complex of BBS proteins cooperates with the GTPase Rab8 to promote ciliary membrane biogenesis. Cell 129(6):1201–1213. https://doi.org/10.1016/j.cell.2007.03.053

Neeha VS, Kinth P (2013) Nutrigenomics research: a review. J Food Sci Technol 50(3):415–428

Niculescu MD, Craciunescu CN, Zeisel SH (2006) Dietary choline deficiency alters global and gene-specific DNA methylation in the developing hippocampus of mouse fetal brains. FASEB J 20:43–49

Nikooyeh B, Zargaraan A, Kalayi A, Shariatzadeh N, Zahedirad M, Jamali A, Khazraie M, Hollis B, Neyestani TR (2020) Vitamin D-fortified cooking oil is an effective way to improve vitamin D status: an institutional efficacy trial. Eur J Nutr 59(6):2547–2555

Nojaba L, Guzman N (2023) Nephrolithiasis, Kidney stones. Complications. Treasure Island (FL): StatPearls Publishing

O'Rahilly S, Gray H, Humphreys PJ, Krook A, Polonsky KS, White A, Gibson S, Taylor K, Carr C (1995) Brief report: impaired processing of prohormones associated with abnormalities of glucose homeostasis and adrenal function. N Engl J Med 333(21):1386–1390

Ocvirk S, O'Keefe SJD (2021) Dietary fat, bile acid metabolism and colorectal cancer. Semin Cancer Biol 73:347–355

Palacios C, Hofmeyr GJ, Cormick G, Garcia CMN, Peña RJP, Betrán AP (2021) Current calcium fortification experiences: a review. Ann N Y Acad Sci 1484(1):55–73

Pearce LR, Joe R, Doche ME, Su HW, Keogh JM, Henning E, Argetsinger LS, Bochukova EG, Cline JM, Garg S, Saeed S, Shoelson S, O'Rahilly S, Barroso I, Rui L, Farooqi IS, Carter-Su C (2014) Functional characterization of obesity-associated variants involving the α and β isoforms of human SH2B1. Endocrinology 155(9):3219–3226

Peña-Romero AC, Navas-Carrillo D, Marín F, Orenes EP (2018) The future of nutrition: nutrigenomics and nutrigenetics in obesity and cardiovascular diseases. Crit Rev Food Sci Nutr 58(17):3030–3041

Perry GH, Dominy NJ, Claw KG, Lee AS, Fiegler H, Redon R, Werner J, Villanea FA, Mountain JL, Misra R, Carter NP, Lee C, Stone AC (2007) Diet and the evolution of human amylase gene copy number variation. Nat Genet 39(10):1256–1260

Pogue AI, Percy ME, Cui JG, Li YY, Bhattacharjee S, Hill JM, Kruck TP, Zhao Y, Lukiw WJ (2011) Up-regulation of NF-kB-sensitive miRNA-125b and miRNA-146a in metal sulfate-stressed human astroglial (HAG) primary cell cultures. J Inorg Biochem 105(11):1434–1437

Porzi M, Burton PKJ, Walther B, Vergères G (2021) Development of personalized nutrition: applications in lactose intolerance diagnosis and management. Nutrients 13(5):1503

Prasad AS (2012) Discovery of human zinc deficiency: 50 years later. J Trace Elem Med Biol 26(2–3):66–69

Puri V, Nagpal M, Singh I, Singh M, Dhingra GA, Huanbutta K, Dheer D, Sharma A, Sangnim T (2022) A comprehensive review on nutraceuticals: therapy support and formulation challenges. Nutrients 14(21):4637

Rajagopal S, Gupta A, Parveen R, Shukla N, Bhattacharya S, Naravula J, Kumar SA, Mathur P, Simlot A, Mehta S, Bihari C, Mehta S, Mishra AK, Nair BG, Medicherla KM, Reddy GB, Sreenivasulu N, Kishor PBK, Suravajhala P (2022) Vitamin K in human health and metabolism: a nutri-genomics review. Trends Food Sci Technol 119:412–427

Rajasekaran A (2017) Nutraceuticals. In: Reference module in chemistry, molecular sciences and chemical engineering, pp 107–134

Ramachandrappa S, Raimondo A, Cali AM, Keogh JM, Henning E, Saeed S, Thompson A, Garg S, Bochukova EG, Brage S, Trowse V, Wheeler E, Sullivan AE, Dattani M, Clayton PE, Datta V, Bruning JB, Wareham NJ, O'Rahilly S, Peet DJ, Barroso I, Whitelaw ML, Farooqi IS (2013) Rare variants in single-minded 1 (SIM1) are associated with severe obesity. J Clin Invest 123(7):3042–3050

Ramos-Lopez O, Panduro A, Martinez-Lopez E, Roman S (2016) Sweet taste receptor TAS1R2 polymorphism (Val191Val) is associated with a higher carbohydrate intake and hypertriglyceridemia among the population of West Mexico. Nutrients 8:101

Rana S, Kumar S, Rathore N, Padwad Y, Bhushana S (2016) Nutrigenomics and its impact on lifestyle associated metabolic diseases. Curr Genomics 17(3):261–278

Rodríguez-Cruz M, Serna DS (2017) Nutrigenomics of ω-3 fatty acids: regulators of the master transcription factors. Nutrition 41:90–96

Rui L (2014) Energy metabolism in the liver. Compr Physiol 4(1):177e197

Sampath H, Ntambi JM (2004) Polyunsaturated fatty acid regulation of gene expression. Nutr Rev 62(9):333–339

Sampson HA (2003) Food allergy. J Allergy Clin Immunol 111(Suppl 2):S540-7

Sellami M, Bragazzi NL (2020) Nutrigenomics and breast cancer: state-of-art, future perspectives and insights for prevention. Nutrients 12(2):512

Shahbaz U, Yu XB, Akhtar W, Ndagijimana R, Rauf H (2020) Golden rice to eradicate the vitamin a deficiency in the developing countries. Eur J Nutr Food Saf 12(1):53–63. ISSN: 2347-5641

Shan S, Niu J, Yin R, Shi J, Zhang L, Wu C, Li H, Li Z (2022) Peroxidase from foxtail millet bran exerts anti-colorectal cancer activity via targeting cell-surface GRP78 to inactivate STAT3 pathway. Acta Pharm Sin B 12(3):1254–1270

Shearer MJ, Newman P (2014) Recent trends in the metabolism and cell biology of vitamin K with special reference to vitamin K cycling and MK-4 biosynthesis. J Lipid Res 55(3):345–362

Singer-Englar T, Barlow G, Mathur R (2019) Obesity, diabetes, and the gut microbiome: an updated review. Expert Rev Gastroenterol Hepatol 13(1):3–15

Sobczak P, Grochowicz J, Łusiak P, Żukiewicz-Sobczak W (2023) Development of Alternative Protein Sources in Terms of a Sustainable System. Sustainability, 15(16):12111

Song Y, Niu T, Manson JAE, Kwiatkowski DJ, Liu S (2004) Are variants in the CAPN10 gene related to risk of type 2 diabetes? A quantitative assessment of population and family-based association studies. Am J Hum Genet 74(2):208–222

Srivastava S, Dubey AK, Madan R, Bala R, Gupta Y, Singh B, Kumar S (2022) Emergence of nutrigenomics and dietary components as a complementary therapy in cancer prevention. Environ Sci Pollut Res Int 29(60):89853–89873

Stoetzel C, Laurier V, Davis EE, Muller J, Rix S, Badano JL, Leitch CC, Salem N, Chouery E, Corbani S, Jalk N, Vicaire S, Sarda P, Hamel C, Lacombe D, Holder M, Odent S, Holder S, Brooks AS, Elcioglu NH, Silva ED, Rossillion B, Sigaudy S, de Ravel TJ, Lewis RA, Leheup B, Verloes A, Amati-Bonneau P, Mégarbané A, Poch O, Bonneau D, Beales PL, Mandel JL, Katsanis N, Dollfus HM (2006) BBS10 encodes a vertebrate-specific chaperonin-like protein and is a major BBS locus. Nat Genet 38(5):521–524

Tain, You-Lin, Chan, Julie YH, Hsu, Chien-Ning (2016) Maternal fructose intake affects transcriptome changes and programmed hypertension in offspring in later life. Nutrients, 8(12):757

Tang G, Qin J, Dolnikowski GG, Russell RM, Grusak MA (2009) Golden Rice is an effective source of vitamin A. Am J Clin Nutr 89(6):1776–1783

Thaker VV (2017) Genetic and epigenetic causes of obesity. Adolesc Med State Art Rev 28(2):379

Valenta R, Hochwallner H, Linhart B, Pahr S (2015) Food allergies: the basics. Gastroenterology 148(6):1120–1131.e4

Verdier C, Ruidavets JB, Bongard V, Taraszkiewicz D, Martinez LO, Elbaz M, Ferrières J, Perret B (2013) Association of hepatic lipase -514T allele with coronary artery disease and ankle-brachial index, dependence on the lipoprotein phenotype: the GENES study. PLoS One 8(7):e67805

Voight BF, Scott LJ, Steinthorsdottir V, Morris AP, Dina C, Welch RP, Zeggini E, Huth C, Aulchenko YS, Thorleifsson G, McCulloch LJ, Ferreira T, Grallert H, Amin N, Wu G, Willer CJ, Raychaudhuri S, McCarroll SA, Langenberg C, Hofmann OM, GIANT Consortium et al (2010) Twelve type 2 diabetes susceptibility loci identified through large-scale association analysis. Nat Genet 42(7):579–589

Wabitsch M, Funcke JB, Lennerz B, Kuhnle KU, Lahr G, Debatin KM, Vatter P, Gierschik P, Moepps B, Fischer PP (2015) Biologically inactive leptin and early-onset extreme obesity. N Engl J Med 372(1):48–54

Woodson K, Tangrea JA, Barrett MJ, Virtamo J, Taylor PR, Albanes D (1999) Serum alpha-tocopherol and subsequent risk of lung cancer among male smokers. J Natl Cancer Inst 91(20):1738–1743

Zahova S, Anthony RI (2018) The role of the Prader-Willi syndrome critical interval for epigenetic regulation, transcription and phenotype. Epigenomes 2(4):18

Zhang Y, Proenca R, Maffei M, Barone M, Leopold L, Friedman JM (1994) Positional cloning of the mouse obese gene and its human homologue. Nature 372(6505):425–432

Zhang F, Basinski MB, Beals JM, Briggs SL, Churgay LM, Clawson DK, Di Marchi RD, Furman TC, Hale JE, Hsiung HM, Schoner BE, Smith DP, Zhang XY, Wery JP, Schevitz RW (1997) Crystal structure of the obese protein leptin-E100. Nature 387(6629):206–209

Zhao M, Lin Y, Chen H (2020) Improving nutritional quality of rice for human health. Theor Appl Genet 133:1397–1413

Zhou H, Urso CJ, Jadeja V (2020) Saturated fatty acids in obesity-associated inflammation. J Inflamm Res 20:1–14

Ziemba JB, Matlaga BR (2017) Epidemiology and economics of nephrolithiasis. Investigative and clinical urology, 58(5):299–306

Food–Drug Interactions

5

Manoj Kumar Tripathi, Nidhi V. Maheshwari, Anil Kumar, Adinath Kate, Rajpal Singh Jadam, Chetna Porwal, Sharad Pandey, Aman Kumar, and Soumya Tripathi

Abstract

Food and drugs interactions may instinctively increase or decrease the effect of drugs. The potential of food and diet ingredients that affect the health is known in the last few years. Consumption of food now not only helps to reduce the hunger but is also involved in numerous health issues, so fluctuating with consumption of pharmaceutical products. This curiosity in the well-being and health sector forces the sales of market foods as functional and health foods. The active components of food products, which affect human health are bioactive compounds. These mentioned products are mainly classified as foodstuffs, but consumers are increasingly drawn to items at the connections of nutrition and pharmaceuticals. A wide range of dietary compounds is found to interact with protein biomolecules involved in drug pharmacokinetics and affecting the process from oral bioavailability and intestinal transport to metabolism, blood circulation, and systemic distribution. Some clinically important food–drug interactions result from food-induced alterations in drug bioavailability.

M. K. Tripathi (✉) · A. Kate · R. S. Jadam · C. Porwal · A. Kumar
ICAR- Central Institute of Agricultural Engineering, Bhopal, Madhya Pradesh, India
e-mail: tripathimanoj007@gmail.com

N. V. Maheshwari
Somaiya Vidyavihar University, Mumbai, Maharashtra, India

A. Kumar
Rani Lakshmi Bai Central Agricultural University, Jhansi, Uttar Pradesh, India

S. Pandey
School of Agriculture, Uttaranchal University, Dehradun, Uttarakhand, India

S. Tripathi
Atal Bihari Vajpayee Govt Medical College, Vidisha, Madhya Pradesh, India

A. Kumar et al. (eds.), *Innovations in Ayurvedic Nutrition*,
https://doi.org/10.1007/978-981-95-1213-3_5

Clinically important food–drug relations that cause likely damages to the patient, may be due to alterations in pharmaceutical properties. Food–drug interactions reduce the effectiveness and may cause toxicity and also sometime reduce bioavailability and alter clearance processes. Food and drugs both are very essential for life but their interactions can cause side effects so very careful identification is needed.

Keywords

Drug efficacy · Bioavailability · Metabolism · Diet · Absorption · Drug interaction

5.1 Introduction

Food–drug interactions refer to physical, chemical, and physiological effects occurring among a medicine and nutrients (Santos and Boullata 2005). An interaction is clinically important if it changes medicine's response or nutritional status, affecting the drug's disposition and therapeutic or nutritional effects. The disposition describes to medicine's or nutrient's absorption rate, delivery, and removal involving transporters and enzymes. Some clinically significant food-drug interactions risk increases in patients with chronic diseases using multiple medications. Elderly individuals are particularly vulnerable due to higher medications use and associated adverse effects and interactions (Salazar et al. 2007).

Individuals at age extremes or with any genetic variations or any poor nutritional status are prone to interactions. Poor nutrition may alter body composition, body function that is mainly caused by imbalances between nutrients need and intake whether from insufficient diet or disrupted nutrient metabolism. Drugs and nutrients can influence the signal transduction pathways, changing drug-metabolizing enzymes' activity and transporters with effect on receptor-mediated gene expression. Pharmacokinetic interactions naturally comprise enzymes and transporters that effect drug absorption, distribution, and elimination, possibly altering therapeutic efficacy or toxicity (Rushmore and Kong 2002; Gillies and Krul 2007).

Drug interactions can root adverse effects and have led to drug withdrawals (Huang and Lesko 2004). Such types of interactions can modify the drug's nature and efficiency, meaningly affecting patient consequences. Clinicians may identify specific drug–food interactions, as calcium with tetracycline but may not recognize these as part of broader interaction categories. Looking at them within a larger classification system can improve thoughtful organization of such interactions in clinical exercise, attractive patient safety, and treatment outcomes.

Drug–drug interactions are regularly known, and accomplished in medical practices, and are a significant emphasis throughout drug advance, as highlighted in regulatory guidance. However, drug–nutrient interactions beyond basic meal effects also permit care during new drug assessments to safeguard complete care and effectiveness valuations (Huang and Lesko 2004).

5.2 Classification of Food–Drug Interactions

Nutrient–drug interactions are broadly classified mainly into five categories (Santos and Boullata 2005) and each group is well-defined by some specific precipitating factor and interaction, permitting systematic identifications and considerate of various interaction types. In nutrient–drug interactions, the drug may act as either the precipitating factor, affecting nutritional status, influenced by nutrients or food. These interactions become clinically important when the causing factor reasons for prominent changes in the object's effect (Fig. 5.1).

In few situations, the medicine is the precipitating factor, while in others the drug is the object of the interaction (i.e. changes in drug's disposition or resulting effects from a nutrient, food, or nutritional status). Drug–nutrient interactions are clinically important if the precipitating factor produces significant changes in the object of the contact (Fig. 5.1).

The interaction process depends on the physicochemical properties of both the drug and the food within a specified environment. The resulting effects altered the disposition of the drug or nutrient and is affected by the specific location where the interaction occurs.

5.3 Nutritional Modulation of Drug's Disposition

Food intake during oral drug administration alters gastrointestinal conditions that affect drug absorption (Cheymol 2000). However, the impact of nutritional status as obesity or micronutrient deficiencies on drug's disposition and the metabolism

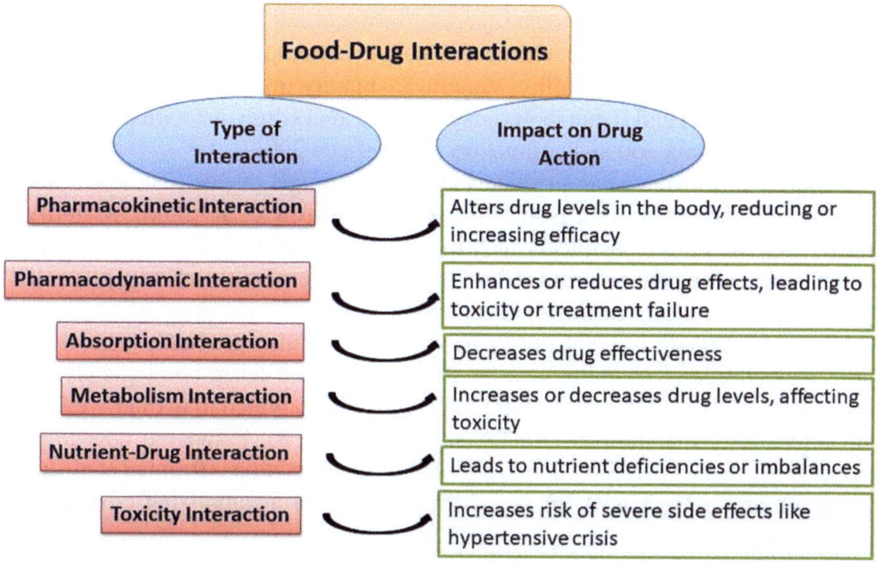

Fig. 5.1 Classification of food–drug interactions

remains underexplored, despite its recognized influence in several pharmacological studies Cheymol 2000). The result of food on a once-daily oral iron chelator and BCS Class II drug, was evaluated by Galanello et al. (2008). Diet, particularly high-fat meals, amplified its bioavailability, possibly due to improved solubilization. However, pharmacodynamically, plasma having high levels of the iron–drug complex in iron-excess patients continued unaffected despite food consumption (Galanello et al. 2008).

The food consumption does not significantly alter the level of the iron–drug complex in iron-overloaded patients (Galanello et al. 2008). Certain food exclusively affects a drug's disposition. For example cow's milk can diminish the bioavailability of drug mercaptopurine because of the presence of xanthine oxidase that alters drug into the inactive metabolite 6-thiouric acid (de Lemos et al. 2007). Cruciferous vegetables contain good amount of glucosinolates and metabolize into isothiocyanates and indole compounds that act as substrates of glutathione-S-transferase enzymes (GSTs). Soy protein isolates can also reduce the cytochrome P450 CYP1A1 expression via posttranslational suppression of the aryl hydrocarbon receptor (AhR) (Singhal et al. 2007; Wang et al. 2009). Numerous types of juices can knowingly mark drug character by interacting with transporter molecules and metabolizing enzymes, basically due to their composition with furanocoumarin, and flavonoid level (Dresser et al. 2002; Bailey et al. 2003). Though, the impact of juices resulting from crushed vegetables on these pathways is not clear and underexplored.

5.4 Role of Dietary Nutrients and Supplements in Modulating Drug's Disposition

Numerous research works state that specific nutrients and non-nutrient food supplement constituents can interact with several drugs. Divalent and trivalent cations may chelate and reduce bioavailability. Vitamin D, mainly in its active form, improves the level of phases I and II metabolic enzymes, and alters drug metabolism (Stargrove et al. 2008; Boullata 2005a, b; Kutuzova and DeLuca 2007).

Majority of nutrients can positively impact on drug's disposition. For example pyridoxine supports prevent isoniazid toxicity (Morrow et al. 2006). Majority of polyphenols and phytochemicals such as flavonoids, phenolic acids, stilbenes, and lignans may cause healing profits (Ramos 2008). Moreover, bioactive peptides have shown possible roles in health and drug interaction (Erdmann et al. 2008).

These compounds are not only parts of diets but also gradually increasing in nutritional additions. Cooking herbs and spices comprise several biologically active compounds such as terpenes and vanilloids, flavonoids, which may offer well-being and affect drug metabolism (Kaefer and Milner 2008). Flavonoid consumption should be evaluated carefully due to possible drug interactions (Erdman et al. 2007), because many polyphenols act as substrates for drug-metabolizing enzymes and transporters.

Many polyphenolic compounds show wide inhibitory effects, although others selectively target specific isoenzymes (Volak et al. 2008). Research reports their impact on efflux transporters than on uptake transporters (Morris and Zhang 2006; Shim et al. 2007). Certain spice-derived phytochemicals may affect CYP3A4 metabolism (Zhang and Lim 2008), and affect the drug's disposition. Flavonoids, specifically quercetin, are effective inhibitors of cytosolic SULT isozymes participating in drug metabolism (Cermak 2008). Daidzein, at 200 mg twice every day, improved theophylline bioavailability by dropping CYP1A2 activity (Peng et al. 2003). Diosmin may improve, although silymarin may decrease, metronidazole bioavailability, and indicate that there are variable effects of flavonoids on drug absorption and metabolism (Rajnarayana et al. 2003, 2004).

5.5 Impact of Drugs on Nutritive Status

Drugs generally impact on food consumption, ingestion, and absorption. A medicine may modify food consumption by direct effects on the gastrointestinal tract or the gut–brain axis. The mechanism for the sensitivity of gastrointestinal function to drugs has not received much attention (Tack 2007). When important, disorders occur in the digestive trait they damage persons' capability to keep or recover their nutritive status. A compromised ability to acquire, prepare, or consume food could contribute to these effects (Halford and Blundell 2000). The usage of some second-generation antipsychotics has been associated with many metabolic adverse effects, including weight gain, hyperglycemia, and dyslipidemia (ADA 2004). An analysis of a comprehensive database unveiled that increased body mass index (BMI) was notably associated with the usage of risperidone, quetiapine, and olanzapine when related to first-generation antipsychotic agents. Conversely, aripiprazole, ziprasidone, and clozapine were linked to a lower likelihood of weight gain (Brixner et al. 2006). Additional medications, such as capecitabine, can induce severe hypertriglyceridemia (>500 mg/dL), especially among individuals predisposed to this condition (Kurt et al. 2006).

5.6 Drug–Nutrient Interactions: Impact on Nutrient Status

Medicines can affect nutrient absorption and rate, delivery, breakdown, and excretion, possibly causing deficiencies. The medical impact depends on some important aspects of nutrients as nutrient's role, quantity, action period, and individual variability. Drug-induced nutrient deficiencies are documented as a subset of opposing effects, dose-dependent, duration-related, or characteristic.

Carbamazepine might harm biotin status by reducing its rate of absorption and enhancing clearance, possibly contributing to certain adverse drug effects (Rathman et al. 2002). Similarly, continued usage of valproic acid can cause to carnitine deficiency, marked by reduced plasma and urinary carnitine levels. In such cases, typical nutrient supplementation might not fully address the primary nutrient imbalances or deficiencies (Venhoff et al. 2002).

Valproic acid's action is related to alterations in acylcarnitine subspecies, suggesting disturbed intermediate metabolism that may contribute to hepatotoxicity (Werner et al. 2007). Addictive substances also affect nutritional status; for example cigarette smoking is linked to reduced levels of folate, pyridoxine, and vitamin B12, and may increase biotin metabolism, potentially leading to marginal deficiency and teratogenic risks in women (Gabriel et al. 2006; Sealey et al. 2004).

5.7 Nutrient–Drug Interactions: Effects on Absorption and Metabolism

For active systemic bioavailability via oral administration, a drug must overcome several barriers, including solubility in GI fluids, dissolution rate, and intestinal permeability. Factors like GI secretions, transit time, first-pass metabolism, and the food's presence also significantly affect drug absorption and overall bioavailability (Dressman et al. 2008).

Many drugs differ in solubility and permeability, influencing their classifications and absorption. Diets effects on absorption depend on drug properties, dosage form, and GI physiology. Key rate-limiting steps include drug dissolution, gastric emptying, and intestinal permeability. Tables 5.1 and 5.2 list meal-timing impacts on common oral drug pharmacokinetics.

Table 5.1 Medicines that should be taken before meals

Basic name	Medical consequence
Azithromycin	Diet declines absorption
Digoxin	Diet reduces absorption, declines peak level
Dextroamphetamine	Acidic diets/juices may hinder drug's absorption
Furosemide	Improved absorption in fasting state
Levothyroxine	Take consistently on an empty stomach for optimal absorption
Phenytoin	Food affects absorption, take consistently in relation to meals
Lansoprazole, omeprazole, pantoprazole, and rabeprazole	Take before meals to enhance absorption and therapeutic effectiveness
Tetracyclines	Iron, milk, and food significantly reduce the drug's absorption
Quinolones	Decreased absorption with antacids, some major cations (Ca, Fe, and Zn), and dairy products
Theophylline	Diet may decline absorption
Zolpidem	Diet delays the action
Warfarin	Diet modifies absorption with respect to meals

Table 5.2 Medicines best taken with food

Basic name	Clinical effect
Carvedilol	Diet drops risk for orthostatic hypotension
Amoxicillin/clavulanate	Diet rises the rate of absorption
Carbamazepine	Diet increases absorption
Divalproex	Diet declines GI upset
Fenofibrate	Diet enhances bioavailability
Glucocorticoids	Diet reduces gastrointestinal upset
Glyburide/metformin	Diet intake helps reduce gastrointestinal side effects
Labetalol	Food enhances absorption
Metformin	Food intake helps minimize gastrointestinal disturbances
Metoprolol	Food improves absorption; take consistently in relation to meals
Niacin	Food consumption reduces GI disturbances
Nitrofurantoin	Food enhances absorption; take consistently with meals
Celecoxib, diclofenac, etodolac, and ibuprofen,	Food consumption minimizes GI disturbances
Potassium chloride	Food consumption minimizes GI disturbances
Venlafaxine	Food consumption minimizes GI disturbances

5.8 Diet and Drug's Absorption

Drug's absorption relies on physicochemical properties of the drug and characteristics of the dosage form containing the active ingredient. The diet's GI absorption is solubility-limited. Effective membrane permeability often correlates with strong lipid solubility (lipophilicity), while exhibiting limited hydrophilicity. Accordingly, the absorption rate of lipophilic drugs is hindered by low closure in the aqueous environment of the gastrointestinal tract.

Many lipophilic drugs show improved absorption when taken with fat-containing meals, with absorption often growing as meal fat content rises. In contrast, hydrophilic drugs dissolve rapidly due to high aqueous solubility but have limited absorption because their passage through lipid membranes is restricted by low permeability rather than dissolution.

5.9 Meals and Their Effects

A meal can impact gastrointestinal transportation and medicine absorption. Although average intestinal transit time is generally consistent between fasting and fed states, certain drugs, excipients, and over-the-counter products can alter absorption by affecting transit. Both quantity and caloric density of a meal show key roles in this effect.

5.10 Diet–Drug Interactions; Effects on Metabolic Pathways

Both nutritious and nonnutritive parts of diets can affect drug metabolism similar to drug–drug interactions. Many drugs originate from plant-based compounds and make drug–nutrient interactions biologically reasonable. The biologically active cytochrome P450 (CYP) enzyme system, specifically in the liver and intestinal mucosa, has as a key role in these interactions. Nutritional components, like drugs, may inhibit or encourage CYP enzymes, varying drug metabolism and clearance. Such effects are well-documented, mainly for drugs metabolized by CYP enzymes in humans.

Some important effects of food on drug metabolism were initially found in animals and later established in humans (Ioannides 2003; Murray 2006). Humans are usually more compliant in short-term, precise studies, permitting dietary changes without varying total energy consumption. In contrast, animal studies require some important approaches as pair feeding to isolate dietary effects without the confounding impact of overall energy consumption. In a sequence of several studies, dietary protein and carbohydrate level were consecutively improved though keeping constant fat and total energy consumption. The rates of metabolic clearance of antipyrine and theophylline improved during consumption of high-protein diets, and faster plasma drug elimination was observed. These medicines were selected due to their dependence on hepatic CYP enzymes, particularly CYP1A2, for metabolism. Improved protein consumption also makes faster the clearance of propranolol, and also possibly aminopyrine and caffeine, in the case of both men and women. In contrast, switching between high-fat and high-carbohydrate diets showed no significant effect. Overall, the intake of protein seems to improve hepatic medicine oxidation. Dietary protein plays a higher role in comparison to carbohydrates or fats in regulating oxidative drug metabolism, inducing drug oxidation even at variable calorie consumptions and under clinical circumstances, as reported in both healthy and patient studies, as well as other clinical settings. Several human studies on dietary protein and drug metabolism align with previous rodent research; however rodent results are complex due to sex differences absent in humans (Anderson and Kappas 1991).

Dietary nutritional composition can suggestively affect drug metabolism and hormone regulation. Increased level of protein and carbohydrate proportion in food is found to rise estrogen 2-hydroxylation and reduce androgen 5α-reduction in well persons. This type of dietary shift may also disturb plasma levels of hormone testosterone and cortisol, along with deviations in their binding globulins and effects similar to as caused by phenobarbital (Anderson et al. 1987). Moreover, dietary protein can impact renal drug clearance by varying renal plasma flow, creatinine clearance, and tubular transport, mainly for basic drugs and their metabolites. Some specific nutritional components may also improve or inhibit drug absorption, further affecting overall drug's disposition and therapeutic outcomes.

Dietary components can impact on dispersal of drugs on target sites. High-protein consumption raises many neutral amino acids that compete for transporting transversely the blood–brain barrier, dropping dopamine levels in brain. Protein redistribution limiting protein during the day time and permitting higher intake at night has shown clinical benefits (Barichella et al. 2006). However, if baseline protein or nutrient intake is inadequate, such dietary adjustments may lead to deficiencies and negative health effects.

5.10.1 Alcohol–Drug Interactions: Mechanisms and Risks

Some adversative responses can happen after alcohol drinking in patients treated with drug tetraethyl thiuram disulfide that is used to care alcohol abstinence. These types of drugs and alcohol collaboration show some unpleasant symptoms (as flushing, headache, nausea, hypotension, vomiting, weakness, dizziness, and blurred vision). Disulfiram drugs work by preventing the action of aldehyde dehydrogenase, an enzyme that oxidizes acetaldehyde, a byproduct in alcohol metabolism. A similar drug, cyanamide, has been prescribed in nations like Japan but they may cause liver harmfulness (Tamai et al. 2000). The disulfiram response, also called "acetaldehyde syndrome", has been reproduced using acetaldehyde alone and may even occur after consuming foods prepared with wine, wine vinegar, or alcoholic desserts.

5.10.2 Vitamins and Drug Interactions: Implications for Health

Vitamin deficiencies can affect hepatic drug metabolism in animals, signifying that supplement may affect drug processing. Though, human data are less, and translating animal discoveries is inspiring due to important species changes in metabolic pathways Murray 2006.

High vitamin quantities may change drug metabolism; vitamin C deficit reduces it, particularly in liver disease. Any supplement in old and diabetic patients enhanced ascorbate levels and reduced antipyrine half-lives; however other nutritional deficiencies may have also affected the metabolism. Studies on some well and healthy persons have shown a very nominal influence of minor vitamin C deficiency on drug metabolism. For example five male volunteers having short-range subclinical vitamin C deficit displayed no significant alteration in antipyrine metabolism, and ten old subjects exhausted of ascorbate for 4 weeks duration displayed no change in caffeine metabolism. These results recommend that only severe shortages may affect drug metabolism. Furthermore, vitamin B6 can improve peripheral conversion of levodopa to dopamine via dopa-decarboxylase, decrease the quantity of levodopa accessible to cross the blood–brain barrier, where it is required. Meanwhile dopamine cannot cross the barrier, this reduces efficacy. Yet, carbidopa inhibits peripheral dopamine decarboxylase, preventing this effect and preserving levodopa's beneficial action.

5.11 Nutrients in Mitigating Drug Toxicity

5.11.1 Folic Acid

Fluorouracil (5-FU) used in treatment of several cancerous conditions by changing to an active metabolite prevents and inhibits thymidylate synthase, disorderly pyrimidine synthesis, and tumor cell spread. Leucovorin, frequently given with 5-FU, increases its antitumor properties by increasing the level of intracellular folates that stabilize the thymidylate synthase–fluorodeoxyuridine monophosphate complex. This process increases the enzyme inhibition; subsequently reduced folate metabolites potentiate 5-FU activity; and folic acid has been suggested as a possible alternative to leucovorin, provided it achieves similar plasma metabolite levels. In rheumatoid arthritis (RA), low amounts (5–25 mg/week) are generally agreed for both short- and long-term supervision (Cutolo et al. 2001). Higher amounts are hardly used, which mainly include bone marrow suppression, gastrointestinal, hepatic, and pulmonary effects.

Methotrexate functions similar to folic acid and blocks an enzyme desirable to turn folic acid into its active form. This drops folate concentrations in cells and stops DNA from being made, which reduces cell growth (Ortiz et al. 1998; Morgan et al. 1994). Low levels of folate can cause side effects like diarrhea, mouth sores, and low white blood cells similar to folic acid deficiency. To decrease these side effects, folate additions are important. Leucovorin (folinic acid) is used to help reverse methotrexate toxicity.

5.12 Dietary Modulation of Pharmacological Activity

5.12.1 Calcitriol and Docetaxel

Docetaxel drug is a mitotic phase inhibitor, which is applied in the treatment of cancers such as breast, ovarian, head and neck, and prostate cancer. Docetaxel's antitumor result might be improved by calcitriol (active vitamin D), which performances at high drug concentrations. The antineoplastic action involves vitamin D receptors and cytoplasmic signaling pathways. It encourages apoptosis, prevents proliferation and differentiation, and decreases angiogenesis and invasiveness, and mechanisms of action change by type of tumor and experimental model.

5.12.2 Phytosterols and Statins

Plant sterols (phytosterols), for example campesterol, sitosterol, and stigmasterol, are natural compounds present in mainly in edible oils, nuts, and seeds. Both sterols and stanols are added to diets as margarine and salad dressing frequently in Europe. Both efficiently low the serum cholesterol and have distinct structural and functional differences (Hallikainen et al. 2000). Combination of statins with plant sterols can affect lowering of LDL cholesterol as efficiently after use of double the statin dose, as reported in a study (Stein 2002). The role of plant sterols was also examined in patients in observations under familial hypercholesterolemia conditions (Neil et al. 2001). Because plant sterols are water-insoluble but liquefy well in fats, so maximum clinical studies of sterol-rich foods have been made on stanol-enriched margarine. Benecol, a marketable invention comprising plant stanol esters, is also accessible in light spreads and chews. It is naturally consumed with foods for cholesterol management.

Numerous multi-ingredient nutritive additions contain plant stanols and sterols are available in the market. Their cholesterol-reducing result is modest due to liver cholesterol synthesis (Turley 2002). High price and regular treating decrease user demand; however emerging reports recommend possible cost-effectiveness of nutritional supplements with plant origin stanols and sterols.

5.13 Interactions of Natural Products

The usage of nutritional supplement is extensive, mainly among middle-aged Caucasian females and old persons who have chronic health circumstances (Sloan 2007; Timbo et al. 2006). Several users also use prescription medicines. Marketing reviews show that aging babies signify the fastest-growing user clusters for supplements,; these results indicate the improved well-being alertness and curiosity in protective health approaches in this population (Sloan 2007).

Extensive usage of nutritional additions, exclusively by persons on many prescription drugs for chronic circumstances, the hazard of drug–nutrient relations is important and can lead to serious opposing effects. Usually used supplements comprise glucosamine/chondroitin, omega-3 fatty acids, cranberry extract, coenzyme Q10, and green tea extracts. Preferably, categorizing these relations by their basic mechanisms, which supports in successfully classifying and managing possible risks (Chan 2000). Specific references for drug–dietary supplement pairs are very rare. A practical basis involves the thorough literature evaluation, valuation of the patient's medical conditions and use of medicines, and also submission of the clinical decision. A suggested strategy is outlined in Table 5.3.

Some current studies advise that some compounds showing possible interactions include garlic, valerian, kava, ginkgo, St. John's Wort (Hypericum perforatum) (SJW), glucosamine, and ginseng. Some common medicines with interaction dangers comprise antithrombotics, sedatives, antidepressants, and antidiabetic agents (Table 5.4).

5.14 Garlic

Garlic has been used as a food flavoring and traditional medicine for sicknesses like headaches, weakness, and epilepsy for a very long time (Mahady et al. 2001a, b). Current uses comprise hypertension, high cholesterol, atherosclerosis,

Table 5.3 Possible interactions between a drug and a dietary supplement

Sr. No.	Drug–nutrient interaction strategy
1.	Identification of symptoms associated with the drug or supplement such as cardiovascular, liver, CNS, or electrolyte effects Align the patient's symptoms with clinical symbols to evaluate probable interaction If expected, stop the cause and give supportive care
2.	Search the data and literature to confirm the interaction using clinical studies or, if report is not available, check for case reports or papers published
3.	In case of no any reports, assess the possibility of interactions between the compounds being reasonable
4.	Use Drug Interaction Probability Scale tools to evaluate interaction possibility (Horn et al. 2007)

Table 5.4 Common dietary supplements that may cause drug interactions

Sr. No.	Dietary supplements	Other dietary supplements
1.	Aloe (Aloe vera)	Elder (Sambucus nigra) - a dietary supplement with potential drug interaction
2.	Alfalfa (*Medicagosativa*)	*Echinacea*
3.	*Angelica* sp. (e.g. *BaiZhi, Dong Quai*)	Fenugreek
4.	Betel nut	Flaxseed
5.	Boldo	*Garcinia*
6.	Black cohosh	Garlic
7.	Bromelain	Ginger
8.	Caffeine	Ginkgo
9.	Camellia	Ginseng
10.	Capsicum	Grape seed extract
11.	Cascara	Hawthorn
12.	Chlorella	Lemon balm
13.	Cocoa	Quercetin
14.	CoEnzyme Q10	Saw palmetto

Boullata (2005a, b), Haller et al. (2008)

improvement in blood circulation, and acting as a blood thinner (Rahman 2007; Allison et al. 2006). Allicin compounds present in garlic are the main active compounds. Other bioactive compounds in garlic also show potential health beneficial effects. Garlic inhibits CYP2E1, an enzyme involved in metabolizing inhalation anesthetics, acetaminophen, and ethanol (Taubert et al. 2006). Garlic oil may also be effective in reducing anesthetic quantity required during the surgery process. It also has effects on some other CYP enzymes, such as CYP2D6 and CYP3A4; it seems nominal with restricted medical significance (Markowitz et al. 2003).

Garlic compounds may bind with antithrombotic medicines by inhibiting platelet aggregation through several mechanisms such as minimization of cyclooxygenase and thromboxane A2 development; minimize intraplatelet calcium mobilization, improve cAMP/cGMP, and inhibit of GPIIb/IIIa receptors. These activities can improve hemorrhage dangers in patients consuming drugs like ticlopidine, clopidogrel, or warfarin (Rahman 2007).

5.15 Conclusions

It is well known and also established that many medicines can cause vitamin deficiencies, it is very less frequently known that nutritional vitamin supplements can affect drug absorption, metabolism, and several pharmacological activities. Nutrients, including vitamins, may interrelate with medicines, possibly changing their therapeutic effects. Though, the available indication extensively arises from reports on isolated circumstances of animal studies, or in vitro experiments, and preventive extensive clinical usages. One prominent example is vitamin E, which has shown the possibility to improve the oral absorption of cyclosporine, mainly in pediatric liver transplant patients. All these interactions highlight the status of seeing nutrient–drug interactions in clinical applications. Greater alertness, more investigation, and cautious clinical valuation are important to know and accomplish these connections for safe and effective medical care.

References

Allison GL, Lowe GM, Rahman K (2006) Aged garlic extract and its constituents inhibit platelet aggregation through multiple mechanisms. J Nutr 136(3 Suppl):782S–788S

American Diabetes Association (2004) Consensus development conference on antipsychotyic drugs and obesity and diabetes. Diabetes Care 27:596–601

Anderson KE, Kappas A (1991) Dietary regulation of cytochrome P450. Annu Rev Nutr 11:141–167

Anderson KE, Rosner W, New MI, Pang S, Wissel PS, Kappas A (1987) Diet-hormone interactions: protein/carbohydrate ratio alters reciprocally the plasma levels of testosterone and cortisol and their respective binding globulins in man. Life Sci 40:1761–1768

Bailey DG, Dresser GK, Bend JR (2003) Bergamottin, lime juice and red wine as inhibitors of CYP3A4 activity: comparison with grapefruit juice. Clin Pharmacol Ther 73:529–537

Barichella M, Marczewska A, De Notaris R, Vairo A, Baldo C, Mauri A, Savardi C, Pezzoli G (2006) Special low-protein foods ameliorate postprandial off in patients with advanced Parkinson's disease. Mov Disord 21(10):1682–1687

Boullata JI (2005a) Influence of medication on nutritional status. In: Bendich A, Deckelbaum RJ (eds) Preventive nutrition, 3rd edn. Humana Press Inc., Totowa, pp 833–868

Boullata JI (2005b) Natural health product interactions with medication. Nutr Clin Pract 20:33–51

Brixner DI, Said Q, Corey-Lisle PK, Tuomari AV, L'italien GJ, Stockdale W, Oderda GM (2006) Naturalistic impact of second generation antipsychotics on weight gain. Ann Pharmacother 40:626–632

Cermak R (2008) Effect of dietary flavanoids on pathways involved in drug metabolism. Expert Opin Drug Metab Toxicol 4:17–35

Chan LN (2000) Redefining drug–nutrient interactions. Nutr Clin Pract 15(5):249–252

Cheymol G (2000) Effects of obesity on pharmacokinetics: implications for drug therapy. Clin Pharmacokinet 39:215–231

Cutolo M, Sulli A, Pizzorni C, Seriolo B, Straub RH (2001) Anti-inflammatory mechanisms of methotrexate in rheumatoid arthritis. Ann Rheum Dis 60:729–735

De Lemos ML, Hamata L, Jennings S, Leduc T (2007) Interaction between mercaptopurine and milk. J Oncol Pharm Pract 13:237–240
Dresser GK, Bailey DG, Leake BF, Schwarz UI, Dawson PA, Freeman DJ, Kim RB (2002) Fruit juices inhibit organic anion transporting polypeptide-mediated drug uptake to decrease the oral availability of fexofenadine. Clin Pharmacol Ther 71:11–20
Dressman JB, Thelen K, Jantratid E (2008) Towards quantitative prediction of oral drug absorption. Clin Pharmacokinet 47:655–667
Erdman JW, Balentine D, Arab L, Beecher G, Dwyer JT, Folts J, Hollman P, Keen CL, Mazza G, Messina M (2007) Flavonoids and heart health: proceedings of the ILSI North America flavonoids workshop. J Nutr 137:718S–737S
Erdmann K, Cheung BWY, Schroder H (2008) The possible roles of food-derived bioactive peptides in reducing the risk of cardiovascular disease. J Nutr Biochem 19:643–654
Gabriel HE, Crott JW, Ghandour H, Ghandour H, Dallal GE, Choi SW, Keyes MK, Jang H, Liu Z, Nadeau M, Johnston A, Mager D (2006) Chronic cigarette smoking is associated with diminished folate status, altered folate form distribution, and increased genetic damage in the buccal mucosa of healthy adults. Am J Clin Nutr 83:835–841
Galanello R, Piga A, Cappellini MD, Forni GL, Zappu A, Origa R, Dutreix C, Belleli R, Ford JM, Riviere GJ, Balez S (2008) Effect of food, type of food, and time of food intake on deferasirox bioavailability: recommendations for an optimal deferasirox administration regimen. J Clin Pharmacol 48:428–435
Gillies PJ, Krul ES (2007) Using genetic variation to optimize nutritional preemption. J Nutr 137:270S–274S
Halford JC, Blundell JE (2000) Pharmacology of appetite suppression. Prog Drug Res 54:25–58
Hallikainen MA, Sarkkinen ES, Gylling H, Erkkilä AT, Uusitupa MIJ (2000) Comparison of the effects of plant sterol ester and plant stanol ester-enriched margarines in lowering serum cholesterol concentrations in hypercholesterolaemic subjects on a low-fat diet. Eur J Clin Nutr 54:715–725
Horn JR, Hansten PD, Chan LN (2007) Proposal for a new tool to evaluate drug interaction cases. Ann Pharmacother 41(4):674–680
Huang SM, Lesko LJ (2004) Drug–drug, drug dietary supplement, and drug-citrus fruit and other food interactions: what have we learned? J Clin Pharmacol 44:559–569
Ioannides C (2003) Drug-phytochemical interactions. Inflammopharmacology 11(1):7–42
Kaefer CM, Milner JA (2008) The role of herbs and spices in cancer prevention. J Nutr Biochem 19:347–361
Kurt M, Babaoglu MO, Yasar U, Shorbagi A, Guler N (2006) Capecitabine-induced severe hypertriglyceridemia: report of two cases. Ann Pharmacother 40:328–331
Kutuzova GD, DeLuca HF (2007) 1, 25-Dihydroxyvitamin D3 regulates genes responsible for detoxification in intestine. Toxicol Appl Pharmacol 218:37–44
Mahady GB, Fong H, Farnsworth NR (2001a) Garlic. In: Botanical dietary supplements: quality, safety and efficacy. Swets & Zeitlinger Group BV, Lisse, pp 97–114
Mahady GB, Fong H, Farnsworth NR (2001b) Ginkobiloba. In: Botanical dietary supplements: quality, safety and efficacy. Swets & Zeitlinger Group BV, Lisse, pp 140–158
Markowitz JS, Devane CL, Chavin KD, Taylor RM, Ruan Y, Donovan JL (2003) Effects of garlic (Allium sativum L.) supplementation on cytochrome P450 2D6 and 3A4 activity in healthy volunteers. Clin Pharmacol Ther 74(2):170–177
Morris ME, Zhang S (2006) Flavonoid-drug interactions: effects of flavonoids on ABC transporters. Life Sci 78:2116–2130
Morrow LE, Wear RE, Schuller D, Malesker M (2006) Acute isoniazid toxicity and the need for adequate pyridoxine supplies. Pharmacotherapy 26:1529–1532
Murray M (2006) Altered CYP expression and function in response to dietary factors: potential roles in disease pathogenesis. Curr Drug Metab 7(1):67–81
Neil HA, Meijer GW, Roe LS (2001) Randomized controlled trial of use by hypercholesterolaemic patients of a vegetable oil sterol-enriched fat spread. Atherosclerosis 156:329–337

Peng WX, Li HD, Zhou HH (2003) Effect of daidzein on CYP1A2 activity and pharmacokinetics of theophylline in healthy volunteers. Eur J Clin Pharmacol 58:237–241
Rahman K (2007) Effects of garlic on platelet biochemistry and physiology. Mol Nutr Food Res 51(11):1335–1344
Rajnarayana K, Reddy MS, Krishna DR (2003) Diosmin pretreatment affects bioavailability of metronidazole. Eur J Clin Pharmacol 58:803–807
Rajnarayana K, Reddy MS, Vidyasagar J, Krishna DR (2004) Study on the influence of silymarin pretreatment on metabolism and disposition of metronidazole. Arzneim Forsch 54:109–113
Ramos S (2008) Cancer chemoprevention and chemotherapy: dietary polyphenols and signaling pathways. Mol Nutr Food Res 52:507–526
Rathman SC, Eisenschenk S, McMahon RJ (2002) The abundance and function of biotin-dependent enzymes are reduced in rats chronically administered carbamazepine. J Nutr 132:3405–3410
Rushmore TH, Kong ANT (2002) Pharmacogenomics, regulation and signaling pathways of phase I and II drug metabolizing enzymes. Curr Drug Metab 3:481–490
Salazar JA, Poon I, Nair M (2007) Clinical consequences of polypharmacy in elderly: expect the unexpected, think the unthinkable. Expert Opin Drug Saf 6:695–704
Santos CA, Boullata JI (2005) An approach to evaluating drug–nutrient interactions. Pharmacotherapy 25:1789–1800
Sealey WM, Teague AM, Stratton SL, Mock DM (2004) Smoking accelerates biotin catabolism in women. Am J Clin Nutr 80:932–935
Shim CK, Cheon EP, Kang KW, Seo KS, Han HK (2007) Inhibition effect of flavonoids on monocarboxylate transporter 1 (MCT1) in Caco-2 cells. J Pharm Pharmacol 59:1515–1519
Singhal R, Badger TM, Ronis MJ (2007) Reduction in 7,12-dimethylbenz[a]anthracene-induced hepatic cytochrome-P450 1A1 expression following soy consumption in female rats is mediated by degradation of the aryl hydrocarbon receptor. J Nutr 137:19–24
Sloan E (2007) Why people use vitamin and mineral supplements. Nutr Today 42(2):55–61
Stargrove MB, Treasure J, McKee DL (2008) Herb, nutrient, and drug interactions: clinical implications and therapeutic strategies. Mosby Elsevier, St. Louis
Stein EA (2002) Managing dyslipidemia in the high risk patient. Am J Cardiol 89(Suppl):50C–57C
Tack J (2007) Chemosensitivity of the human gastrointestinal tract in health and disease. Neurogastroenterol Motil 19:241–244
Tamai H, Yokoyama A, Okuyama K, Takahashi H, Maruyama K, Suzuki Y, Ishii H (2000) Comparison of cyanamide and disulfiram in effects on liver function. Alcohol Clin Exp Res 24(4 Suppl):97S–99S
Taubert D, Glockner R, Muller D, Schomig E (2006) The garlic ingredient diallyl sulfide inhibits cytochrome P450 2E1 dependent bioactivation of acrylamide to glycidamide. Toxicol Lett 164(1):1–5
Timbo BB, Ross MP, McCarthy PV, Lin CTJ (2006) Dietary supplements in a national survey: prevalence of use and reports of adverse events. J Am Diet Assoc 106:1966–1974
Turley SD (2002) State of the art in cholesterol management: targeting multiple pathways. Am J Manag Care 8:S29–S32
Venhoff N, Setzer B, Lebrecht D, Walker UA (2002) Dietary supplements in the treatment of nucleoside reverse transcriptase inhibitor-related mitochondrial toxicity. AIDS 16:800–802
Volak LP, Ghirmai S, Cashman JR, Court MH (2008) Curcuminoids inhibit multiple human cytochromes P450, UDP-glucuronosyltransferase, and sulfotransferase enzymes, whereas piperine is a relatively selective CYP3A4 inhibitor. Drug Metab Dispos 36:1594–1605
Wang G, Xiao CQ, Li Z, Guo D, Chen Y, Fan L, Qian RH, Penj XJ, Hu DL, Zhou HH (2009) Effect of soy extract administration on losartan pharmacokinetics in healthy female volunteers. Ann Pharmacother 43:1045–1049
Werner T, Treiss I, Kohlmueller D, Mehlem P, Teich M, Longin E, Gerstner T, Koenig SA, Schulze A (2007) Effects of valproate on acylcarnitines in children with epilepsy using ESI-MS/MS. Epilepsia 48:72–76
Zhang W, Lim LY (2008) Effects of spice constituents on P-glycoprotein-mediated transport and CYP3A4-mediated metabolism in vitro. Drug Metab Dispos 36:1283–1290

Foodomics: Recent Trends in Food and Omics

6

Rahul Dev and Mahesh Gupta

Abstract

Safe, nutritious, and sustainable food is crucial for maintaining human health and well-being, particularly in view of the growing global challenges such as nutrition security, climate change, and biodiversity loss. The COVID-19 pandemic has heightened awareness of healthy eating, sustainability, and the importance of food quality and safety. Advancements in food technologies, such as foodomics, have revolutionized our understanding of food, not only as a source of energy and nutrients but as a preventative tool for future diseases. Foodomics integrates genomics, transcriptomics, proteomics, and metabolomics (omics tools), offers a comprehensive approach to the analysis of food composition, nutritional properties, and their impact on health. This approach aligns with the tenets of Ayurvedic nutrition, which emphasize food as a medicine, promoting balance and wellness. By employing multi-omics techniques, it is possible to develop personalized nutrition solutions that are tailored to address specific health challenges. Furthermore, foodomics has potential to influence the circular economy by promoting sustainable food production practices. This chapter provides an overview of foodomics, exploring its tools, applications, and future potential in achieving safer, more sustainable, and personalized nutrition in the new food era.

Keywords

Foodomics · Foodomics tools · Proteomics · Metabolomics · Health and wellness

---

R. Dev · M. Gupta (✉)
Food and Nutraceutical Laboratory, Dietetics and Nutrition Technology Division, CSIR-Institute of Himalayan Bioresource Technology, Palampur, Himachal Pradesh, India
e-mail: mgupta@ihbt.res.in

A. Kumar et al. (eds.), *Innovations in Ayurvedic Nutrition*,
https://doi.org/10.1007/978-981-95-1213-3_6

6.1 Introduction

In contemporary food science and nutrition, a major goal is to improve our knowledge of the molecular functions of nutritional compounds (i.e. their interactions with genes and subsequent effects on metabolites and proteins) to rationally design dietary manipulation strategies that are expected to have profound effects on our health. Additionally, nutritional molecules can be viewed as signaling molecules that the body's specific sensory systems can detect, which is why thousands of substances are examined simultaneously to study various temporal and spatial reactions (Garcia-Cañas et al. 2012). To prove that food is healthy, researchers must uncover the mechanisms that influence the human metabolome. This new way of thinking about food is known as "foodomics", and it pushes researchers to think in new ways about food.

In this context, "foodomics" was first introduced in 2009 as a unique concept based on advanced analytical tools (omics) and an understanding of bioinformatics to study food composition and its impact on nutrition and health. Foodomics is therefore designed to be a useful concept able to focus on the food ingredient using qualitative and quantitative data with all the omics, but more importantly, it is intended to help a researcher to identify the specific effects of foods on the human body, health, and diet. Figure 6.1 depicts the omics tools employed under foodomics and their applications. For instance, foodomics understates the interaction of food with the human body using tools: genomics, transcriptomics, proteomics, and metabolomics (Ghahary and Abiri 2021). It is an interdisciplinary field that requires fundamental research in a broad range of disciplines; biology, physics, mathematics, and many branches of chemistry (organic, inorganic, and analytical chemistry), with a variety of omics subdisciplines (epigenomics, lipidomics, nutrigenomics, toxigenomics, metallomics, etc.). In food and nutrition science, foodomics offers

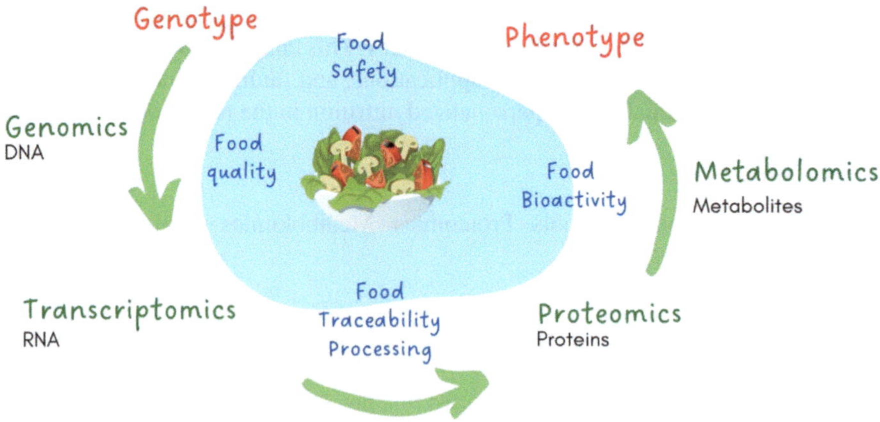

Fig. 6.1 Representation of foodomic tools

researchers new analytical approaches by combining genomics, transcriptomics, proteomics, and metabolomics, to solve a myriad of current challenges.

The interaction of food with various aspects, such as nutritional values, safety, bioactivity, quality, and traceability through the use of advanced food strategies, all these issues are well established under the Foodomics concept, defined as "a study of the food science and nutrition domain by integrating leading omics technologies to improve wellbeing, health, and knowledge of the consumers" (Cifuentes 2009). Foodomics' main objective is to work in tandem with medicine and biosciences to avoid diseases in the future by ensuring proper food consumption and the creation of so-called functional foods and nutraceuticals by identifying and characterizing bioactive compounds (Cifuentes 2013).

In this regard, foodomics is considered an accessible method for preventing a variety of diseases by investigating the biochemical, molecular, and cellular mechanisms associated with certain bioactive food components; individual gene variations in response to a specific dietary pattern that might lead to personalized nutrition; identification of genes involved in an early stage before the onset of a disease, which could lead to the molecular biomarkers' discovery (Álvarez-Rivera et al. 2021). In addition to identifying possible bioactive compounds, it is also important to understand how these molecules act on cells, tissues, and organs.

6.2 Foodomics Tools

The term "Omics" refers to the comprehensive study of biological systems. The discipline of Foodomics includes four major areas: genomics, transcriptomics, proteomics, and metabolomics (Casas-Agustench and Andres-Lacueva 2020) as shown in Fig. 6.2.

6.2.1 Genomics

As humans consume food every day there is a strong relationship between human genes and food. In this instance, interactions between genes and exposure to the environment, particularly diet, lead to changes in human health. Therefore, without genomics research, it is challenging to explore the link between food nutrition and health (Zheng and Chen 2014). As part of genomics, researchers examine every genetic profile and the specifics of the genome, such as how it is structured and functions. The use of genomics in nutrition research is a vast issue, with a particular focus on the connection between genetics, hereditary factors, and dietary patterns. It would greatly facilitate individual nutrigenomic studies and diet plan recommendations for certain people (Ghahary and Abiri 2021). This ought to promote the development of food-derived medications and nutrient-modified foods to improve health.

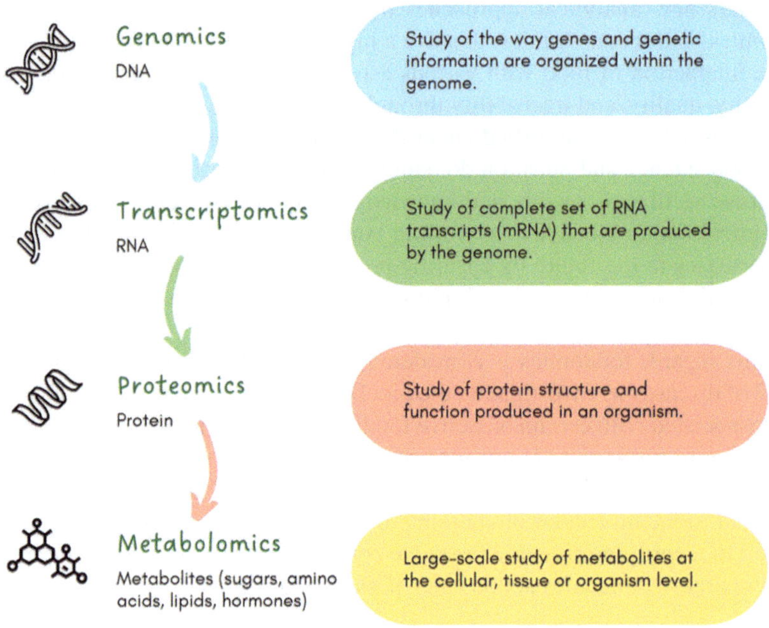

Fig. 6.2 Definition of omics technologies

6.2.2 Transcriptomics

Transcriptomics study covers the whole set of gene expressions, usually the full expression of mRNAs (Zheng and Chen 2014). The entire collection of RNA molecules in one organism is referred to as the transcriptome. Transfer (tRNA), ribosomal (rRNA), and messenger (mRNAs) RNA that code for proteins, and a variety of noncoding RNAs, including short (sRNAs), make up the majority of its RNAs. In transcriptomics, three essential approaches can be applied to identify and quantify changes in the transcriptome: microarrays, real-time RT-PCR, and next-generation RNA sequencing (Lamas et al. 2019). Meals' nutrients and other bioactive substances may regulate a number of processes involved in how genetic information is expressed. As a result, one of the primary objectives in foodomics research is to examine messenger RNA (mRNA) expression alterations brought on by bioactive food components. This is often the beginning of examining the various aspects of food's effects, from the genome to proteome and metabolome (García-Cañas et al. 2010). The use of transcriptomics allows researchers to measure the effects of harmful chemicals, toxic ingredients in food and nutritious foods on transcription. It is also found useful for determining the behavior of microbes under various environmental conditions (Ghahary and Abiri 2021).

6.2.3 Proteomics

In Proteomics, proteins are studied, particularly their structure and function and changes in the metabolism under different stress conditions. Proteomics is the next logical step after the development and success of genomics in understanding how cells function. It is the study of proteins that are encoded by the genome (the entire set of genetic information (DNA) in food is translated into a protein via transcription (mRNA)). Proteomics can complement genomics in a way that it cannot otherwise (Chandrasekhar et al. 2014). Proteomics is a powerful method of identifying and analyzing the composition of proteins (proteome) in plants to understand their function under certain time and environmental conditions. Identification, cataloging, and functional classification of gene products from cells, tissues, and organs are the main objectives of proteome profiling (or mapping). Proteins build or control every component of the cell, and the proteome's particular state determines the phenotype. Understanding phenotype is one of biology's primary objectives (Labuschagne 2018).

In proteomic analysis, four key steps are involved: (i) extraction of protein, (ii) separation and quantification of protein, (iii) identification of protein, and (iv) characterization (data analysis and interpretation) of protein. The analytical sample is employed as the source for the protein extraction (Gallardo et al. 2013). The separation of proteins can be done using two methods, a bottom-up proteomic method and the top-down proteomic method where the digestion stage is skipped and mass spectrometry is used to analyze the peptides from fragmented proteins (McLafferty et al. 2007). After this, proteins are quantified and identified using mass spectrometric methods such as MALDI-TOF MS, LC-MS, or MS/MS. Protein identification is done using MALDI-TOF MS, while identification, quantification, and characterization of protein can be done using LC-MS/MS or MS/MS. An analytical technique that is performed by using 2D electrophoresis and thereafter mass spectrometry in the digestion of protein in a gel is called peptide mass fingerprinting (Afzaal et al. 2022). Proteomics enables assessments of the proteomes in specific tissues of a plant at certain physiological and developmental phases on a qualitative, quantitative, and functional level. In qualitative proteomics, proteins in a food product are identified and characterized; this may involve all proteins or just a particular subset of proteins that are of interest. During quantitative proteomics, both relative quantitation and absolute quantitation are performed to determine the concentration of proteins in various samples. Comparatively, functional proteomics investigates how proteins interact with each other and with other molecules as well as the effects of these interactions (Geisslitz and Scherf 2021). Proteomics workflows are shown in Fig. 6.3.

Currently, consumers are interested in more than just the sensory attributes of food products; they demand safe, nutritious, minimally processed, and additive-free food (Saeed et al. 2021). Foods are identified by their proteins as indicators of their origin, properties, and processes. The use of proteomics is to study food components, the development of quick and accurate methods for the quantification and detection of adulterants and spoilage or pathogenic microorganisms, changes in

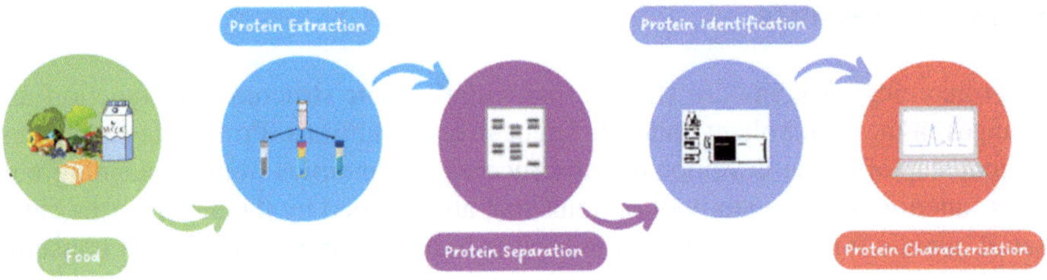

Fig. 6.3 A typical workflow in proteomics

food proteins as a result of food processing, rates of protein synthesis, degradation, and steady-state abundance, protein modification (e.g. post-translational modifications (PTMs) such as phosphorylation), protein movement across subcellular compartments, protein involvement in metabolic pathways, and protein interactions. By using multiple mass spectrometry techniques on food (tandem MS, LC-MS, and MALDI-TOF MS) (Ortea et al. 2016), in addition to proving the authenticity and safety of food products, proteomic analysis is integral to tracking the food product from raw to final product. The study performed in the area of proteomics to characterize or identify potential beneficial compounds in food matrixes can be observed in Table 6.1.

6.2.4 Metabolomics

Metabolism means the chemical reaction that is happening inside the system that includes anabolism and catabolism (synthetic reactions and degradation or breakdown reactions). All these chemical reactions produced different small molecules and these molecules form the metabolome. It includes peptides, lipids, starch, amino acids, fatty acids, organic acids, hormones, and vitamins called metabolites. Metabolomics, the study of the metabolome of a system, offers a systematic and comprehensive approach to determine, quantify, and identify food components influencing the characteristics of the final product. Metabolomics aims to investigate all endogenous or exogenous metabolites in a biological sample (cell, tissue, or organism) (Cubero-Leon et al. 2013; Rizo et al. 2020). To understand the metabolic activity status for genetic expression and genetic variation, a specific metabolomics profile must be able to recognize the interactions between the environmental agents and host molecules, such as proteins, lipids, deoxyribonucleic acid (DNA), ribonucleic acid (RNA), and other enzymes (Kettunen et al. 2013).

Metabolomics approach has had great success in solving a variety of issues, including food fraud or authenticity as well as biomedical, biological, nutritional, and agricultural sciences, such as disease diagnoses, drug discoveries, and plant phenomena (Pinu et al. 2019). There are two types of metabolomics approaches: untargeted and targeted. Untargeted metabolomics evaluates the total metabolite profile without knowing what kinds of compounds are responsible for changes in

Table 6.1 Applications of proteomics in food

Study	Food compound	Analyzed sample	Reference
To study the goat and ewe cheeses adulteration with cow milk.	Caseins	Cheese	Špoljarić et al. (2013)
To study the rapid detection of food adulterants using MALDI-TOF-MS on peptidomic and proteomic profiling.	Several milk proteins	Milk samples	Sassi et al. (2015)
To assess the origin of floral honey using proteomic approach.	Honey proteins	Honey	Girolamo et al. (2012)
A comparative study on proteomic analysis of two varieties of bean.	Grain proteome	GM and non-GM common bean	Balsamo et al. (2015)
The detection of gluten by MS using grain-specific peptide markers.	Gluten	Wheat, barley, rye, and oat flour	Fiedler et al. (2014)
Determination of authenticity in bread by peptide biomarkers.	Peptides	Bread: wheat, spelt, barley, maze, oat, and rye	Bönick et al. (2017)
To examine the presence of gluten in fermented vinegar and soy sauce.	Peptides and gluten proteins	Vinegar and soy sauce	Lia et al. (2018)
To study a comparison between modern and old varieties of wheat.	Gluten peptides	Modern and old *Triticum* varieties	Prandi et al. (2017)
Analysis using proteomics and suppression subtractive hybridization (Suppression Subtractive Hybridization (SSH)) of ALA-induced fruit coloring and proof of MdMADS1 and MADS-Box gene involvement.	5-aminolevulinic acid (ALA)	Apple	Feng et al. (2016)
Proteomic study of phytase in maize transgenic and non-transgenic seeds.	Proteins	Maize	Tan et al. (2017)
Analyses of transcriptomic, proteomic, and LC-MS data demonstrate anthocyanin biosynthesis during browning of the litchi pericarp.	Anthocyanin	Litchi pericarp	Qu et al. (2021)
Proteomic analysis reveals that the purple sweet potato's tuberous root anthocyanin buildup is caused by starch degradation.	Starch and anthocyanin	Purple and yellow sweet potato	Wang et al. (2016)

the system and that facilitate the new compounds discovery (Selamat et al. 2021). A complete scan with a high-resolution MS quantifies the metabolite, and tandem MS determines the metabolite's structure. Due to the untargeted nature of metabolite in food, it is possible to identify food fraud (Jia et al. 2020). Conversely, targeted metabolomics uses analytical methods with high accuracy, selectivity, and precision to identify and quantify the chemical characteristics of the metabolites in a sample under specific conditions. Once metabolites have been identified chemically,

Table 6.2 Comparison of untargeted and targeted metabolomics

Untargeted metabolomics	Targeted metabolomics
Global analysis of metabolic changes in response to disease, environment.	Predefined set of metabolites to quantify.
Typically carried out for hypothesis generation, followed by targeted profiling.	Typically carried out in diagnostics.
Enables discovery of unexpected new compounds in the sample.	Simpler data interpretation and analysis.
Technically challenging (both the analysis and the bioinformatics), risk of getting too many unknowns.	Limited compounds can be assessed.

biological information can be extracted from the collected data. Biochemical pathways, metabolic enzymes, and kinetics are utilized in this approach. Comparisons of consecutively targeted and untargeted approach are tabulated below (Table 6.2) (Selamat et al. 2021). However, because only a limited number of known substances may be examined, the application of targeted metabolomics in global metabolomics research is constrained.

Researchers have recently focused on the concept of pseudo targets, which combines the benefits of untargeted and targeted approaches. In pseudo targeted metabolomics large number of auto-MS/MS spectra are acquired from a pool of biological samples in the untargeted mode and as many targeted ion pairs as possible are measured in a biological sample in the targeted mode (Xu et al. 2020). Currently, MS and NMR are the two primary analytical techniques used in metabolomics. MS spectrometry technique uses high-resolution instruments designed to detect metabolites of either a nonpolar or a polar nature with high speed, sensitivity, and efficiency, while NMR spectroscopy offers a "holistic view" of metabolites, due to its ability to measure both micro- and macromolecules with minimal sample preparation under specified conditions (Li et al. 2021).

One of the main objectives of metabolomics studies is the identification of biomarkers. Biomarkers can be defined as compounds whose presence or abundance indicates the existence or disturbance of the metabolism or more specifically a metabolic pathway in a living organism (Cevallos-Cevallos and Reyes-De-Corcuera 2012). Effective statistical tools, such as multivariate analysis, are required to reduce the data complexity because untargeted metabolomics generates enormous datasets (Lacalle-Bergeron et al. 2021). The two types of untargeted analysis are fingerprinting and metabolite profiling. Fingerprinting involves the detection and statistical analysis of the results, without identifying and quantifying the compounds within the matrix. It is usually done on samples directly injected into the detector system, traditionally mass spectrometry (MS), whereas metabolite profiling enables the identification and quantification of each compound in a sample by using databases or software applications (Utpott et al. 2022). Metabolite profiling requires a separation of each metabolite prior to detection. Fingerprinting can be applied when the identity or characteristics of the compounds are not a priority. In food science, applications of metabolomics study the areas of food quality, safety, processing, and microbiology (Table 6.3).

Table 6.3 Applications of metabolomics in food

Study	Food compound	Analyzed sample	Reference
Metabolomic and proteomic approaches in investigating the impact of the drying process on nonvolatile compounds of white tea	Amino acids, flavonoids, nucleosides, nucleotides, peptides, and phenolic acids.	Tea	Chen et al. (2020)
Metabolomic modifications caused by the length of storage time of fresh-cut iceberg lettuce	Phenolic compounds, amino acids, lactones fatty acids, and lysophospholipids,	Iceberg lettuce	Garcia et al. (2016)
To study the lemon juice component profile affected by heat processing	Amino acids, organic acids, and carbohydrates (arabinose).	Lemon juice	Mabuchi et al. (2018)
To study the changes in milk during fermentation using metabolomics approach	Proteins, sugars (lactose, galactose), lactate, citrate, acetate, pyruvate, and alanine	Yoghurt	Trimigno et al. (2020)
To study the impact of various industrial and preprocessing techniques on tomato paste, puree, and pulp	Lycopene, flavonoids, phenylpropanoids, and lignans	Tomato products	Lucini et al. 2017)
To identify the metabolomic biomarkers in minor dairy animals and Holstein cow's milk	Metabolite profiles	Milk	Yang et al. (2015)
To study the relationship between technological properties of two dairy breeds' bovine milk with metabolite profile	Choline, carnitine, citrate, and lactose	Milk	Sundekilde et al. (2011)
Identification and measurement of the phytochemicals in watermelons	L-citrulline, glucose, fructose, and sucrose	Watermelon	Jayaprakasha and Patil (2016)
Comparative study using non-targeted metabolomics of normal and discolored red pepper	Carotenoids, metabolites	Red pepper	Feng et al. (2022)
Combined study of carotenoid metabolites and transcription to determine the molecular mechanism behind the coloration of zucchini fruit	Carotenoid metabolites	Zucchini peel	Xu et al. (2021)
Untargeted metabolomic analysis of capsicum species	Amino acids, sugars, and organic acids	Capsicum species	Aranha et al. (2017)

6.3 Foodomics for Health and Wellness

Foodomics technologies have already been used for the study of process development in food processing and essentially correspond to the quality and safety of raw and finished products. Nutrition intake plays a significant role in a person's health. Poor diet, use of tobacco, excessive alcohol consumption, and physical inactivity, are the main contributors to NCDs (noncommunicable diseases). These illnesses place a significant socioeconomic burden on society and cause close to 74% of all deaths worldwide (https://www.who.int/news-room/fact-sheets/detail/noncommunicable-diseases). Among the major goals of foodomics is the expansion of our understanding of how diet affects disease prevention. As a result, we can understand how food interacts with genes, proteins, and metabolites. This leads to the identification and development of molecular biomarkers that link diet to health. Following that, researchers could then also examine why different people react differently to food. It could potentially aid in the creation of individualized interventions.

Additionally, foodomics plays an important role in identifying potentially hazardous compounds within foods. Protein constituents and the byproducts of protein decomposition can cause food allergies, which have a significant negative impact on public health. In terms of allergen sources, some of the most significant ones are wheat, peanuts, milk, soya, fish, shellfish, eggs, and tree nuts. Traditional ELISA-based antigen–antibody/nucleic acid detection, mass spectrometry-based proteomics can detect food allergens effectively (Croote and Quake 2016).

Considering that foods are nowadays produced and distributed throughout the world, foodomics can also become useful for identifying adulterants and ensuring quality. Foodomics can aid both industry and inspection agencies to monitor and assess food authenticity to ensure food safety and stop the spread of food fraud. One study, for instance, identified the metabolic fingerprint of fruit juice using various analytical tools, such as mass spectrometry and chromatography (Dasenaki and Thomaidis 2019). Foodomics has an enormous potential to address new issues in the area of food science, as evidenced by the usage of both metabolomics and proteome profiling to distinguish conventional food from organic foods (Vallverdu-Queralt and Lamuela-Raventos 2016). Also researchers can use foodomics to aid the discovery of genes responsible for producing desirable metabolites and produce healthy foods.

6.4 Current Aspects and Future Trends

A decisive acceleration has been observed in the transition from mass production toward enhancing the nutritional value of food for the entire global population in the twenty-first century. Additionally, a steady shift is seen in nutrition research that has traditionally been concerned with feeding people enough food to sustain them, toward an understanding of diet as a creative tool to enhance or restore health. This increases the possibility to produce functional foods and nutraceuticals from plants, or their byproducts (Braconi et al. 2018). Human metabolome and digestive processes play a vital role in the relationship between nutrition and health. Therefore, finding biomarkers for food consumption and health status is crucial and NMR spectroscopy is a vital tool. Six subclasses for the classification of food biomarkers are proposed, based on their intended use: component intake biomarkers, compound intake biomarkers, impact biomarkers, compound status biomarkers, health or physiological state biomarkers, and dietary pattern biomarkers (Picone et al. 2022).

The complexity of food, the variety of nutrients and bioactive food components, their varying quantities, and a large number of potential targets present significant challenges for foodomics analysis. In this context, the analytical tools proteomics and metabolomics provide a strong analytical framework designed for the study of proteins and metabolites, along with transcriptomics. In the future, a key challenge will be understanding how certain diets, nutrients, and environmental factors affect the function of cells and organs. Using the differential response from these systems, logical intervention strategies can be developed to prevent diseases such as obesity, diabetes, inflammatory bowel diseases, and metabolic syndrome, or by modifying nutrition. Overall, foodomics has proven to be a great way to produce foods that contain biomolecules and help the development of high-quality foods based on science. To stay up with food innovations foodomics methodologies need to be improved, as well as promote the future development of food-based quality evaluation methods.

6.5 Conclusions

As the demand for healthier, minimally processed, and sustainable foods increases, foodomics leads the way in scientific advancement, providing tools for the design of balanced diets and the development of nutraceuticals made to individual genetic and metabolic profiles. This comprehensive approach to food science integrates advanced omics technologies to enhance our comprehension of the intricate interrelationships between food, nutrition, and health. The combination of genomics, transcriptomics, proteomics, and metabolomics within this interdisciplinary field facilitates not only the identification of bioactive compounds and the creation of functional foods but also advances personalized nutrition and disease prevention. Furthermore, foodomics plays a pivotal role in ensuring food safety, authenticity, and quality, addressing critical challenges such as food fraud and allergen detection. The convergence of omics technologies with food science marks the beginning of a new era where the promise of improved health through diet becomes a reality.

References

Afzaal M, Saeed F, Hussain M, Shahid F, Siddeeg A, Al-Farga A (2022) Proteomics as a promising biomarker in food authentication, quality and safety: a review. Food Sci Nutr 10:2333–2346. https://doi.org/10.1002/fsn3.2842

Álvarez-Rivera G, Valdés A, León C, Cifuentes A (2021) Foodomics: Omic strategies and applications in food science. RSC Publishing, London

Aranha BC, Hoffmann JF, Barbieri RL, Rombaldi CV, Chavesa FC (2017) Untargeted metabolomic analysis of Capsicum spp. by GC–MS. Phytochem Anal 28:439–447. https://doi.org/10.1002/pca.2692

Balsamo GM, Valentim-Neto PA, Mello CS, Arisi ACM (2015) Comparative proteomic analysis of two varieties of genetically modified (GM) Embrapa 5.1 common bean (Phaseolus vulgaris L.) and their non-GM counterparts. J Agric Food Chem 63:10569–10577. https://doi.org/10.1021/acs.jafc.5b04659

Bönick J, Huschek G, Rawel HM (2017) Determination of wheat, rye and spelt authenticity in bread by targeted peptide biomarkers. J Food Comp Analysis 58:82–91. https://doi.org/10.1016/j.jfca.2017.01.019

Braconi D, Bernardini G, Millucci L, Santucci A (2018) Foodomics for human health: current status and perspectives. Expert Rev Proteomics 15(2):153–164. https://doi.org/10.1080/14789450.2018.1421072

Casas-Agustench P, Andres-Lacueva C (2020) Principles of nutrigenetics and nutrigenomics. In: A broader view on omics and systems biology. https://doi.org/10.1016/B978-0-12-804572-5.00012-4

Cevallos-Cevallos JM, Reyes-De-Corcuera JI (2012) Metabolomics in food science. Adv Food Nutr Res 67:1–24. https://doi.org/10.1016/B978-0-12-394598-3.00001-0

Chandrasekhar K, Dileep A, Lebonah DE, Kumari JP (2014) A short review on proteomics and its applications. Int Lett Nat Sci 12(1):77–84. https://doi.org/10.18052/www.scipress.com/ILNS.17.77

Chen Q, Shi J, Mu B, Chen Z, Dai W, Lin Z (2020) Metabolomics combined with proteomics provides a novel interpretation of the changes in nonvolatile compounds during white tea processing. Food Chem 332:127412. https://doi.org/10.1016/j.foodchem.2020.127412

Cifuentes A (2009) Food analysis and foodomics. J Chromatography A 1216:7109–7110. https://doi.org/10.1016/j.chroma.2009.09.018

Cifuentes A (2013) Foodomics: advanced mass spectrometry in modern food science and nutrition. In: Foodomics: principles and applications. Wiley

Croote D, Quake SR (2016) Food allergen detection by mass spectrometry: the role of systems biology. Systems Biol Appl 2:16022. https://doi.org/10.1038/npjsba.2016.22

Cubero-Leon E, Peñalver R, Maquet A (2013) Review on metabolomics for food authentication. Food Res Int 60. https://doi.org/10.1016/j.foodres.2013.11.041

Dasenaki ME, Thomaidis NS (2019) Quality and authenticity control of fruit juices-a review. Molecules 24:1014. https://doi.org/10.3390/molecules24061014

Feng X, An Y, Zheng J, Sun M, Wang L (2016) Proteomics and Suppression Subtractive Hybridization (SSH) analyses of ALA-promoted fruit coloration and evidence for the involvement of a MADS-box gene, MdMADS1. Front Plant Sci 7:1615. https://doi.org/10.3389/fpls.2016.01615

Feng X, Yu Q, Li B, Kan J (2022) Comparative analysis of carotenoids and metabolite characteristics in discolored red pepper and normal red pepper based on non-targeted metabolomics. LWT Food Sci Tech 153:112398. https://doi.org/10.1016/j.lwt.2021.112398

Fiedler KL, McGrath SC, Callahan JH, Ross MM (2014) Characterization of grain-specific peptide markers for the detection of gluten by mass spectrometry. J Agric Food Chem 62(25):5835–5844. https://doi.org/10.1021/jf500997j

Gallardo JM, Ortea I, Carrera M (2013) Proteomics and its applications for food authentication and food-technology research. Trends Analytical Chem 52:135–141. https://doi.org/10.1016/j.trac.2013.05.019

García-Cañas V, Simó C, León C, Cifuentes A (2010) Advances in nutrigenomics research: novel and future analytical approaches to investigate the biological activity of natural compounds and food functions. J Pharma Biomed Anal 51:290–304. https://doi.org/10.1016/j.jpba.2009.04.019

Garcia-Cañas V, Simó C, Herrero M, Ibañez E, Cifuentes A (2012) OMICs technologies: tools for food science. CRC Press, New York

Garcia CJ, García-Villalba R, Garrido Y, Gil MI, Tomás-Barberán FA (2016) Untargeted metabolomics approach using UPLC-ESI-QTOF-MS to explore the metabolome of fresh-cut iceberg lettuce. Metabolomics 12(8):138. https://doi.org/10.1007/s11306-016-1082-x

Geisslitz S, Scherf KA (2021) Comprehensive foodomics, vol 1. Academic, pp 699–717. https://doi.org/10.1016/B978-0-08-100596-5.22762-5

Ghahary A, Abiri R (2021) Foodomics; principles, challenges, and applications - a promising tool for food analysis. Acta Sci Nutr Health 5(3):01–05

Girolamo FD, D'Amato A, Righetti PG (2012) Assessment of the floral origin of honey via proteomic tools. J Proteome 75:3688–3693. https://doi.org/10.1016/j.jprot.2012.04.029

Jayaprakasha GK, Patil BS (2016) A metabolomics approach to identify and quantify the phytochemicals in watermelons by quantitative HNMR. Talanta 153:268–277. https://doi.org/10.1016/j.talanta.2016.02.060

Jia W, Dong X, Shi L, Chu X (2020) Discrimination of Milk from different animal species by a foodomics approach based on high-resolution mass spectrometry. J Agric Food Chem 68(24):6638–6645. https://doi.org/10.1021/acs.jafc.0c02222

Kettunen J, Tukiainen T, Sarin AP, Alonso AO, Tikkanen E, Lyytikäinen LP, Kangas AJ, Soininen P, Würtz P, Silander K, Dick DM, Rose RJ, Savolainen MJ, Viikari J, Kähönen M, Lehtimäki T, Pietiläinen KH, Inouye M, McCarthy MI, Jula A, Eriksson J, Raitakari OT, Salomaa V, Kaprio J, Järvelin MR, Peltonen L, Perola M, Freimer NB, Korpela MA, Palotie A, Ripatti S (2013) Genome-wide association study identifies multiple loci influencing human serum metabolite levels. Nat Genet 44(3):269–276. https://doi.org/10.1038/ng.1073

Labuschagne MT (2018) A review of cereal grain proteomics and its potential for sorghum improvement. J Cereal Sci 84:151–158. https://doi.org/10.1016/j.jcs.2018.10.010

Lacalle-Bergeron L, Izquierdo-Sandoval D, Sancho JV, López FJ, Hernández F, Portolés T (2021) Chromatography hyphenated to high resolution mass spectrometry in untargeted metabolomics for investigation of food (bio)markers. TrAC Trends Anal Chem 135:116161. https://doi.org/10.1016/j.trac.2020.116161

Lamas A, Regal P, Vázquez B, Miranda JM, Franco CM, Cepeda A (2019) Transcriptomics: a powerful tool to evaluate the behavior of foodborne pathogens in the food production chain. Food Res Int 125:108543. https://doi.org/10.1016/j.foodres.2019.108543

Li S, Tian Y, Jiang P, Lin Y, Liu X, Yang H (2021) Recent advances in the application of metabolomics for food safety control and food quality analyses. Critic Rev Food Sci Nutri 61(9):1448–1469. https://doi.org/10.1080/10408398.2020.1761287

Lia H, Byrne K, Galiamov R, Mendoza-Porras O, Bose U, Howitt CA, Colgrave ML (2018) Using LC-MS to examine the fermented food products vinegar and soy sauce for the presence of gluten. Food Chem 254:302–308. https://doi.org/10.1016/j.foodchem.2018.02.023

Lucini L, Rocchetti G, Kane D, Trevisan M (2017) Phenolic fingerprint allows discriminating processed tomato products and tracing different processing sites. Food Control 73:696–703. https://doi.org/10.1016/j.foodcont.2016.09.020

Mabuchi R, Zhao H, Tanimoto S (2018) Effect of heat processing on the constituent profile of lemon juice. Jpn Soc Food Sci Technol 65(4):183–191. https://doi.org/10.3136/nskkk.65.183

McLafferty FW, Breuker K, Jin M, Han X, Infusini G, Jiang H, Kong X, Begley TP (2007) Top-down MS, a powerful complement to the high capabilities of proteolysis proteomics. FEBS J 274:6256–6268. https://doi.org/10.1111/j.1742-4658.2007.06147.x

Ortea I, O'Connor G, Maquet A (2016) Review on proteomics for food authentication. J Proteome 147:212–225. https://doi.org/10.1016/j.jprot.2016.06.033

Picone G, Mengucci C, Capozzi F (2022) The NMR added value to the green foodomics perspective: advances by machine learning to the holistic view on food and nutrition. Magn Reson Chem 60:590–596. https://doi.org/10.1002/mrc.5257

Pinu FR, Goldansaz SA, Jaine J (2019) Translational metabolomics: current challenges and future opportunities. Meta 9. https://doi.org/10.3390/metabo9060108
Prandi B, Tedeschi T, Folloni S, Galaverna G, Sforza S (2017) Peptides from gluten digestion: a comparison between old and modern wheat varieties. Food Res Int 91:92–102. https://doi.org/10.1016/j.foodres.2016.11.034
Qu S, Li M, Wang G, Yu W, Zhu S (2021) Transcriptomic, proteomic and LC–MS analyses reveal anthocyanin biosynthesis during litchi pericarp browning. Sci Hortic 189:110443. https://doi.org/10.1016/j.scienta.2021.110443
Rizo J, Guillén D, Farrés A, Díaz-Ruiz G, Sánchez S, Wacher C, Rodríguez-Sanoja R (2020) Omics in traditional vegetable fermented foods and beverages. Critic Rev Food Sci Nutri 60(5):791–809. https://doi.org/10.1080/10408398.2018.1551189
Saeed F, Afzaal M, Hussain M, Tufail T (2021) Food losses, sustainable postharvest and food technologies. Academic, pp 191–218. https://doi.org/10.1016/B978-0-12-821912-6.00003-1
Sassi M, Arena S, Scaloni A (2015) MALDI-TOF-MS platform for integrated proteomic and Peptidomic profiling of Milk samples allows rapid detection of food adulterations. J Agric Food Chem 63:6157–6171. https://doi.org/10.1021/acs.jafc.5b02384
Selamat J, Rozani NAA, Murugesu S (2021) Application of the metabolomics approach in food authentication. Molecules 26:7565. https://doi.org/10.3390/molecules26247565
Špoljarić J, Mikulec N, Plavljanić D, Radeljević B, Havranek J, Antunac N (2013) Proving the adulteration of ewe and goat cheeses with cow milk using the reference method of isoelectric focusing of γ-casein. Mljekarstvo 63(3):115–121
Sundekilde UK, Frederiksen PD, Clausen MR, Larsen LB, Bertram HC (2011) Relationship between the metabolite profile and technological properties of bovine milk from two dairy breeds elucidated by NMR-based metabolomics. J Agric Food Chem 59:7360–7367. https://doi.org/10.1021/jf202057x
Tan Y, Tong Z, Yang Q, Sun Y, Jin X, Peng C, Guo A, Wang X (2017) Proteomic analysis of phytase transgenic and non-transgenic maize seeds. Sci Rep 7(1):1–11. https://doi.org/10.1038/s41598-017-09557-8
Trimigno A, Bøge Lyndgaard C, Atladóttir GA, Aru V, Balling Engelsen S, Harder Clemmensen LK (2020) An NMR metabolomics approach to investigate factors affecting the yoghurt fermentation process and quality. Meta 10(7):293. https://doi.org/10.3390/metabo10070293
Utpott M, Rodrigues E, Oliveira Rios A, Mercali GD, Flôres SH (2022) Metabolomics: an analytical technique for food processing evaluation. Food Chem 366:130685
Vallverdu-Queralt A, Lamuela-Raventos RM (2016) Foodomics: a new tool to differentiate between organic and conventional foods. Electrophoresis 37:1784–1794. https://doi.org/10.1002/elps.201500348
Wang S, Pan D, Lv X, Song X, Qiu Z, Huang C, Huang R, Chen W (2016) Proteomic approach reveals that starch degradation contributes to anthocyanin accumulation in tuberous root of purple sweet potato. J Proteome 143:298–305. https://doi.org/10.1016/j.jprot.2016.03.010
World Health Organization (WHO) Newsroom Non-communicable diseases. https://www.who.int/news-room/fact-sheets/detail/noncommunicable-diseases
Xu L, Xu Z, Wang X, Wang B, Liao X (2020) The application of pseudotargeted metabolomics method for fruit juices discrimination. Food Chem 316:126278. https://doi.org/10.1016/j.foodchem.2020.126278
Xu X, Lu X, Tang Z, Zhang X, Lei F, Hou L, Li M (2021) Combined analysis of carotenoid metabolites and the transcriptome to reveal the molecular mechanism underlying fruit colouration in zucchini (Cucurbita pepo L.). Food Chem Mol Sci 2:100021. https://doi.org/10.1016/j.fochms.2021.100021
Yang Y, Zheng N, Zhao X, Zhang Y, Han R, Yang J, Zhao S, Li S, Guo T, Zang C (2015) Metabolomic biomarkers identify differences in milk produced by Holstein cows and other minor dairy animals. J Proteome 136:174–182. https://doi.org/10.1016/j.jprot.2015.12.031
Zheng C, Chen A (2014) System biological research on food quality for personalised nutrition and health using foodomics techniques: a review. J Food Nutri Res 2(9):608–616. https://doi.org/10.12691/jfnr-2-9-13

Nutraceuticals: Nutritionally Functional Foods

7

Manoj S. Aroor, Tanvi Phull, and Mahesh Gupta

Abstract

Nutraceuticals and functional foods are popular topics in the current day, owing to consumer knowledge of the health-beneficial aspects of foods. Nutraceuticals are food items or parts of foods that include bioactive chemicals in the form of tablets or capsules, such as vitamin supplements, fish oil, and plant extracts that aid in the prevention or reduction of serious illnesses. Berries, asparagus, broccoli, and nuts are examples of functional foods that include bioactive chemicals in their food matrixes. Fruits and vegetables contain several bioactive chemicals, such as phenolic acids and flavonoids, which have anticancer and anti-inflammatory properties. Cereals, grains, legumes, and spices have secondary plant metabolites, which have health-beneficial characteristics. *Lactobacillus* species are prevalent in dairy products such as yoghurt and fermented milk, which contribute to maintaining gut health. Ayurveda, an ancient Indian medicinal system, has stated the health benefits of several plants and spices. Algae contain long-chain fatty acids like PUFA and polysaccharides and can be explored for future functional foods.

Keywords

Nutraceuticals · Functional foods · Fruits and vegetables · Dairy products

M. S. Aroor · T. Phull · M. Gupta (✉)
Food and Nutraceutical Laboratory, Dietetics and Nutrition Technology Division, CSIR-Institute of Himalayan Bioresource Technology, Palampur, Himachal Pradesh, India
e-mail: mgupta@ihbt.res.in

A. Kumar et al. (eds.), *Innovations in Ayurvedic Nutrition*,
https://doi.org/10.1007/978-981-95-1213-3_7

7.1 Introduction

"No disease that can be treated by diet should be treated with any other means", wrote the twelfth century philosopher Maimonides, which still holds true today. In the last decade, there has been a significant increase on interest in nutraceuticals and functional foods that fulfill basic nutritional requirements as well as provide additional health advantages and may be a superior alternative to contemporary medicine (Santini 2022). The subject of functional foods is the result of the fusion of two significant occurrences in our lives, food and health. The foundation of preventative nutrition is the well-accepted link between diet and illness. The idea of "nutraceuticals and functional foods" is frequently mentioned as a recently developing area. The idea to create functional meals is in line with the eastern notion that "medicine and food have a shared genesis" (Henry 2010). However, the earliest log, "*Ebers Papyrus*", an Egyptian traditional medical record from 2900 BC, comprises 700 plant-derived medicines (Prasathkumar et al. 2021). The Atharvaveda, the finest organized traditional health care system still in use today with preventatives and treatments as essential aspects, marks the beginning of Indian medicine, roughly in 6000 BC. The earliest known Hindu writings that record the precise categorization, pharmacology, and medicinal characteristics of over 700 plants are the Charak Samhita and Sushrut Samhita (100–500 BC) (Saggar et al. 2022). Ayurvedic herbal compounds such as reserpine, embelin, azadirachtin, and curcumin have gone on to become medications or nutraceuticals (Patwardhan 2005).

Although functional foods have been described several times, no universally agreed-upon definition exists for this concept. Additionally, there is no scientific consensus on how to differentiate between functional foods, nutraceuticals, and dietary supplements (Damián et al. 2022). The Japanese government is credited with introducing the phrase "functional food" in 1991. It describes a diet that has been fortified with additional nutrients such as proteins, dietary fiber, probiotics, vitamins, or other food additives that improve human health and wellness (Min et al. 2019). Stephen De Felice is credited with coining the phrase "nutraceutical" that he defines as "food or a component of food that delivers medical or health advantages, including the prevention and/or treatment of a disease" (DeFelice 1995). Because of the significant growth in the consumption of nutraceuticals and functional foods, there has been an upsurge in research interests on functional foods. Figure 7.1 indicates the number of publications related to nutraceuticals and functional foods from 2005 to 2023. Consumption of plant-based food items, such as fruits, vegetables, nuts, whole grains, and cereals as well as marine foods with their long-chain fatty acids, is widely established to help promote health and lower the risk of diseases (Shahidi 2009). Glucosinolates, sulfur-containing molecules like allicin, allyl isothiocyanates, which are found in *Allium* species, terpenoids like phytosterols, carotenoids, monoterpenes, and various phenolic compounds like anthocyanins, flavones, isoflavones, and stilbenoids are examples of phytochemicals found in fruits and vegetables that have been associated with health benefits (Gul et al. 2016; Kumari et al. 2021). Some of the secondary metabolites like quercetin a flavonoid widely present in fruits and vegetables, are noted for their

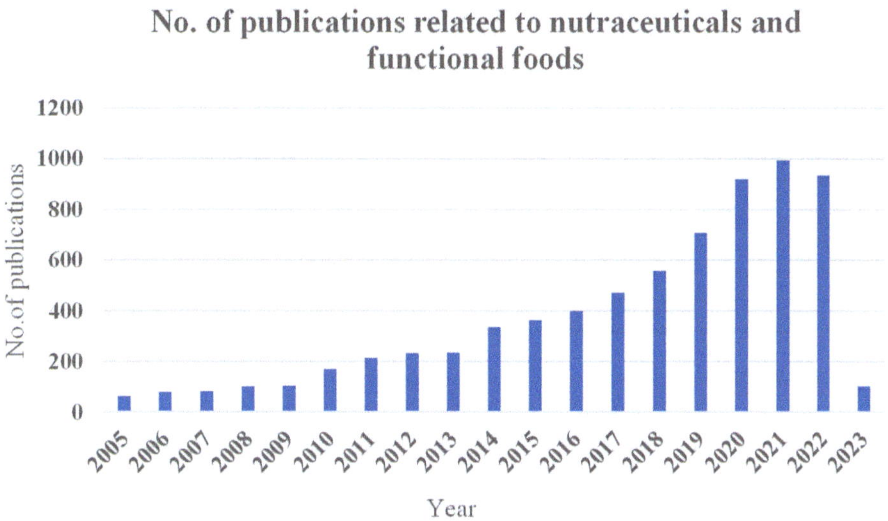

Fig. 7.1 Number of publications related to nutraceuticals and functional foods

anti-inflammatory, anti-microbial, antiviral, and antioxidant properties (Di Petrillo et al. 2022). Resveratrol is a compound that naturally occurs in many fruits, including blueberries, peanuts, grapes, and beverages made from them like red wine is reported to prevent a wide variety of disorders like cardiovascular diseases (CVDs), various kinds of cancers, liver diseases, diabetes mellitus, obesity, cancer, neurological diseases like Alzheimer's disease, and Parkinson's disease (Meng et al. 2020).

Probiotics are live microorganisms and can be classified into functional foods or nutraceuticals. If the probiotics are present in the food matrix, they will be considered functional foods; if they are present in the form of a pill or a capsule, they are considered as nutraceuticals (Zeisel 1999). Probiotics are thought to be one of the primary mechanisms causing positive effects. It has been demonstrated that the host's ability to get energy depends critically on the activity of the gut microbiota. Therefore, adding living microorganisms to the diet, like probiotics, aids in regulating the gut microbiota (Damián et al. 2022). Approximately there are 10^{10}–10^{12} live microorganisms per gram in the human colon according to the previous literature (Collins and Reid 2016). *Lactobacillus reuteri* is a well-known probiotic agent and one of the few indigenous *Lactobacillus* species present in the human gut. It is the most common *Lactobacillus* species found in mammals. A few yeasts, such as *Saccharomyces cerevisiae* and *Saccharomyces boulardii*, may also exhibit probiotic properties (Figueroa-González et al. 2011). Probiotic bacteria can also produce vitamins, immunomodulatory proteins, and a variety of peptides with inhibitory properties, which are of a huge benefit to human health (Spinler et al. 2008). Prebiotics are a class of compounds that the gut microbes break down. The interest in their connection to general human health has grown in the last decade. They can nourish the gut flora as they degrade short-chain fatty acids that are released into the bloodstream, impacting the gastrointestinal tracts and other major organs. The two

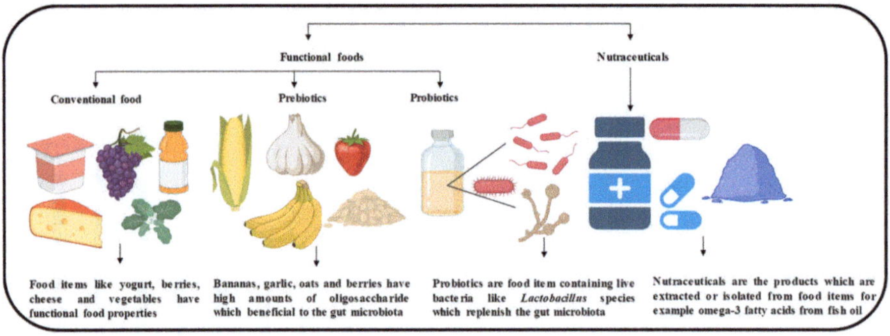

Fig. 7.2 Classification of nutraceuticals and functional foods

significant prebiotic subgroups having positive effects on human health are fructo-oligosaccharides and galacto-oligosaccharides (Davani-Davari et al. 2019). The classification of functional foods and nutraceuticals is depicted in Fig. 7.2. This chapter's primary focus is on functional foods and nutraceuticals. It intends to give more contemporary scientific and technological insights into fortified food products. In addition, an overview of traditional Indian medicine systems like Ayurveda and future functional foods has been discussed.

7.2 Functional Foods

7.2.1 Fruits and Vegetables

Fruits, vegetables, and nuts are part of the human diet since prehistoric times even before the advent of agriculture. These food items provide basic nutritional requirements along with health-beneficial properties. These properties are mostly attributable to secondary metabolites found in fruits and vegetables (Yahia et al. 2019). These secondary metabolites can be roughly divided into proanthocyanidins, phenolic acids, stilbenes, lignans, and flavonoids. Phenolic acids, commonly found in fruits and vegetables, are reported to have anti-inflammatory activity in humans, which is supported by a significant reduction in pro-inflammatory markers like cytokine and interleukins. The antioxidant property of phenolic acids is attributed to their chemical structure that can quench free radicals produced during oxidative stress. Similarly, flavonoids like rutin, hesperidin, and naringin are known to have cardioprotective properties and anticarcinogenic activity (Maleki et al. 2019). Around the world, cardiovascular disease (CVD) has been a leading cause of mortality. There is a lot of data to support the idea that the nutrients found in fruits and vegetables reduce the risk of CVD. Vegetables and fruits with pectin and fiber and nuts can reduce blood lipid levels in people by preventing the production of cholesterol and reducing the absorption of fat. Preclinical studies show strong evidence for polyphenols having prebiotic properties. Pomegranate juice is a rich source of polyphenols with a high potential for antioxidant activity. Additionally, human investigations have demonstrated its antiatherogenic, antihypertensive, and anti-inflammatory properties. Clinical and preclinical research, as well as epidemiological data, indicate that the flavanones found in the citrus genus have a favorable effect on cardiometabolic parameters and lower the risk of cardiovascular disease. (Asgary et al. 2018) The detailed bioactive properties of different fruits, vegetables and nuts are mentioned in Table 7.1.

Table 7.1 Biological effects of fruits, vegetables, and nuts

Food items	Functional compounds	Biological effects	References
Fruits			
Apple (*Malus domestica* and *Malus baccata*)	Phloretins and chlorogenic acids	Antioxidant effects, anti-inflammatory effects, and cytotoxic and apoptotic effects on cancer cell lines.	Behzad et al. (2017)
Blueberry (*Vaccinium* species)	Malvidin, chlorogenic acids, quercetin, and glycosides	Antioxidant effects, hepatoprotective effects, and prevents prediabetic progression.	Nunes et al. (2021), Stevenson and Scalzo (2012)
Cherry (*Prunus padus* and *Prunus serotina)*	Cyanidin-3-glucoside, coumaric acid, and chlorogenic acid	Antidiabetic effects and cardioprotective.	Telichowska et al. (2020)
Orange *Citrus sinensis, citrus reticulate*, and *Citrus maxima*	Hesperetin, naringin, and tangeritin	Antihypertensive, cardioprotective, and antioxidant.	Chhikara et al. (2018), Dadwal et al. (2022)
Vegetables			
Asparagus (*asparagus officinali)*	Rutin, quercetin, and anthocyanins	Antitumor, antioxidant, immunomodulatory, hypoglycaemic and anti-hypertensive activity.	Guo et al. (2020)
Broccoli (*Brassica oleracea var. italica*)	Kaempferol and glucosinolates	Immunity modulation, bone health, and antimicrobial and antioxidant properties.	Nagraj et al. (2020)
Celery (*Apium graveolens*),	Apigenin, caffeic acid, and dietary fibers	Antitumor, antioxidant	Al Aboody (2021)
Onion (*Allium cepa*)	Quercetin and thiosulfates	Antitumor, antioxidant, and antimicrobial activity.	Kumar et al. (2022)
Nuts			
Walnuts (*Juglans* species)	Polymeric procyanidins, oleanic and pomolic acids	Improves glycaemic status in subjects with type-2 diabetes mellitus.	Wojdyło et al. (2022)
Hazelnuts (*Corylus* species)	α-Tocopherol, Pomolic acids	Inhibitory effect against intestinal α-glucosidase.	Wojdyło et al. (2022)

7.2.2 Cereal Grains, Legumes, and Spices

Commonly consumed cereal grains including wheat, maize, oats, and barley consist of a class of dietary fiber-phenolic compounds with ester linkages that can be fractioned by the fermentation process, to release the bound phenolic acids like ferulic acid, thereby enhancing therapeutic values, including several beneficial physiological effects on the gut (Capozzi et al. 2012; Vitaglione et al. 2008). Fermentation of wheat bran fiber can be an effective method for inculcating the merits of probiotics and prebiotics (Katina et al. 2007). Rice protein is hypoallergenic with a good quantity of lysine and may be a suitable ingredient for infant food formulations (Das et al. 2012). Diabetes mellitus, one of today's main illnesses, can be managed through the concept of food functionality. Whole grains (rye, oats, barley, and wheat) offer antidiabetic properties as they contain non-digestible complex polysaccharides such as total dietary fibers, inulin, β-glucan, and resistant starches, which have potential prebiotic effects (Ballali and Lanciai 2012). Prebiotics are non-digestible components, which positively impact their host by stimulating bacterial growth, count, and thriving the gut and enhancing consumer wellness, these compounds are present in cereal grains and legumes. Soy, a popular source of protein also constitutes polyunsaturated fats, fibers, minerals, and vitamins. Flavones in soy interact with estrogen receptors, primarily interacting with α and β- forms, and therefore largely responsible for soybean's antidiabetic benefits. The estrogen α receptor is an important regulator of glucose and lipid metabolism, with additional functions like insulin production, secretion, and β-cell survival. Cinnamaldehyde and its *trans* isomer, a chemical compound typically identified in cinnamon, might help prevent diabetes (Sikand et al. 2015). The detailed bioactive properties of different spices and grains are mentioned in Table 7.2.

7.3 Dairy-Based Products

7.3.1 Fermented Dairy Products

Probiotic food items have stimulated the consumer market due to scientific indications relative to the positive health impact brought on by them. A probiotic is a dietary supplement made of living microbial organisms, which improves health by influencing the intestinal system. The majority of probiotics are members of a bacterial group that produces lactic acid as the major end product (LAB bacteria), usually present in products such as yoghurt, fermented milk, and other fermented foods (Fazilah et al. 2018). The nutritional value of many foods is often increased by fermentation procedures that also boost the nutrient bioavailability. The most commonly employed LAB strains for fermenting milk comprise *Streptococcusphilus* species, coupled with *Bifidobacteri* species (*Bifidobacterium breve, Bifidobacterium lactis, Bifidobacterium longum*, and *Bifidobacterium animalis),* or with *Lactobacilli* (*Lactobacillus acidophilus, Lactobacillus rhamnosus, Lactobacillus johnsonii*, and *Lactobacillus casei*) (Granier et al. 2013), which are usually considered "Generally

Table 7.2 Biological effects of spices, cereals, and legumes

Food items	Functional compounds	Biological effects	References
Spices			
Black pepper *(Piper nigrum)*	α-pinene, camphene, sabinene, β-pinene, limonene, and caryophyllene	Antibacterial, antispasmodic, antiasthmatic, antitumor, and hepatoprotective	Li et al. (2007)
Long pepper *(Piper longum)*	Piperine, piplartine, piper longumine, and dihydro-stigmasterol	Anti-inflammatory, antitussive rheumatoid, antifungal, antimicrobial, antidiabetic, and hepatoprotective	Yende et al. (2010)
Ginger *(Zingiber officinale)*	Zingiberol, zingiberene, phellandrene, and linalool and gingerol (diarylheptanoids)	Hypolipidemic, antiemetic, chemoprotective, antiviral, and antiulcerogenic	Kikuzaki et al. (1991)
Cereals			
Finger millet *(Eleusine coracana)*	Arabinoxylans, coumaric acid, and sinapic acid	Antioxidant, antiobesity, antidiabetic, Anticarcinogenic, and antiviral	Himanshu et al. (2018)
Buckwheat *(Fagopyrum esculentum* and *Fagopyrum tartaricum)*	Protocatechuicand syringic acids, caffeic acid, rutin, quercetin, and quercitrin	Antioxidant, anti-inflammatory, antihaemorrhagic, and vasculoprotector	Martín-García et al. (2019)
Quinoa *(Chenopodium quinoa)*	Gallic acid, protocatechuic, and cinnamic acids	Anti-inflammatory, anticancer, and antiviral	Shahbaz et al. (2022), Al-Qabba et al. (2020)
Chia (*Salvia hispanica)*	Fiber and ω-3 fatty acids	Antiobesity, anticancerous, and antidiabetic	Shahbaz et al. (2022)
Legumes			
Lentil *(Lens culinaris)*	Lectins, phytates, and oligosaccharides	Anticarcinogenic, and anti-hyperglycemic	Shahwar et al. (2017)
Chickpea *(Cicer arietinum)*	Sterols, tocopherols, and toco-trienols	Anti-ulcerative, anti-bacterial, anti-fungal, antitumor, and anti-inflammatory	Akihisa et al. (2000)
Pigeon pea *(Cajanus cajan)*	Dietary fiber and folate	Vasodilator and anticholesteremic	Gai et al. (2021)

Recognized as Safe" (GRAS) by the respective regulatory organizations. Although different LAB creates various fermentation products, they all share the characteristic feature of being alive in the product and having the ability to engage with the gut microflora at the time of intestinal transit (Granier et al. 2013). In addition, antinutritional components may be eliminated from milk through the fermentative activity of certain LAB species for preventing lactose intolerance and buildup (Shiby and

Mishra 2013). During the fermentation process of milk, *Lactobacillus helveticus* synthesizes the bioactive peptides that can be utilized to control other bacterial infections due to its antibacterial and immune-stimulating qualities (Matar et al. 2001). The major types of fermented milk include yoghurt, kefir, and kumis, with minor and regional numbers of other products (Fox 2011). The main approaches for incorporating probiotic microorganisms into foods are still done using yoghurt and fermented milk, with several novel approaches entering global market, including dairy-based desserts and products, dried functional powders, for newborns, in capsules to be consumed directly or powder forms that are to be reconstituted first (Granato et al. 2010).

7.3.2 Yoghurt

Yoghurt is available in a range of flavors (natural, fruit, and cereal), textures (flowable, set, smooth) and fat contents (extravagance, low-fat, practically fat-free) traditionally produced by fermenting milk with lactic acid either naturally or artificially. It can assist digestion, increase immunity, relieve diarrhea, and protect against cancer (Fazilah et al. 2018) as yoghurt is claimed to be more nutritious than milk since it contains more protein, calcium, vitamin B2, B6, and B12. Yoghurt with added probiotics, in comparison to regular yoghurt comprising *Lactobacillus acidophilus* and *Bifidobacterium lactis,* significantly lowers serum cholesterol levels (Ataie-Jafari et al. 2009). Yoghurt consumption has also been linked to reduced risks of hip fracture, bone wearing and boosting bone mass density (Bian et al. 2018). Moreover, yoghurt has demonstrated control of tumor growth by lowering the response of inflammation by up surging the count of cells that secrete IL-10, the process of apoptosis and decreasing procarcinogenic enzymes (De LeBlanc and Perdigón 2010).

7.3.3 Kefir

Kefir is produced from the fermentation of milk by kefir grains and milk along with a yeast population rendering it with health benefits such as immunomodulatory, anti-allergen, cholesterol-lowering, angiotensin-converting enzyme (ACE) inhibition, wound healing, anticarcinogenic, gastrointestinal with antimicrobial activities, majorly due to the presence of marker metabolites like kefiran and exopolysaccharides (Bourrie et al. 2016). The bioactive peptides in kefir promote phagocytosis, nitric oxide (NO) generation, and macrophage activation (Sharifi et al. 2017). Milk, fermented using kefir functions equivalent to some of the well-known antibiotics such as ampicillin, amoxicillin, azithromycin, ceftriaxone, and cetoconazol. In an animal model, kefir or kefiran ingestion increased the population of useful bacteria, primarily *Lactobacillus* and *Bifidobacterium*, while decreasing the number of pathogenic microbial species like *Clostridium perfringens.* Kefir intake has proven to lessen the effect of infection caused by *Giardia intestinalis* in mice due to immune system regulation (Bourrie et al. 2016). Kefir inhibits cell proliferation in a time and dose-dependent manner, by inducing apoptosis in tumor cells, without damaging healthy cells in individuals with leukemia patients (Rafie et al. 2015). Patients with osteoporosis who consume kefir have also been linked to exhibit improved bone health and short-term alterations in bone turnover indices (Tu et al. 2015).

7.3.4 Koumis

Koumis is a naturally fermented, acidic-alcoholic, dairy beverage from the Mediterranean region (Meybodi et al. 2021). Both lactic acid bacteria (LAB) and yeast species have been employed in the acidification process, along with species including *L. casei*, *L. helveticus*, and *L. plantarum* having a particular dominance among the *lactobacilli* species. However, these have been found less frequently than *Lactobacillus fermentum*, *Lactobacillus coryniformis*, *L. paracasei*, *L. kefiranofaciens*, and others (Hati et al. 2019). In addition to vitamins A, B2, B5, B12, and E; koumis also includes significant amounts of vitamin C, linoleic and linolenic acids, and bacteriocins (Orlandi et al. 2003). Koumis has been demonstrated to aid in the treatment of cardiovascular disease, tuberculosis and diarrhea nourishing the arteries, relieving depression, and aiding digestion. Furthermore, probiotics from Koumis are believed to decrease tumor growth by enhancing the immune system and reducing the generation of cancer-causing substances (Leite et al. 2013). Regular intake of koumis lowers blood cholesterol levels and regulates the production of blood lipids.

7.3.5 Cheese

Cheese can be defined as a food item whose whey to casein ratio is lesser than that of milk. The starter cultures of healthy bacteria, added to the cheese, produce lactic acid along with the typical flavor and aroma, in addition to appropriate enzymes. It has been found that cheese promotes muscle growth, lowers blood pressure, and LDL cholesterol, and is beneficial against obesity, diabetes, cancer, and tooth decay (Tunick and Van Hekken 2015). Bioactive compounds that provide health benefits in functional foods and nutraceuticals are shown in Fig. 7.3.

7.4 Meat-Based Products

Meat supplies well-balanced necessary amino acids, specifically sulfated amino acids like cysteine and methionine as it offers an ample supply of proteins with great biological significance (Stadnik and Kęska 2015). Meat provides bioactive metabolites like carnosine, anserine, L-carnitine, conjugated linoleic acid, glutathione, taurine, creatine, iron, zinc, and B-vitamins that have already been investigated for their physiological properties. Conjugated linoleic acid (CLA) is a fatty acid extracted from grilled beef and has been reported to show anticarcinogenic, antioxidant, and immunomodulatory capabilities (Jiménez-Colmenero et al. 2001).

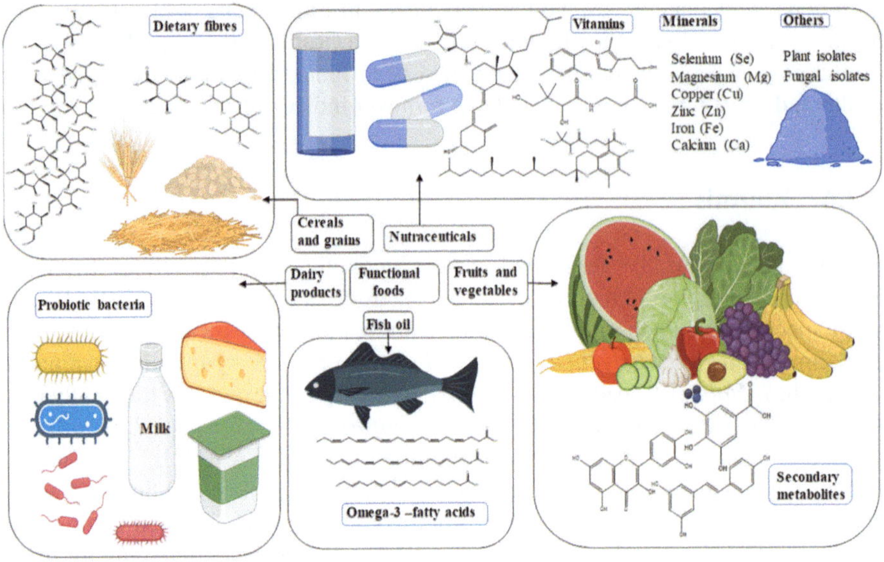

Fig. 7.3 The bioactive compounds present in nutraceuticals and functional foods

7.4.1 Meat as Probiotic

Lactobacillus lactis and *Lactobacillus plantarum* are two possible probiotics having applications in fermented meat products and are mainly extracted from fresh, cooked, and fermented meat and its products (Moreno et al. 2018). Additionally, the strains of *Staphylococcus* species are the proposed probiotics from the fermented meat produced in India (Borah et al. 2016). Recent developments in scientific studies have proven that meat can be a potent probiotic as after three days of intake of fermented sausage, containing *Lacticaseibacillus paracasei*, effective colonization of the intestinal environment in healthy participants was observed. A slight activation of the immune response was revealed in a subsequent study using the same strain in a probiotic sausage (antibodies against LDL and CD4 cells) (Munekata et al. 2022).

7.5 Traditional Functional Foods

Ancient India appears to have recognized the significance of food and nutrition far before its time. The Indian dietary pattern and traditional foods emerged from the indigenous Ayurvedic medical system. Ayurveda recommends a balanced diet that considers the food's qualities, the individual's characteristics, and the body's absorption (Srinivasan 2010). Some of the spices used by Ayurveda are *Piper nigrum*, *Piper longum*, *Zingiber officinale*, and *Terminalia arjuna*, which are used to treat a variety of disorders. Traditional Indian food formulations demonstrate creativity in the selection of ingredients and additions, with a focus on nutritious nourishment such as "Chyawanprasha" that is a mixer of multiple ingredients like herbs and spices and it is still consumed to this day (Narayana et al. 2017).

7.6 Future Functional Foods

Algae are gaining popularity as nutritional and functional foods because of their high protein content, long-chain PUFAs such as α-linolenic acid, linoleic acids, and polysaccharides like alginate and sulfated heteroglycans. Algal foods are one of the few vegetarian sources of cobalamin (vitamin B12) and also they can be potential prebiotics because of the high concentration of polysaccharides (Wells et al. 2017). Fungal metabolites are also a trending topic; mushrooms have provided foods for thousands of years because of a common dietary protein source with a wide range of specialized metabolites having positive benefits to humans (Strong et al. 2022). Additionally, advances in techniques like the encapsulation of bioactive compounds and bioactive nanoparticles and the controlled release of compounds will help boost the efficiency and bioaccessibility of nutraceuticals.

7.7 Conclusions

The classification and types of functional foods and their importances were discussed. Fruits, vegetables, and nuts contain secondary metabolites like phenolic acids and flavonoids, which are reported to have antioxidant and anticarcinogenic activities. Cereals and legumes are rich in polysaccharides, which act as prebiotics and are helpful to the human gut microbiota. Spices and herbs contain biologically active molecules, which are shown to have health benefits. Dairy products like yoghurt contain live bacteria like *Lactobacillus* species which are also important for gut health. Meat products also contain important compounds, which are beneficial to muscle health and meat is shown to have probiotic properties. Increasing research shows that functional foods containing biologically active components derived from plants or animals may improve health. Nutraceuticals and functional foods may be able to help lower the strain on the healthcare system by emphasizing prevention over treatment.

References

Akihisa T, Yasukawa K, Yamaura M, Ukiya M, Kimura Y, Shimizu N, Arai K (2000) Triterpene alcohol and sterol ferulates from rice bran and their anti-inflammatory effects. Agri Food Chem 48(6):2313–2319. https://doi.org/10.1021/jf000135o

Al Aboody MS, (2021) Cytotoxic, antioxidant, and antimicrobial activities of Celery (*Apium graveolens L.*). Bioinformation 17(1):147. https://doi.org/10.6026/97320630017147

Al-Qabba MM, El-Mowafy MA, Althwab, SA, Alfheeaid HA, Aljutaily T, Barakat H (2020) Phenolic profile, antioxidant activity, and ameliorating efficacy of *Chenopodium quinoa* sprouts

against CCl4-induced oxidative stress in rats. Nutrients 12(10):2904. https://doi.org/10.3390/nu12102904
Asgary S, Rastqar A, Keshvari M (2018) Functional food and cardiovascular disease prevention and treatment: a review. J Am Coll Nutr 37(5):429–455. https://doi.org/10.1080/07315724.2017.1410867
Ataie-Jafari A, Larijani B, Majd HA, Tahbaz F (2009) Cholesterol-lowering effect of probiotic yogurt in comparison with ordinary yogurt in mildly to moderately hypercholesterolemic subjects. Ann Nutr Metab 54(1):22–27. https://doi.org/10.1159/000203284
Ballali S, Lanciai F (2012) Functional food and diabetes: a natural way in diabetes prevention? Int J Food Sci Nutr 63(sup1):51–61. https://doi.org/10.1080/10408398.2014.903384
Behzad S, Sureda A, Barreca D, Nabavi SF, Rastrelli L, Nabavi SM (2017) Health effects of phloretin: from chemistry to medicine. Phytochem Rev 16:527–533. https://doi.org/10.1007/s11101-017-9500-x
Bian S, Hu J, Zhang K, Wang Y, Yu M, Ma J (2018) Dairy product consumption and risk of hip fracture: a systematic review and meta-analysis. BMC Public Health 18:1–16. https://doi.org/10.1186/s12889-018-5041-5
Borah D, Gogoi, O, Adhikari, C, Kakoti, BB (2016) Isolation and characterization of the new indigenous Staphylococcus sp. DBOCP06 as a probiotic bacterium from traditionally fermented fish and meat products of Assam state. Egypt J Basic Appl Sci 3(3):232–240. https://doi.org/10.1016/j.ejbas.2016.06.001
Bourrie BC, Willing BP, Cotter PD (2016) The microbiota and health-promoting characteristics of the fermented beverage kefir. Front Microbiol 647. https://doi.org/10.3389/fmicb.2016.00647
Capozzi V, Russo P, Dueñas MT, López P, Spano G (2012) Lactic acid bacteria producing B-group vitamins: a great potential for functional cereals products. Appl Microbiol Biotechnol 96:1383–1394. https://doi.org/10.1007/s00253-012-4440-2
Chhikara N, Kour R, Jaglan S, Gupta P, Gat Y, Panghal A (2018) *Citrus medica*: nutritional, phytochemical composition and health benefits–a review. Food Funct 9(4):1978–1992. https://doi.org/10.1039/C7FO02035J
Collins S, Reid G (2016) Distant site effects of ingested prebiotics. Nutrients 8(9):523. https://doi.org/10.3390/nu8090523
Dadwal V, Joshi R, Gupta M (2022) A comparative metabolomic investigation in fruit sections of *Citrus medica L.* and *Citrus maxima L.* detecting potential bioactive metabolites using UHPLC-QTOF-IMS. Food Res Int 157:111486. https://doi.org/10.1016/j.foodres.2022.111486
Damián MR, Cortes-Perez NG, Quintana ET, Ortiz-Moreno A, Garfias Noguez C, Cruceño-Casarrubias CE, Sánchez Pardo ME, Bermúdez-Humarán LG (2022) Functional foods, nutraceuticals and probiotics: a focus on human health. Microorganisms 10(5):1065. https://doi.org/10.3390/microorganisms10051065
Das A, Raychaudhuri U, Chakraborty R (2012) Cereal based functional food of Indian subcontinent: a review. J Food Sci Technol 49:665–672. https://doi.org/10.1007/s13197-011-0474-1
Davani-Davari D, Negahdaripour M, Karimzadeh I, Seifan M, Mohkam M, Masoumi SJ, Berenjian A, Ghasemi Y (2019) Prebiotics: definition, types, sources, mechanisms, and clinical applications. Foods 8(3):92. https://doi.org/10.3390/foods8030092
De LeBlanc ADM, Perdigón G (2010) The application of probiotic fermented milks in cancer and intestinal inflammation. Proc Nutr Soc 3:421–428. https://doi.org/10.1017/S002966511000159X
DeFelice SL (1995) The nutraceutical revolution: its impact on food industry R&D. Trends Food Sci Technol 6(2):59–61. https://doi.org/10.1016/S0924-2244(00)88944-X
Di Petrillo A, Orrù G, Fais A, Fantini MC (2022) Quercetin and its derivates as antiviral potentials: a comprehensive review. Phytother Res 36(1):266–278. https://doi.org/10.1002/ptr.7309
Fazilah NF, Ariff AB, Khayat ME, Rios-Solis L, Halim M (2018) Influence of probiotics, prebiotics, synbiotics and bioactive phytochemicals on the formulation of functional yogurt. J Funct Foods 48:387–399. https://doi.org/10.1016/j.jff.2018.07.039

Figueroa-González I, Quijano G, Ramirez G, Cruz-Guerrero A (2011) Probiotics and prebiotics—perspectives and challenges. J Sci Food Agric 91(8):1341–1348. https://doi.org/10.1002/jsfa.4367
Fox PF (2011) History of dairy products and processes. In: Fuquay JW, Fox PF, McSweeney PLH (eds) Encyclopedia of dairy sciences. Elsevier Academic Press, London. https://doi.org/10.1016/B978-0-12-374407-4.00541-0
Gai QY, Jiao J, Wang X, Fu YJ, Lu Y, Liu J, Wang ZY, Xu XJ (2021) Simultaneous quantification of eleven bioactive phenolic compounds in pigeon pea natural resources and in vitro cultures by ultra-high performance liquid chromatography coupled with triple quadrupole mass spectrometry (UPLC-QqQ-MS/MS). Food Chem 335:127602. https://doi.org/10.1016/j.foodchem.2020.127602
Granato D, Branco GF, Cruz AG, Faria JDAF, Shah NP (2010) Probiotic dairy products as functional foods. Compr Rev Food Sci Food Saf 9(5):455–470. https://doi.org/10.1111/j.1541-4337.2010.00120.x
Granier A, Goulet O, Hoarau C (2013) Fermentation products: immunological effects on human and animal models. Pediatr Res 74(2):238–244. https://doi.org/10.1038/pr.2013.76
Gul K, Singh AK, Jabeen R (2016) Nutraceuticals and functional foods: the foods for the future world. Crit Rev Food Sci Nutr 56(16):2617–2627. https://doi.org/10.1080/10408398.2014.903384
Guo Q, Wang N, Liu H, Li Z, Lu L, Wang C (2020) The bioactive compounds and biological functions of *Asparagus officinalis L.*–A review. J Funct Foods 65:103727. https://doi.org/10.1016/j.jff.2019.103727
Hati S, Das S, Mandal S (2019) Technological advancement of functional fermented dairy beverages. In: Engineering tools in the beverage industry, pp 101–136. Woodhead Publishing. https://doi.org/10.1016/B978-0-12-815258-4.00004-4
Henry CJ (2010) Functional foods. Eur J Clin Nutr 64(7):657–659. https://doi.org/10.1038/ejcn.2010.101
Himanshu K, Sonawane SK, Arya SS (2018) Nutritional and nutraceutical properties of millets: a review. Clin J Nutr Diet 1(1):1–10. https://doi.org/10.33309/2639-8761.010107
Jiménez-Colmenero F, Carballo J, Cofrades S (2001) Healthier meat and meat products: their role as functional foods. Meat Sci 59(1):5–13. https://doi.org/10.1016/S0309-1740(01)00053-5
Katina K, Laitila A, Juvonen R, Liukkonen KH, Kariluoto S, Piironen V, Landberg R, Åman P, Poutanen K (2007) Bran fermentation as a means to enhance technological properties and bioactivity of rye. Food Microbiol 24(2):175–186. https://doi.org/10.1016/j.fm.2006.07.012
Kikuzaki H, Usuguchi J, Nakatani N (1991) Constitutents of Zingiberaceae. I. Diarylheptanoids from the rhizomes of ginger (*Zingiber officinale* Roscoe). Chem Pharm Bull 39(1):120–122. https://doi.org/10.1248/cpb.39.120
Kumar M, Barbhai MD, Hasan M, Punia S, Dhumal S, Rais N, Chandran D, Pandiselvam R, Kothakota A, Tomar M, Satankar V (2022) Onion (*Allium cepa L.*) peels: a review on bioactive compounds and biomedical activities. Biomed Pharmacother 146:112498. https://doi.org/10.1016/j.biopha.2021.112498
Kumari R, Dadwal V, Agrawal H, Gupta M (2021) Recent trends in functional and nutraceutical foods. In: Advances in processing technology, pp 123–141. CRC Press. https://doi.org/10.1201/9781003245513
Leite AMDO, Miguel MAL, Peixoto RS, Rosado AS, Silva JT, Paschoalin VMF (2013) Microbiological, technological and therapeutic properties of kefir: a natural probiotic beverage. Braz J Microbiol 44:341–349. https://doi.org/10.1590/S1517-83822013000200001
Li S, Wang C, Li W, Koike K, Nikaido T, Wang MW (2007) Antidepressant-like effects of piperine and its derivative, antiepilepsirine. J Asian Nat Prod Res 9(5):421–430. https://doi.org/10.1080/10286020500384302
Maleki SJ, Crespo JF, Cabanillas B (2019) Anti-inflammatory effects of flavonoids. Food Chem 299:125124. https://doi.org/10.1016/j.foodchem.2019.125124

Martín-García B, Pasini F, Verardo V, Gómez-Caravaca AM, Marconi E, Caboni MF (2019) Distribution of free and bound phenolic compounds in buckwheat milling fractions. Foods 8(12):670. https://doi.org/10.3390/foods8120670

Matar C, Valdeze JC, Medina M, Rachid M, Perdigon G (2001) Immunomodulating effects of milks fermented by lactobacillus helveticus and its non-proteolytic variant. Res J Dairy Sci 68(4):601–609. https://doi.org/10.1017/S0022029901005143

Meng X, Zhou J, Zhao CN, Gan RY, Li HB (2020) Health benefits and molecular mechanisms of resveratrol: a narrative review. Foods 9(3):340. https://doi.org/10.3390/foods9030340

Meybodi NM, Nasab SS, Khorshidian N, Mortazavian AM (2021) Probiotic beverages: health benefits and current trends in the Middle East. In: Probiotic beverages, pp 99–126. Academic Press. https://doi.org/10.1016/B978-0-12-818588-9.00011-5

Min M, Bunt CR, Mason SL, Hussain MA (2019) Non-dairy probiotic food products: an emerging group of functional foods. Crit Rev Food Sci Nutr 59(16):2626–2641. https://doi.org/10.1080/10408398.2018.1462760

Moreno I, Marasca ETG, de Sá PBZR, de Souza Moitinho J, Marquezini MG, Alves MRC, Bromberg R (2018) Evaluation of probiotic potential of bacteriocinogenic lactic acid bacteria strains isolated from meat products. Probiotics Antimicro 10:762–774. https://doi.org/10.1007/s12602-018-9388-9

Munekata PE, Pateiro M, Tomasevic I, Domínguez R, da Silva Barretto AC, Santos EM, Lorenzo JM (2022) Functional fermented meat products with probiotics—a review. J Appl Microbiol 133(1):91–103. https://doi.org/10.1111/jam.15337

Nagraj GS, Chouksey A, Jaiswal S, Jaiswal AK (2020) Broccoli. In: Nutritional composition and antioxidant properties of fruits and vegetables, pp 5–17. Academic Press. https://doi.org/10.1016/B978-0-12-812780-3.00001-5

Narayana DA, Durg S, Manohar PR, Mahapatra A, Aramya AR (2017) Chyawanprash: a review of therapeutic benefits as in authoritative texts and documented clinical literature. J Ethnopharmacol 197:52–60. https://doi.org/10.1016/j.jep.2016.07.078

Nunes S, Vieira P, Gomes P, Viana SD, Reis F (2021) Blueberry as an attractive functional fruit to prevent (pre) diabetes progression. Antioxidants 10(8):1162. https://doi.org/10.3390/antiox10081162

Orlandi M, Goracci J, Curadi MC (2003) Fat composition of mare's milk with reference to human nutrition. Annali della Facolta di Medicina veterinaria 56:97–106. https://doi.org/10.1002/fsn3.2595

Patwardhan B (2005) Ethnopharmacology and drug discovery. J Ethnopharmacol 100(1–2):50–52. https://doi.org/10.1016/j.jep.2005.06.006

Prasathkumar M, Anisha S, Dhrisya C, Becky R, Sadhasivam S (2021) Therapeutic and pharmacological efficacy of selective Indian medicinal plants–a review. Phytomed Plus 1(2):100029. https://doi.org/10.1016/j.phyplu.2021.100029

Rafie N, Hamedani SG, Ghiasvand R, Miraghajani M (2015) Kefir and cancer: a systematic review of literatures. Arch Iran Med 18(12). https://doi.org/10.51812/aim.0011

Saggar S, Mir PA, Kumar N, Chawla A, Uppal J, Kaur A (2022) Traditional and herbal medicines: opportunities and challenges. Pharm Res 14(2). https://doi.org/10.5530/pres.14.2.15

Santini A (2022) Nutraceuticals and functional foods: is it possible and sustainable for bridging health and food? Foods 11(11):1608. https://doi.org/10.3390/foods11111608

Shahbaz M, Raza N, Islam M, Imran M, Ahmad I, Meyyazhagan A, Pushparaj K, Balasubramanian B, Park S, Rengasamy KR, Gondal TA (2022) The nutraceutical properties and health benefits of pseudocereals: a comprehensive treatise. Crit Rev Food Sci Nutr 1-13. https://doi.org/10.1080/10408398.2022.2071205

Shahidi F (2009) Nutraceuticals and functional foods: whole versus processed foods. Trends Food Sci Technol 20(9):376–387. https://doi.org/10.1016/j.tifs.2008.08.004

Shahwar D, Bhat TM, Ansari MYK, Chaudhary S, Aslam R (2017) Health functional compounds of lentil (*Lens culinaris* Medik): a review. Int J Food Prop 20(sup1):S1–S15. https://doi.org/10.1080/10942912.2017.1287192

Sharifi M, Moridnia A, Mortazavi D, Salehi M, Bagheri M, Sheikhi A (2017) Kefir: a powerful probiotic with anticancer properties. Clin Oncol 34:1–7. https://doi.org/10.1007/s12032-017-1044-9

Shiby VK, Mishra HN (2013) Fermented milks and milk products as functional foods—a review. Crit Rev Food Sci Nutr 53(5):482–496. https://doi.org/10.1080/10408398.2010.547398

Sikand G, Kris-Etherton P, Boulos NM (2015) Impact of functional foods on prevention of cardiovascular disease and diabetes. Curr Cardiol Rep 17:1–16. https://doi.org/10.1007/s11886-015-0593-9

Spinler JK, Taweechotipatr M, Rognerud CL, Ou CN, Tumwasorn S, Versalovic J (2008) Human-derived probiotic lactobacillus reuteri demonstrates antimicrobial activities targeting diverse enteric bacterial pathogens. Anaerobe 14(3):166–171. https://doi.org/10.1016/j.anaerobe.2008.02.001

Srinivasan K (2010) Traditional Indian functional foods. Funct Foods East, Nutraceut Sci Technol Ser 10:51–76. https://doi.org/10.1201/b10264-4

Stadnik J, Kęska P (2015) Meat and fermented meat products as a source of bioactive peptides. Acta Scientiarum Polonorum Technologia Alimentaria 14(3):181–190. https://doi.org/10.17306/J.AFS.2015.3.19

Stevenson D, Scalzo J (2012) Anthocyanin composition and content of blueberries from around the world. J Berry Res 2(4):179–189. https://doi.org/10.3233/JBR-2012-038

Strong PJ, Self R, Allikian K, Szewczyk E, Speight R, O'Hara I, Harrison MD (2022) Filamentous fungi for future functional food and feed. Curr Opin Biotechnol 76:102729. https://doi.org/10.1016/j.copbio.2022.102729

Telichowska A, Kobus-Cisowska J, Szulc P (2020) Phytopharmacological possibilities of bird cherry *Prunus padus L.* and *Prunus serotina L.* species and their bioactive phytochemicals. Nutrients 12(7):1966. https://doi.org/10.3390/nu12071966

Tu MY, Chen HL, Tung YT, Kao CC, Hu FC, Chen CM (2015) Short-term effects of kefir-fermented milk consumption on bone mineral density and bone metabolism in a randomized clinical trial of osteoporotic patients. PLoS One 10(12):0144231. https://doi.org/10.1371/journal.pone.0144231

Tunick MH, Van Hekken DL (2015) Dairy products and health: recent insights. J Agric Food Chem 63(43):9381–9388. https://doi.org/10.1021/jf5042454

Vitaglione P, Napolitano A, Fogliano V (2008) Cereal dietary fibre: a natural functional ingredient to deliver phenolic compounds into the gut. Trends Food Sci 19(9):451–463. https://doi.org/10.1016/j.tifs.2008.02.005

Wells ML, Potin P, Craigie JS, Raven JA, Merchant SS, Helliwell KE, Smith AG, Camire ME, Brawley SH (2017) Algae as nutritional and functional food sources: revisiting our understanding. J Appl Phycol 29:949–982. https://doi.org/10.1007/s10811-016-0974-5

Wojdyło A, Turkiewicz IP, Tkacz K, Nowicka P, Bobak Ł (2022) Nuts as functional foods: variation of nutritional and phytochemical profiles and their *in vitro* bioactive properties. Food Chem X 15:100418. https://doi.org/10.1016/j.fochx.2022.100418

Yahia EM, García-Solís P, Celis MEM (2019) Contribution of fruits and vegetables to human nutrition and health. In: Postharvest physiology and biochemistry of fruits and vegetables 19–45. Woodhead Publishing. https://doi.org/10.1016/B978-0-12-813278-4.00002-6

Yende SR, Sannapuri VD, Vyawahare NS, Harle UN (2010) Antirheumatoid activity of aqueous extract of *Piper longum* on freund's adjuvant-induced arthritis in rats. Int J Pharm Sci Res 1(9):129–133. https://doi.org/10.13040/IJPSR.0975-8232.1(9-S).129-33

Zeisel SH (1999) Regulation of" nutraceuticals". Science 285(5435):1853–1855. https://doi.org/10.1126/science.285.5435.1853

Nutri-Ayur Components: Millets, Fruits and Vegetables, Spices, Pulses, Cereals, Nuts and Seeds, Herbs

8

Adinath Kate and Manoj Kumar Tripathi

Abstract

As per Ayurveda, nutrition is not only related to performing metabolic activities and various functions of the body, but also often referred to as medicine in terms of playing a crucial role in the prevention and cure of various chronic diseases. The appropriate and balanced diet always maintains overall health, strengthens the immune system, supports essential body functions appropriately, and lowers the risk of diseases like heart disease, diabetes, and cancers. Various sources of food provide particular types of nutritional attributes to the body. Millets, coming under pseudocereals, mainly provide carbohydrates, fiber, proteins, and minerals like calcium, magnesium, and iron. However, fruits and vegetables are rich in vitamins, minerals, phenolic compounds, phytochemicals, and antioxidants. Various spices and herbs are mainly consumed in very small quantities, but they are very essential due to the presence of valuable aromatic compounds, pigments, essential oils, etc. They have a special role in immunity boosting. The staple food mainly includes cereals and pulses that are the major source of carbohydrates and proteins required for basic body metabolism, energy generation, and growth.

Keywords

Millets · Antioxidants · Phytochemicals · Ayurveda · Nutrition

A. Kate (✉) · M. K. Tripathi
ICAR- Central Institute of Agricultural Engineering, Bhopal, Madhya Pradesh, India

A. Kumar et al. (eds.), *Innovations in Ayurvedic Nutrition*,
https://doi.org/10.1007/978-981-95-1213-3_8

8.1 Introduction

The food is essential for fulfillment of the nutritional requirements of the human body. All the physical activities involve energy requirement, including metabolic activities that require particular types of nutritional constituents. The nutritional constituents include macronutrients like carbohydrates, protein, fats, and micronutrients mainly include minerals and vitamins. Besides these, food material contains various other bioactive constituents like phytochemicals, phenolic compounds, antioxidants, etc., which also play a key role in various body functions. Besides these, all these compounds also play a vital role in maintaining the immune system and fighting against diseases, infections, and disorders found in the human body. Many times these compounds act as medicine in therapeutic and ayurvedic applications. There are diverse sources of such nutri-ayur compounds in daily consumption like cereals, pulses, oilseeds, fruits, vegetables, nuts, spices, and herbs. The specific type of compounds and their nutritional, therapeutic, and ayurvedic properties are elaborated in this chapter.

8.2 Nutritional and Ayurvedic Components in Millets

Millet is one of the ancient crops that comes under cereals and pseudocereals and is consumed by humans. The type of millets includes Sorghum (jawar), Pearl millet, finger millet (ragi), barnyard millet, proso millet, kodo millet, foxtail millet, etc. The millets were the staple food for the ancient population; however, after the advancement in cultivation technologies in agriculture, millets remained as the food for the poor group of the population, mainly living in rural areas. However, in recent days, due to the health benefits and nutritional value, demand has increased in urban areas in developed countries also (Table 8.1).

Millets are not only cost-effective for production but also highly nutritious in nature. Millet grains are dense with proteins, vitamins, nutrients, fiber, minerals, and specialized phytochemicals. The glycemic index of millets is also low, which means when we ingest the millets, they release a lower amount of glucose for a longer period of time (Geetha et al. 2020). This is because millets have high fiber and complex carbohydrates, which take longer to digest and absorb. The glycemic index (GI) value of the millets is quite lower than the other staple cereal grains like wheat, corn, rice, etc. The low GI characteristics of millet are very much effective for diabetic, prediabetic, and other metabolic disorders found in humans. They also play a vital role in the situations of celiac disease or gluten allergy or gluten intolerance (Jacob et al. 2024). The iron found in millets is also helpful for managing the situation of iron deficiency, anemia, etc. (Krishnan et al. 2022).

In Ayush Dietary Advisory for *KuposhanMukta Bharat,* region-specific millets such as Aata of Jowar (sorghum), Bajra (pearl millet), Ragi (finger millet), Konidhan (tiny rice), Sava (Barnyard Millet), Kodo (Paspalum), etc., are mentioned and they maintain dietary diversification. In Ayurveda, millets are known as *KshudraDhanya* based on the smaller size of the grains (Jacob et al. 2024).

Table 8.1 Nutritional and nutraceutical potential of millets (Tripathi et al. 2021)

S.no.	Disease/clinical conditions	Benefits	Helpful factors
1	Diabetes	Helpful in diabetes	Low glycemic index grain
2	Anemia	Increase the level of hemoglobin	Higher levels of iron and zinc
3	Constipation	Help in decreasing constipation	High fiber amount
4	Cancer	Anticancerous property	Prevent tumor formation
5	Bone growth, development, and repair	High phosphorus amount for bone growth. In ATP synthesis	Presence of phosphorus.
6	Stomach ulcer	Helpful in the treatment of stomach ulcers. Control stomach alkaline conditions and prevent the formation of ulcers.	Helpful in the control of excess acidity.
7	Heart health	Phytonutrients and lignin act as strong antioxidants, preventing heart disease. High content of magnesium useful in blood pressure and heart stress control.	As a strong antioxidant.
8	Respiratory problems for asthma patients	High amount of magnesium decreases the respiratory problems (asthma patients). Reduce migraine attacks.	High amount of magnesium
9	Weight loss (obesity)	Useful in weight loss, contains high fiber content. Reduces the overall consumption of food.	High fiber content
10	Prevention gall stones	Decreases the risk of gall bladder stone. Decreases the production of excessive bile juice.	High fiber content
11	Antiallergic properties	Highly digestible Low allergic response.	Due to hypoallergic property

8.2.1 Various Health Benefits: Nutrition and Therapeutic Properties of Millets (Saleh et al. 2013)

- Millets are rich in micronutrient profile and bioactive flavonoids.
- Rich source of quality minerals like iron, zinc, and calcium.
- Millets have a low Glycemic Index (GI) and thus are helpful in the prevention and management of diabetes and other related disorders.
- Rich in antioxidants, and its consumption decreases triglycerides and C-reactive protein, thereby preventing cardiovascular disease.
- Millets are helpful in the reduction of weight, BMI, and high blood pressure.
- Millets have gluten-free properties; therefore, they can be consumed by celiac disease (gluten allergy) and IBS patients.
- Millet is typically complemented with legumes, creating a balanced intake of protein that improves the overall protein digestibility.

8.3 Nutritional and Ayurvedic Components in Fruits and Vegetables

Fruits and vegetables are the basic dietary requirement for the fulfillment of the nutritional requirements of the human body. The various nutritional as well as dietary constituents of the fruit and vegetables include fibers, vitamins, minerals, phenolic compounds including flavonoids, phytoestrogens, sulfur compounds, monoterpenes, and bioactive peptides. The presence of particular element and their content in the particular commodity varies with its type and many more cultivation-related factors. Nutrients are essential molecules needed for the survival and growth of organisms (Joshi et al. 2018). Dietary Reference Intakes (DRIs) are established guidelines for these nutrients. Fruits and vegetables are often rich in fiber, minerals (especially potassium), and vitamins, particularly vitamins C and K. Among them, dark green leafy vegetables like spinach and cabbage provide at least 50% of the DRI for vitamins C and K. Legumes and Allium family bulbs offer 50% of the DRI for vitamin K, while tomatoes and other red fruits supply 50% of the DRI for vitamin C. Dark green leafy vegetables and legumes contribute over 25% of the DRI for folate, and Allium family bulbs provide notable amounts of manganese and vitamin B6 (Septembre-Malaterre et al. 2018). While all fruits contribute significantly to vitamin C intake, citrus fruits may account for up to 40% of the DRI. Nutrient composition tables often highlight which foods are a "good source of" or "contribute to" specific nutrients. In addition to nutrients, phytochemicals are bioactive, nonnutrient compounds found in plant-based foods, mainly fruits and vegetables. There are over 5000 identified phytochemicals found in fruits and vegetables. Fruits and vegetables contain a variety of nutritional compounds like vitamins, minerals, fiber, and bioactive phytochemicals like flavonoids, carotenoids, and phenolic acids, while in Ayurveda, they are categorized based on their "*rasa*" (taste) and "*guna*" (qualities) with specific health benefits depending on their properties like cooling, heating, or balancing, with prominent examples including mango, amla, and bitter melon. Some of the key nutritional compounds found in different types of fruits and vegetables include (Liu 2013):

1. Vitamins: Vitamin C (citrus fruits), Vitamin A (carrots, sweet potatoes), Vitamin K (leafy greens), Vitamin B complex (whole grains, legumes).
2. Minerals: Potassium (bananas, potatoes), Calcium (broccoli, kale), Magnesium (almonds, spinach).
3. Fiber: Insoluble fiber (whole grains, legumes), Soluble fiber (apples, oats).
4. Flavonoids: Antioxidants found in berries, citrus fruits, and onions.
5. Carotenoids: Antioxidants found in carrots, tomatoes, and sweet potatoes.
6. Polyphenols: Antioxidants with anti-inflammatory properties found in tea, grapes, and berries.
7. Sulforaphane: Found in cruciferous vegetables like broccoli and cabbage, with potential anticancer properties.

8.3.1 Ayurvedic Perspective on Fruits and Vegetables

Rasa (Taste) means Sweet (madhura), sour (amla), salty (celery), pungent (ginger), bitter (bitter melon) while *Guna* (Qualities) includes Sattvic means Cooling, calming (cucumber, coconut), Rajasic means Heating, stimulating (ginger, chili peppers), and Tamasic means Heavy, dulling (heavy starchy vegetables).

8.3.2 Ayurvedic Importance of Different Fruits and Vegetables (Vincente et al. 2014)

Mango (Mangifera indica): Considered the "king of fruits" in Ayurveda, balancing Pitta and Vata when ripe.

Amla (Phyllanthus emblica): High in Vitamin C, considered a rejuvenating fruit with a sour taste.

Bottle Gourd (Lagenaria siceraria): Cooling and soothing, good for digestion.

Spinach (Spinacia oleracea): Rich in iron, considered a blood purifier.

Ash Gourd (White pumpkin): This vegetable contains plenty of water with zero fat content. It has enormous medicinal properties. Being low in calories, it is an ideal vegetable for diabetic patients and it is good for weight control. In Ayurveda, the juice of ash gourd is used effectively in mercury poisoning and snakebites.

Eggplant (Brinjal): It contains some essential nutrients that are highly beneficial for the human body. It is light in digestion, acts as a purgative, and helps in obesity. It is rich in dietary fiber, vitamins, and minerals, especially in vitamin C, thiamine, riboflavin, niacin, etc.

Baby Corn: Low in fat, baby corn is a good source of potassium, vitamin C, and fiber. It prevents constipation and colon cancer. It holds a great degree of nutritional value and has numerous health benefits. Baby corn contains some carotenoids which help in the promotion of eye health.

Banana: It is very good for people who are anemic because it contains a high level of iron and can stimulate the production of hemoglobin in the blood. It is extremely high in potassium yet low in salt, which is good for blood pressure. It also helps to overcome constipation.

Banana Stem: This is supposed to be the waste of the plant yet it is very good for health. It has very high nutritive value. It adds bulk to the food and it is very good for weight reduction. The fiber in it helps to overcome constipation and it also helps to detoxify the body.

Beetroot: High in nutrients like vitamin C and iron. It is best eaten raw. If you cook the beetroot, it loses its vitamin content.

Bitter Gourd: This is one vegetable that can help your body be disease-free, due to its disease-preventing and health-promoting phytochemical compounds. As its name suggests, it is one of the most bitter of all culinary vegetables. It is very low in calories, but rich in dietary fiber, minerals, vitamins, and antioxidants.

Black Carrot: It has a high therapeutic value and contains a complex of vitamins, like vitamin C, potassium salts, and essential oils. This fruit is also considered to be an elixir of youth. It is a good diuretic and has antirheumatic effects and helps in the elimination of uric acid.

Bottle Gourd: One of the most common vegetables in India, bottle gourd has a lot of health benefits. It is very good for high blood pressure and heart disease. It is considered to be good for weight reduction as it contains 90% water and it is very low in calories.

Broccoli: It belongs to the same family as cauliflower, and it is also low in fat and can fight against cancer. Broccoli contains vitamin C and K. It also provides fiber, folate, manganese, and beta carotene. This vegetable helps to protect from prostate cancer, stroke risks, and eye diseases.

Cabbage: It is an excellent source of vitamin C, which is one of the best antioxidants and helps in reducing the aging process. It is also good for constipation. It helps in stomach ulcers, excess weight, skin disorders, eczema, rheumatism, arthritis, gout and eye disorders, and in the proper functioning of the nervous system.

Capsicum: It holds a great degree of nutritional value and has numerous health benefits. Capsicum is a very good source of vitamins A, B, and C and minerals like calcium and potassium. It is also good for weight reduction.

Carrot: As a good source of fiber, carrot is an amazing vegetable, easy to add to your diet. It slows down the aging of cells, is excellent for the eyes, and contains a large quantity of vitamin A in the form of beta-carotene. It also has cancer-curing properties.

Cauliflower: It is low in fat and carbohydrates but high in dietary fiber. Folate and vitamin C. Possessing high nutritional value, cauliflower is beneficial to human health. It is very helpful to those suffering from prostate, breast, cervical, colon, and ovarian cancer as it contains several anticancer phytochemicals.

Coconut: This fruit has many benefits with amazing medicinal properties. Coconut water is a natural drink for hydration, and it is high in energy. Its edible flesh is a part of the daily diet of people in Kerala and it is used in most of the dishes. It is rich in fiber, minerals, and vitamins and has more than 90% saturated fats.

Coriander Leaves: These leaves, when digested, turn sweet and alleviate irritation in the intestine. They have magnesium, potassium, and fiber in plenty. Regular consumption boosts immunity and purifies blood. This is one herb that is widely cultivated in India. It is also a great herb for skin, to treat pimples and blackheads.

Cucumber: It has many health benefits and that is why it is a very important part of the food diet and also the skin diet. It is soothing and softening for the skin and cooling for eyes. Regular intake of cucumber juice is very beneficial both internally and externally. It contains almost 90% of water; hence is good for weight reduction.

Curry Leaves: As an aromatic herb, curry leaves are a unique flavoring agent. The leaves' benefits are not just for their taste, but it is also used as a natural remedy for many health conditions and disorders. It is believed that eating a few fresh curry leaves daily manages diabetes, reduces cholesterol, aids weight loss, and prevents the development of cataracts.

Drumstick: Many of the medicinal and nutritional properties of drumsticks have long been known in India. Due to its high iron content, it is very beneficial for many ailments. It contains digestible protein, calcium, iron, vitamin C, and carotenoids. Almost all parts of the drumstick tree have medicinal value.

Drumstick Leaves: The drumstick leaves are not only relished as a vegetable, but they are used in treatments too for their medicinal value. They are good for the treatment of rheumatism and as a circulatory stimulant. The leaves are also used in the poultice for reducing glandular swelling.

French Beans: Very low in fat and a good source of vitamins and minerals. They act as a laxative and help in good digestion. These beans are very good antioxidants and contain excellent levels of vitamins A and C which help the body to develop resistance against infection.

Grapes: This fruit has a great medicinal value and it is rich in nutrients. It prevents blood clots and the antioxidants in the grapes help to stop the oxidation of the bad cholesterol. Grapes contain flavonoids, which help to reduce the effects of aging. Grapes are sweet and slightly sour, making them a useful liver tonic.

Green Peas: One of the most nutritious, leguminous vegetables, rich in minerals, vitamins, and antioxidants. Green peas are relatively low in calories and have no cholesterol. They are a good source of protein and contain soluble as well as insoluble fiber. Green peas are an excellent source of folic acid, vitamins C, K, and A.

Guava: It is one of the richest sources of dietary fiber. Guava seeds serve as an excellent laxative. It is also rich in iron, which is proven to be preventive against cold and viral infections. It contains a lot of vitamins, keeps the skin glowing, and prevents aging.

Lime: This fruit is not only used for culinary purposes but also for cosmetic and medicinal purposes. It contains water-soluble vitamin C, which is very good for the blood vessels, muscles, and cartilage. It also has anticancer properties and it is a natural cure for diseases like scurvy.

Long Beans: This is one vegetable that is available throughout the year. They are low in calories and hence can be consumed by those on a diet. It is considered to be an energy food. Being green in color, it is rich in phytochemicals and antioxidants and can fight cancer and delay aging.

Mint: This is an herb with remarkable medicinal properties. It is used in various products from toothpastes to candies and also in our daily food. It promotes digestion and it is a good appetizer. The strong and refreshing aroma of mint is an excellent quick remedy for nausea, respiratory disorders, cold, and cough. It is an excellent skin cleanser.

Okra: This is a very low-calorie vegetable containing no saturated fats or cholesterol. It is rich in dietary fiber, minerals, and vitamins, and it is highly recommended for weight reduction and cholesterol control programs. As a good source of calcium and potassium, okra helps to stabilize blood sugar.

Onion: Its nutritional value has been evident for many generations and has been used for thousands of years. It is used as a diuretic, for digestion, for the heart, eyes, and joints. It is low in fat, calories, and is cholesterol-free. Onion extract is very good for prevention of arthritis, cough and cold, asthma, and bronchitis.

Papaya: It is a rich and powerful source of antioxidants and contains carotenes, vitamin C, B, and E, and minerals like potassium and magnesium. It helps to prevent cancer and it is very good for digestive disorders. It is believed to be one of the best for premature aging.

Pomegranate: This fruit has been widely used in Ayurveda for various remedies down the ages. It is very effective in reducing heart diseases, in lowering blood pressure and it has antioxidant properties. It also lowers the risk of cancer and controls weight. Pomegranate is a good blood thinner.

Potato: It is rich in vitamin C and iron. Vitamin C promotes iron absorption. It is a good source of vitamins B1, B3, and B6 and minerals such as potassium, phosphorus, etc. Potato also contains antioxidants which may play a part in preventing diseases related to aging.

Raw Banana: Like potato, raw banana is used as a good source of carbohydrates. The dietary fiber helps in normal bowel movements and in reducing constipation. The potassium in it helps to control heart rate and blood pressure, countering negative effects of sodium. It is also beneficial for our brain and kidneys.

Spinach: Spinach is very low in calories and very high in vitamins, minerals, and other phytonutrients. It is an excellent source of vitamin K, vitamin A, magnesium, iron, calcium, vitamin C, vitamin B2, potassium, and vitamin B6. It is also a good source of protein, phosphorus, vitamin E, and zinc. It contains a lot of fiber and has omega-3 fatty acids. The various nutrients help in protecting against diseases.

Star Fruit: Rich in vitamin A and C, potassium, phosphorus, iron, and calcium, star fruit is a good source of fiber, amino acids, and antioxidants. The skin of the fruit is rich in tannin, which regulates the intestine. It is also known to be effective in hormone regulation. Star fruit is a popular remedy for curing hangovers.

Tomato: This vegetable is routinely used in the Indian kitchen. It not only has nutrients like calcium and sulfur with medicinal values, but it is full of micronutrients and minerals that are essential for the maintenance of the body and its growth. It is very low in fat content and has zero cholesterol levels.

Watermelon: It is an excellent source of vitamins A and C. Vitamin A is important for healthy eyes. Vitamin B6 found in watermelon helps the immune system produce antibodies which are needed to fight diseases. It is an important fruit to be added to the weight reduction diet.

8.4 Nutritional and Ayurvedic Components in Spices

In Ayurveda, various spices are known for their health benefits. Ginger is recognized for its anti-inflammatory properties, while cumin supports digestion. Cardamom also offers anti-inflammatory effects, and coriander is valued for its antioxidant properties. Fennel serves as a cooling spice that aids digestion, and cloves provide both antimicrobial and anti-inflammatory benefits. Fenugreek is believed to help regulate blood sugar levels, and ajwain (bishop's weed) is commonly used to relieve gas. Turmeric is renowned for its strong anti-inflammatory and antioxidant activity (Spence 2025). Many of these spices are staples in Indian cuisine.

1. *Ashwagandha*
   Ashwagandha (*Withania somnifera*) is a small woody plant native to India and North Africa. Its root and berries are used to make a well-known Ayurvedic remedy. Often classified as an adaptogen, ashwagandha is believed to help the body better manage stress. Studies have shown that it can reduce cortisol levels, a hormone produced by the adrenal glands in response to stress. There is also evidence suggesting that ashwagandha may help lower anxiety and improve sleep in individuals dealing with stress and anxiety disorders. Additionally, research indicates that ashwagandha may boost muscle growth, enhance memory, improve male fertility, and reduce blood sugar levels. However, more extensive studies are needed to fully confirm these potential benefits.
2. *Boswellia*
   Boswellia, also called Indian frankincense or olibanum, is derived from the resin of the Boswellia serrata tree and is known for its distinctive spicy, woody aroma. Research suggests that Boswellia may be especially effective in reducing inflammation by inhibiting the release of leukotrienes, compounds that trigger inflammation. Studies on humans have linked Boswellia to reduced pain, improved mobility, and increased range of motion in people with osteoarthritis and rheumatoid arthritis. It may also help prevent oral infections and combat gingivitis. Additionally, Boswellia shows promise in improving digestion for those with ulcerative colitis and Crohn's disease, and it may assist in improving breathing for individuals with chronic asthma.
3. *Triphala*
   Triphala is an Ayurvedic remedy consisting of the following three small medicinal fruits: amla (*Emblica officinalis*, or Indian gooseberry), bibhitaki (*Terminalia bellirica*), haritaki (*Terminalia chebula*). Test-tube and animal studies show that triphala may reduce inflammation caused by arthritis, as well as prevent or limit the growth of certain types of cancer. It may also function as a natural laxative, reducing constipation, abdominal pain, and flatulence while improving the frequency and consistency of bowel movements in people with gut disorders. In addition, a limited number of studies suggest that a mouthwash containing triphala may reduce plaque build-up, decrease gum inflammation, and prevent the growth of bacteria in the mouth.
4. *Brahmi*
   Brahmi (*Bacopa monnieri*) is a key herb in Ayurvedic medicine. Test-tube and animal studies suggest that it has powerful anti-inflammatory properties. Research has also shown that brahmi may enhance learning, attention, memory, and information processing. It has been linked to improvements in symptoms of attention deficit hyperactivity disorder (ADHD), such as inattention, impulsivity, poor self-control, and restlessness. Additionally, some animal studies suggest that brahmi may possess adaptogenic properties, which means it could help the body better manage stress and anxiety.

5. *Cumin*
   Cumin is one of the important spices with various health benefits. It is made from the seeds of the *Cuminum cyminum* plant, which are known for their distinctive earthy, nutty, and spicy flavor. Some studies show cumin to be beneficial in controlling blood lipids and protecting the liver from a high-fat diet. Cumin may also protect against type 2 diabetes by lowering blood sugar levels and improving insulin sensitivity. It may also protect against heart disease by increasing HDL (good) cholesterol while reducing triglycerides and LDL (bad) cholesterol.
6. *Turmeric*
   Turmeric, the spice that gives curry is vibrant yellow color, is a well-known Ayurvedic remedy. Its primary active compound, curcumin, has powerful antioxidant and anti-inflammatory effects. Research suggests that curcumin may be just as effective, or even more so, than some anti-inflammatory drugs, but without their side effects. Additionally, turmeric may help protect against heart disease by improving blood flow, working as effectively as exercise or certain medications. Furthermore, compounds in turmeric may support brain health by boosting levels of brain-derived neurotrophic factor (BDNF), a protein linked to cognitive function. Low BDNF levels have been associated with conditions such as Alzheimer's disease and depression.
7. *Licorice root*
   Licorice root, native to Europe and Asia, comes from the *Glycyrrhiza glabra* plant and is a key herb in Ayurvedic medicine. Studies suggest that licorice root may help reduce inflammation and fight against viruses and bacteria. It also seems to provide relief from sore throats and promote oral health by protecting against dental cavities and Candida. Additionally, this Ayurvedic herb may help manage or prevent heartburn, bloating, nausea, belching, and stomach ulcers. When applied topically, licorice root may help alleviate skin rash symptoms, including redness, itching, and swelling.
8. *Gotu kola*
   Gotu kola (*Centella asiatica*), or "the herb of longevity," is another popular Ayurvedic remedy. It is made from a tasteless, odorless plant with fan-shaped green leaves that grows in and around water. One small study suggests that gotu kola supplements may improve people's memory after they have had a stroke (Spence 2025). This herb may help prevent stretch marks, reduce varicose veins, help wounds heal faster, and diminish symptoms of eczema and psoriasis.
9. *Cardamom*
   Cardamom (*Elettaria cardamomum*), often referred to as the "queen of spices," has been used in Ayurvedic medicine for centuries. Cardamom powder may help lower diastolic blood pressure in individuals with elevated levels. Inhaling cardamom essential oil has been shown to alleviate nausea during pregnancy. Additionally, cardamom may offer protection against *Helicobacter pylori*, a common bacterium responsible for stomach ulcers, and has been found to reduce the size of gastric ulcers by up to 50%, or even eliminate them entirely (Spence 2025).

8.5 Nutritional and Ayurvedic Components in Cereal Food Grains

Cereals contain many nutritional compounds, including carotenoids, phytosterols, and vitamin B. They also contain minerals like magnesium, iron, and potassium. The various staple cereal food grains like rice, wheat, etc., have a *sattvic* quality, which means they promote clarity, calmness, and mental balance for their consumption. Therefore, there is a key place in Ayurveda for these crops. Among the cereals, rice is one of the highly consumed cereal grains with respect to diversified culture and geographical locations. Rice also has a cooling effect on the body, which can be beneficial during hot weather for better metabolism and homeostasis. The various nutritional and therapeutic constituents found in the cereals in the various categories are:

Carotenoids: In this group, α- and β-carotene are commonly found in whole grains. Besides these, β-cryptoxanthin, Zeaxanthin, and Lutein are also found in whole grains.

Phytosterols: This is a type of plant sterols and stanols, which are structurally similar to cholesterol found in various food grains.

Vitamin B: Cereals are a good source of vitamin B, including folate, thiamin, niacin, and riboflavin.

Minerals: Cereals consist of minerals like iron, magnesium, copper, phosphorus, and zinc.

8.6 Nutritional and Ayurvedic Compounds in Pulses

Pulses are a rich source of macronutrients like protein (typically 21–26%), carbohydrates, and are low in both calories and fat. Their protein content makes them valuable for gluten-free products, such as muffins and biodegradable edible films (Singh et al. 2017). While the health benefits of pulses have traditionally been linked to their macronutrients, there is now growing evidence that nonnutritional compounds in pulses also play a significant role in supporting human health. Pulses are abundant in bioactive compounds like polyphenols, phytosterols, and nondigestible carbohydrates, all of which contribute to various physiological and metabolic functions (Amarowicz and Pegg 2008). These compounds vary in concentration across different pulse species and varieties. The seed coats of pulses are particularly rich in water-insoluble fibers and polyphenols with strong antioxidant properties, while the cotyledons are higher in soluble fibers, oligosaccharides, and slowly digestible or resistant starches. Among the phenolic compounds in pulses, ferulic acid is the most abundant, while flavonol glycosides, anthocyanins, and tannins give the seed coat its color. The major phytosterols in pulses include sitosterol (the most prevalent), stigmasterol, and campesterol (Balasundram et al. 2006). The fibers, resistant starch, and oligosaccharides in pulses function as prebiotics, offering several health benefits, including anti-inflammatory, antitumor effects, and the ability to reduce blood glucose and lipid levels. Beans and peas, in particular, contain higher amounts of oligosaccharides than other pulses. Processing methods can alter the composition of resistant starch and polyphenols in pulses, often enhancing their antioxidant activity.

Bioactive compounds are typically nonnutrient constituents found in small quantities (compared to macronutrients) in foods like cereals, legumes, fruits, and vegetables. Pulses are rich in these bioactive substances, which, although not considered nutrients, can still have significant metabolic effects on the human body when consumed (Amarowicz and Pegg 2008). Some of these compounds help protect plants from environmental stressors or predators, while others serve as energy reserves in seeds, primarily for germination. Notable bioactive components in pulses include phytates, lectins, and enzyme inhibitors, which are often viewed as antinutritional factors. However, these substances are mainly concentrated in the hulls of pulses and have been suggested to offer protective health benefits. Dehulling pulses can be a valuable method for extracting specialized phytochemicals from the seed coats, which can be used in the development of nutraceuticals, while the cotyledons provide a rich source of vegetable protein. Polyphenols in pulses are particularly noteworthy for their role in seed color and sensory qualities, as well as their wide range of biological properties, including antioxidant, anti-inflammatory, antiatherogenic, and antimicrobial effects. Additionally, phytosterols have gained attention as important nutraceuticals and functional foods, as they are key components of the lipid membrane in all plant tissues and exhibit antibacterial, anti-inflammatory, antitumor, and antiulcer properties (Girish et al. 2012). While other nonnutritional substances in pulses may also offer physiological benefits, further research is needed to determine the safe and effective concentrations required for optimal effects.

8.7 Nutritional and Ayurvedic Potential in Nuts

Nuts have become an important part of the diet thanks to their unique nutritional profile, distinct flavor, and health benefits, which include high-quality proteins, fiber, minerals, tocopherols, phytosterols, and phenolic compounds. Typically classified as dry fruits with an edible seed and a hard shell, the most widely produced nuts include cashews (*Anacardium occidentale*), walnuts (*Juglans regia*), almonds (*Prunus dulcis*), chestnuts (*Castanea sativa*), pistachios (*Pistacia vera*), and hazelnuts (*Corylus avellana*). Nuts are widely recognized for their rich nutrient content, including monounsaturated and polyunsaturated fatty acids, vitamins E and K, essential minerals like magnesium, copper, potassium, and selenium, dietary fibers, carotenoids, and phytosterols, many of which have potential antioxidant properties (Goncalves et al. 2023). The compact size of nuts also makes them easy to transport, making them an ideal snack for any occasion. Furthermore, regular nut consumption is linked to a reduced risk of chronic diseases, thanks to their beneficial fatty acid profiles, squalene, fibers, plant proteins, vitamins, minerals, carotenoids, and phytosterols. Interestingly, most of the antioxidants in nuts are concentrated in the skin or pellicle, as seen in almonds and peanuts, and these are often lost when the skin is removed. In the case of pistachios, the antioxidants are mostly destroyed when the hard shell is cracked.

In Ayurveda, nuts are regarded as tonics that positively impact the body, mind, and spirit. They are considered nourishing, strengthening, and rejuvenating, promoting the growth of fat, marrow, nerve, and reproductive tissues, as well as supporting the development of blood and muscle. Nuts are also believed to enhance immunity (ojas) and are classified as Sattvic, which is considered pure and harmonious. In addition to their nutritional benefits, tree nuts contain phytochemicals that give them antioxidant, anti-inflammatory, and antiviral properties. However, nuts are high in calories, heavy, and oily, making them harder to digest, so they should be eaten in moderation, particularly for those with a Pitta or Kapha constitution. Soaking nuts and seeds can reduce their heat and phytic acid/tannins, improving their digestibility and absorption. Blanching and peeling nuts also remove the outer covering, making them easier to digest. Nuts are an excellent source of fiber and provide a wide range of nutrients, including vitamins E, B, calcium, selenium, copper, magnesium, riboflavin, iron, potassium, zinc, niacin, thiamine, and folate (Milbury et al. 2006). They are believed to protect against chronic diseases like diabetes and heart conditions. Typically, nuts have a sweet and astringent taste, which is beneficial for Vata and Pitta doshas, while the astringent taste is especially good for Pitta and Kapha doshas. Nuts are also generally heating in nature, which makes them suitable for Vata and Kapha types. Vatas benefit most from nuts due to their high-fat content, with almonds being the best option, especially raw and salted. Roasted almonds should be avoided as they are dry. Pittas thrive on sunflower seeds, pine nuts, and coconut, with blanched and peeled almonds offering a cooling effect. Kapha types should limit nut intake due to their heavy and astringent qualities, which can increase Ama (toxins). Walnuts, with their heating nature, are the most suitable for Kapha, while sunflower and pumpkin seeds are considered tri-doshic (beneficial for all doshas). Nuts can be an excellent snack for weight loss because their high protein and fiber content promote satiety and help regulate blood sugar levels. However, they are not recommended for individuals with poor gut health, digestive issues, bloating, acidity, GERD, diarrhea, IBS, ulcerative colitis, or nut allergies.

According to Ayurveda, nuts are considered as heavy to digest due to their high content of healthy fats, protein, and fiber, and are considered hot in potency; key nutritional compounds in nuts include healthy fats, protein, fiber, magnesium, copper, vitamins E and B, and various antioxidants like phenols and flavonoids, which are considered beneficial in ayurvedic practice (Goncalves et al. 2023). The role of key nutritional compounds found in the nuts includes:

Healthy Fats: Primarily unsaturated fatty acids, considered beneficial for heart health.
Protein: A good source of plant-based protein.
Fiber: Provides digestive support and helps with satiety.
Magnesium: Important for muscle function and nerve health.
Copper: Plays a role in iron absorption and enzyme function.
Vitamin E: A potent antioxidant.
Vitamin B: Important for energy metabolism.

Due to their high fat and protein content, nuts are considered to be heavier on the digestive system and should be consumed in moderation. Ayurveda classifies nuts as having a heating quality, which may not be suitable for individuals with "pitta" dominance. To improve digestibility, Ayurveda often recommends soaking nuts before consumption.

8.8 Specific Nut Compounds and Their Potential Benefits

Walnuts: Rich in omega-3 fatty acids and antioxidants, potentially beneficial for brain health.
Almonds: High in vitamin E and magnesium, considered good for skin and bone health.
Cashews: Contain zinc and copper, important for immune function.
Brazil Nuts: Excellent source of selenium, an important antioxidant.

8.9 Nutritional and Ayurvedic Importance of Herbs

Herbs have been used as food and for medicinal purposes for centuries. Various herbs possess hypolipidemic, antiplatelet, antitumor, or immune-stimulating properties that can be useful adjuncts in helping reduce the risk of cardiovascular disease and cancer. Different herbs are a rich source of a wide variety of active phytochemicals, including flavonoids, terpenoids, lignans, sulfides, polyphenolics, carotenoids, coumarins, saponins, plant sterols, curcumins, and phthalides (Peter 2006). Several of these phytochemicals either inhibit nitrosation or the formation of DNA adducts or stimulate the activity of protective enzymes such as the Phase-II enzyme glutathione transferase. Many of these herbs contain potent antioxidant compounds that provide significant protection against chronic diseases. These compounds may protect LDL cholesterol from oxidation, inhibit cyclooxygenase and lipoxygenase enzymes, inhibit lipid peroxidation, or have antiviral or antitumor activity (Craig 1999). The volatile essential oils of commonly used culinary herbs, spices, and herbal teas inhibit mevalonate synthesis and thereby suppress cholesterol synthesis and tumor growth. A variety of herbs and herbal extracts contain different phytochemicals with biological activity that can provide therapeutic effects. Several herbs can help to reduce high blood cholesterol concentrations, provide some protection against cancer, and stimulate the immune system. Furthermore, a diet in which culinary herbs are used generously to flavor food provides a variety of active phytochemicals that promote health and protect against chronic diseases (Crozier et al. 2009). The discriminate and proper use of some herbal products is safe and may provide some therapeutic benefits, but the indiscriminate or excessive use of herbs can be unsafe and even dangerous.

8.10 Conclusion

Ayurveda places a strong emphasis on the importance of a proper diet for maintaining and enhancing health, as well as preventing and treating diseases. For every condition, specific guidelines for beneficial (pathya) and harmful (apathya) foods are provided. By strictly adhering to dietary recommendations, a person may not need medication, but if the guidelines are ignored, even medicine may not be effective. Eating in the right amounts helps build strength, vitality, and a healthy complexion, and supports tissue health. To live a healthy life, one must align with their environment and follow a diet that suits their unique bodily constitution.

References

Amarowicz R, Pegg RB (2008) Legumes as a source of natural antioxidants. Eur J Lipid Sci Technol 110:865–878

Balasundram N, Sundram K, Samman S (2006) Phenolic compounds in plants and Agri-industrial by-products: antioxidant activity, occurrence, and potential uses. Food Chem 99(1):191–203

Craig WJ (1999) Health-promoting properties of common herbs. Am J Clin Nutr 70(3):491S–499S

Crozier A, Jaganath IB, Clifford MN (2009) Dietary phenolics: chemistry, bioavailability and effects on health. Nat Prod Rep 26(8):1001–1043

Geetha K, Yankanchi GM, Hulamani S, Hiremath N (2020) Glycemic index of millet based food mix and its effect on pre diabetic subjects. J Food Sci Technol 57:2732–2738

Girish TK, Pratape VM, Rao UP (2012) Nutrient distribution, phenolic acid composition, antioxidant and alpha-glucosidase inhibitory potentials of black gram (Vigna mungo L.) and its milled by-products. Food Res Int 46(1):370–377

Goncalves B, Pinto T, Aires A, Morais MC, Bacelar E, Anjos R, Ferreira-Cardoso J, Oliveira I, Vilela A, Cosme F (2023) Composition of nuts and their potential health benefits—an overview. Foods 12(5):942

Jacob J, Krishnan V, Antony C, Bhavyasri M, Aruna C, Mishra K, Nepolean T, Satyavathi CT, Visarada KB (2024) The nutrition and therapeutic potential of millets: an updated narrative review. Front Nutr 11:1346869

Joshi S, Jadhav V, Kadam V (2018) Exotic fruits and vegetable food as nutritional supplement for diabetes, obesity and metabolic diseases. Int J Curr Pharm Res 10(2):51–55

Krishnan V, Verma P, Saha S, Singh B, Vinutha T, Kumar RR, Kulshreshta A, Singh SP, Sathyavathi T, Sachdev A, Praveen S (2022) Polyphenol-enriched extract from pearl millet (Pennisetumglaucum) inhibits key enzymes involved in post prandial hyper glycemia (α-amylase, α-glucosidase) and regulates hepatic glucose uptake. Biocatal Agric Biotechnol 43:102411

Liu RH (2013) Health-promoting components of fruits and vegetables in the diet. Adv Nutr 4(3):384S–392S

Milbury PE, Chen CY, Dolnikowski GG, Blumberg JB (2006) Determination of flavonoids and phenolics and their distribution in almonds. J Agric Food Chem 54(14):5027–5033

Peter KV (ed) (2006) Handbook of herbs and spices. Volume 3. Woodhead Publishing, Cambridge

Saleh AS, Zhang Q, Chen J, Shen Q (2013) Millet grains: nutritional quality, processing, and potential health benefits. Compr Rev Food Sci Food Saf 12(3):281–295

Septembre-Malaterre A, Remize F, Poucheret P (2018) Fruits and vegetables, as a source of nutritional compounds and phytochemicals: changes in bioactive compounds during lactic fermentation. Food Res Int 104:86–99

Singh B, Singh JP, Shevkani K, Singh N, Kaur A (2017) Bioactive constituents in pulses and their health benefits. J Food Sci Technol 54:858–870

Spence C (2025) Unveiling the health-promoting power of bioactive compounds in herbs and spices. Curr Food Sci Technol Rep 3(1):1–9

Tripathi MK, Mohapatra D, Jadam RS, Pandey S, Singh V, Kumar V, Kumar A (2021) Nutritional composition of millets. In: Kumar A, Tripathi MK, Joshi D, Kumar V (eds) Millets and millet technology. Springer Nature Singapore, pp 101–119, eBook ISBN 978-981-16-0676-2

Vincente AR, Manganaris GA, Ortiz CM, Sozzi GO, Crisosto CH (2014) Nutritional quality of fruits and vegetables. In: Postharvest handling. Academic press, pp 69–122

Forest Product Utilization for Development of Nutri-Ayur Components

9

Ankesh Tiwari, Mohineeta Pandey, Astha Tirkey, Roshan Lal Sahu, Rashmi Dubey, and Sudhir Kumar Pandey

Abstract

Nutrition is important for a healthy body and mind. Ayurveda defines how nutritious food can be prepared from forest products, what the components of good food are, and how we can incorporate it into our daily routines. Moreover, consuming an adequate quantity of food is a key principle of Ayurveda for maintaining a healthy life. Ayurveda is a 5000-year-old science that seeks to help individuals understand what is best for them. Its primary goal is to keep a person healthy and cure disease. According to Ayurveda, digestion is more important than merely eating food. Our health completely depends on what we eat and how well we digest it. Ayurveda has always emphasized the importance of easily digestible food. Nowadays, people focus more on consuming processed and fast foods, which can have negative consequences. According to Ayurveda, food should be eaten attentively and with gratitude. It should be fresh, of the highest quality, digestible, flavorful, carefully prepared, and satisfying to the senses. Ayurvedic plants are commonly found in forests, but information about them remains relatively limited. Due to the lack of information and research, these resources are not fully integrated into people's daily lives. Forest-derived raw

A. Tiwari · M. Pandey · S. K. Pandey (✉)
Department of Botany, Guru Ghasidas Vishwavidyalaya, (A Central University) Koni, Bilaspur, Chhattisgarh, India

A. Tirkey
Department of Botany, Government Sant Rameshwar Gahira Guruji Mahavidyalaya, Jashpur, Chhattisgarh, India

R. L. Sahu
Department of Botany, Government Naveen College, Mainpat, Chhattisgarh, India

R. Dubey
Department of Chemistry, Lal Bahadur Shastri College, Shaheed Nandkumar Patel Vishwavidyalaya, Raigarh, Chhattisgarh, India

A. Kumar et al. (eds.), *Innovations in Ayurvedic Nutrition*,
https://doi.org/10.1007/978-981-95-1213-3_9

products are of very high quality and have specific significance. Every living and nonliving thing in the cosmos is made up of five basic elements known as the Pancha Mahabhootas: Earth (Prithvi), Water (Ap), Fire (Teja), Air (Vayu), and Ether (Akasha). The Pancha Mahabhoota components of ingested food sustain their corresponding tissue elements in the body. This chapter provides an overview of the nutri-ayur components derived from forests, including plants and insects. Forest products are rich in nutrition and possess numerous medicinal properties. This chapter also highlights the potential of forest products as a source of income.

Keywords

Panchmahabhoota · Ayurveda · Nutrition · Fibers · Insects

9.1 Introduction

Ayurveda is a 5000-year-old science that aims to assist a person in understanding what is best for them as a unique individual (Rao 2002). It is a kind voyage of self-discovery that equips you with the skills you need to be your own doctor. Ayurveda's name literally translates as "science of life," reflecting the importance of the patient and his disease in the ancient Indian medical system (Pandey et al. 2013). The Sanskrit word Ayur, which means "life" in English, is a component of the word Ayurveda, which means "life knowledge." The art of Ayurveda teaches us about living. Ayurveda claims that maintaining a healthy balance of trayopasthambha is the key to a long and healthy life (three pillars of life). Ahara (diet), Nidra (sleep), and Brahmacharya are explained by Trayopasthambha (abstinence) (Sharma et al. 2022). The importance of Ahara (diet) is highest among these three pillars. The forest is the sole source of the nutri-ayur components used in Ayurveda (Subrat et al. 2002). It has been noted that people in good health are those whose metabolism is in harmony. As it provides a comprehensive approach for living a long, healthy life, Ayurveda is frequently referred to as the "science of longevity." It provides plans for body renewal through diet and nutrition. It provides strategies for treating a variety of common illnesses, including food allergies, which have few effective modern remedies (Pandey et al. 2013). One should be aware that ayurvedic diet is not a "magic bullet" method and that it necessitates the patient's entire cooperation in order to be successful. It is an engaging, user-friendly, interactive system. It teaches the patient to assume personal accountability. Ayurveda is not a nutritional strategy for people seeking an escape or a defense for continuing to mistreat their bodies or brains. It is a long-lasting, independent, and empowering system (Pandey et al. 2013).

The Food and Agriculture Organization of the United Nations (FAO) and the Ministry of Agriculture and Forestry (MAF) presented the significance of a high proportion and high variety of harvested forest products in the daily diet of rural Lao families (Wakdikar 2004). Because they have no side effects and are readily available at reasonable prices, the demand for forest plant-based therapies and medications is rising now in both industrialized and developing nations. According to an ethnobiological survey conducted all over India, there are 8000 plant species used by the population and about 25,000 potent plant-based medicines used in traditional medicine (Wakdikar 2004; Sen and Chakraborty 2017).

In times of adversity, forest resources are frequently exploited to increase household food supplies (Falconer and Arnold 1989). One out of every four people living in poverty around the world is said to be dependent on forests, either directly or indirectly. For a sustainable way of life, the forest supplies the necessary inputs for subsistence needs (food, fuel, fodder, medicine, and shelter), income, and vulnerability (Shukla and Chakravarty 2012). Traditional Ecological Knowledge (TEK) depicts how indigenous people view their environment as well as significant facets of their history, culture, and socioeconomic structure (Urso et al. 2016). In India's rural areas, about 85% of people used wild herbs to treat a range of illnesses (Fransworth 1992; Jain 1992). Ayurvedic medicines, nutritional components, a source of revenue, and fundamental means of subsistence are all provided by the forest. The importance of forests and their products has been covered in this chapter. It has been explained how forests support peasant subsistence, self-insurance, vital food items, the production of ayurvedic medicines, and a fundamental source of revenue.

9.2 Forest Peasant Livelihood

Activities, strategies, policies, assets, and other factors related to survival are essential for a decent livelihood (Chen et al. 2013). It has been widely accepted and discussed globally that forest provides various advantages to adjacent rural communities and society at large (Shackleton et al. 2007). These benefits can be summed up in the form of consumption, aesthetic, employment, and ecological means. Millions of human population living in rural areas depend on forest products and their resources for their daily day-to-day activities. Forest provides valued services of substantial use, which can be implemented through policies. Effective strategies should be adopted by the people to make efficient use of the forest and ecosystem services. The implementation of policies can benefit the social, economic, cultural, and daily activities of people living in and around the forests. People living in forest communities often involve themselves in different forest-related activities which help in the survival of their livelihood (Porro et al. 2015). Forest products such as timber and other woody and nonwoody products have been proved to be of vital importance to humans in providing a daily source of income (Zenteno et al. 2013). Forest livelihood is also crucial in providing safety and security in times of emergency and distress (De Sherbinin et al. 2008). Thus, generating income from forest resources has become a possible strategy for improving rural livelihoods. However, sole dependency on forest resources may limit future development of the environment and society (Zenteno et al. 2013). Therefore, understanding the role of forests in generating income from rural commodities is important in initiating effective strategies for sustainable livelihood.

Forest is located mainly in the remote and rural areas, which means such areas are underdeveloped with limited or no facilities found. The people living in such areas or adjacent areas lack suitable living standards and are poor. So, their source of livelihood depends only on forest products and resources (Sunderlin et al. 2005). Research documents have emphasized that forest resources and their utilization can be effective in reducing poverty and enhancing rural livelihoods (Zada et al. 2019). Forests can support livelihoods by providing food, fodder, income, environmental, and agricultural benefits (Rasmussen et al. 2017). These benefits can help rural people and inhabitants in sustaining decent livelihoods by utilizing the forest products in an effective manner for the return of cash. Therefore, measuring forest contributions in a comprehensive manner is necessary to improve the peasant poverty, and their livelihood (Nerfa et al. 2020).

Various approaches and startup initiatives have been developed for understanding and promoting the role of forest resources in peasant livelihood. In China, people-centered resource and community-related partnership-based initiative has been developed called as community-based co-management (CBCM). CBCM emphasizes the role of community and stakeholders in a positive manner for the development of peasant livelihood and forest resource management (Ting et al. 2011). In India, it is estimated that more than 53 million tribal population and around 60% of rural inhabitants depend on forest products directly or indirectly (Dinda et al. 2020). This can help in improving the livelihood and reducing poverty, especially in underdeveloped countries (Aggarwal and Brockington 2020). People depend on a variety of products for their livelihood, which includes collection of forest commodities such as flowers, roots, shoots, tubers, and leaves for food, agriculture, medicines, lightning fire, construction, and grazing (Atrayee and Chowdhury 2013). Moreover, forest also provides employment to the poor, making a significant contribution to the development of rural livelihood. Besides timber products, non-timber products obtained from forests also provide the essential means for livelihood in times of emergency. According to the Government of India, around 35 million employments were generated in nontimber-related works such as collection and processing, making it an easy source of livelihood in rural areas (Pandey et al. 2016). Furthermore, it is reported that in India, around 275 million people in rural areas (accounting for about 27% of the population) are dependent on the trading of nontimber forest products for the survival of their livelihood (Pandey et al. 2016). Thus, it can be acknowledged that the relationship between forest and rural population has been an important source for peasants' livelihood in providing basic necessities among the village population.

9.3 Forest Food Provides Insurance

Forest provides many nutritious foods, and forest food acts as a safety net in times of food scarcity, reducing food insecurity and malnutrition. Forest food may provide nutrients that humans would not otherwise acquire and may aid in survival during times of famine, war, or drought. In certain circumstances, forest food is the primary source of sustenance, such as for those suffering from human immunodeficiency virus (HIV)/acquired immunodeficiency syndrome (AIDS) and unable to work because of their diseases (Colfer et al. 2006; Vincenti et al. 2008; Johns and Maundu 2006). Forest food does not always contain benefits; sometimes it also contains unhealthy components and toxins. Their actual knowledge is very important for consuming food. Typical forest foods contain wild nuts, leaves, fruits, wild roots, tubers, many mushrooms, and insects. All these include rich protein, carbohydrate, essential amino acids, vitamins, minerals, and fat. They also contain some phytochemicals such as carotenoids and phenolics (Vincenti et al. 2008). Forest foods, such as mushrooms and berries, are also popular in Western countries, owing to their flavor or nutritional and health-promoting properties. Berries from the wild forest and manicured gardens are common in European diets because they are rich in important elements. Phenolic acids, flavonoids, stilbenes, and lignans are phenolic chemicals found in berries (Häkkinen et al. 1999). However, improved understanding of the consumption and bioavailability of dietary bioactive chemicals is required in order to properly evaluate their significance in disease prevention and establish science-based dietary recommendations.

Forest provides mental health, good food, natural resources, medicines, and many income resources. Forest provides many products related to pharmaceuticals. Trees and plants of the forest provide their extract, which contains a variety of bioactive compounds such as polyphenols, phytoestrogens, stilbenes, carotenoids, sterols, etc. (Holmbom et al. 2007; Moutsatsou 2007). All of these components have antioxidant, antiatherogenic, and anticancer action (Kris-Etherton et al. 2002). After all, the forest provides humanity with insurance on behalf of their investment in forest protection. If humans commit their time to protecting the forest, the forest will always defend human life.

9.4 Nutri-Ayur Components from Forest

9.4.1 Component from Plants

All plants contain a variety of rich nutrients, yet we are unaware of what these nutrients are. From the perspective of ayurvedic nutrition, each and every part of the plant is valuable and significant. Forest nontimber products are crucial to household subsistence plans. It gives us vital macronutrients, micronutrients, minerals, proteins, carbohydrates, and fats. A variety of plant parts that are used in nutri-ayur components are described below.

9.4.2 Rhizome or Roots

Ayurveda believes that every plant root has medicinal value, so there is no concept of good and bad food. We need to design an appropriate diet for optimal nutrition and good health (Guha 2006). Rhizomes play a crucial role in ayurvedic nutrition.

For instance, *Curcuma longa* is an important plant used in Ayurveda. Rhizome of this plant is very useful and used as a spice in Indian foods. Rhizome of *Curcuma longa* is full of antibacterial, antifungal, and anti-inflammatory properties. In the form of spice, the rhizome of *Curcuma longa* plays very important role. An appropriate amount of *Curcuma longa* in our food promotes the digestion of food by enhancing the secretion of gastric juice. Another plant is *Gingiber officinalis,* used as a spice in food which is very common in Ayurveda. The nutritional properties of *Gingiber officinalis* are similar to *Curcuma longa,* but it has a lot of other medicinal properties, such as rhizome of *Gingiber officinalis* used as a stimulant, antiemetic drug, analgesic, carminative, decongestant, and as a nervine. Rhizome of *Gingiber officinalis* is a good source of essential amino acids (Ogbuewu et al. 2014). *Maranta arundinacea,* commonly known as West Indian arrowroot, is well-known highly starch-containing medicinal plant used by forest peasants as traditional food and medicine (Pradeepkumar and Pradeep 2008). Tuberous rhizome of *Maranta arundinacea* is used in confectionery and preparation of weaned foods (Jayakumar and Suganthi 2017). *Maranta arundinacea* is mild, so it is a good source of neutral diets. *Maranta arundinacea* is especially helpful for nausea. Due to the very high level of starch, it is used in the preparation of barium meals and tablets (Nishaa et al. 2013). It was also reported that flour of *Maranta arundinacea* is a good source of prebiotics (Harmayani et al. 2011). Similarly, *Dryopteris cochleata* is a herbaceous pteridophyte belonging to the family Dryopteridaceae that exhibit many therapeutic values to treat epilepsy, leprosy, wounds, ulcers, swelling, etc. (Kathirvel et al. 2014). *Nelumbo nucifera* is one of the very common Indian aquatic angiosperms whose rhizome possesses a lot of nutrients such as vitamin C, minerals, and antioxidants (Chen and Tengku 2020). It is also a good source of food due to the high protein and carbohydrate content of the rhizome. Rhizome of *Nelumbo nucifera* is full of minerals such as potassium, copper, and zinc.

9.4.3 Stem

Like other plant parts, stems of many plants are also used as medicine and spices. *Swertia chirayita* is a very unique plant in the traditional medicine system. The stem of this plant is used as an antihelminthic, febrifuge, anticarcinogenic, stomachic, and diuretic. This plant is extensively used in Ayurveda and Unani system of medicine (Williamson 2002). Stem of *Swertia chirayita* is widely used in the treatment of liver-related disorders (Reen et al. 2001). Similarly, *Cinchona* is known for its effective cure of malaria disease. Bark of *Cinchona* produces many alkaloids out of which quinine is the most important alkaloid and has febrifuge properties. Quinine is an infallible drug for the treatment of malaria (Kacprzak 2013). *Boswellia* is another plant belonging to the family Burseraceae is very frequently used in ayurveda system of medicine for inflammatory conditions. Resin of *Boswellia* contained more than 200 compounds (Hamm et al. 2005).

9.4.4 Leaf

Ocimum sp. is very common in traditional medicine system belonging to family Lamiaceae. *Ocimum canum* is used for lowering blood glucose and for treating cold, fever, and parasitic infection. Oils obtained from the leaves possess antibacterial and insecticidal properties. Seeds of *Ocimum canum* is full of fibers (Venkateshappa and Sreenath 2013). Besides, it is also used in common cold, fever, and parasitic infection, and it has antibacterial, insecticidal, and antihelminthic properties. *Adhatoda vasica* is a very important medicinal plant that belongs to the family Acanthaceae and is commonly known as vasaca. Its root, stem, and leaves all have medicinal properties. *Adhatoda vasica* contains many alkaloids. One important alkaloid is vasin found in the leaf of *Adhatoda vasica,* which is used in the treatment of chronic bronchitis and asthma. Leaf juice of *Adhatoda vasica is* also used in the treatment of dysentery and diarrhea. Moreover, this plant has antibacterial, antiviral, antifungal, and antituberculosis activity (Singh et al. 2017).

9.4.5 Fruits

Terminella chebula, Terminella bellirica, and *Phyllanthus emblica* have great medicinal properties. A combination of these three plant products is known as "Triphala." In Ayurveda, triphala is known for its laxative properties. Moreover, triphala is potentially known for its antioxidant, anti-inflammatory, antibacterial, antimutagenic, and reduction of hyperacidity. Besides, phenolics of triphala modulate the human gut microbiota (Peterson et al. 2017). In Ayurveda, *Citrus lemon* is an indispensable part of ahara. Lemon juice works as a stimulant for digestive system. *Citrus lemon* is an important medicinal plant of the family Rutaceae and contains a rich amount of vitamin C (ascorbic acid) and effectively cures vitamin-C deficiency scurvy (Aronson 2001). All parts of this plant have medicinal properties. *Citrus lemon* is mainly known for its alkaloid content which exhibits anticancer, antifungal, antidiabetic, antiviral, and antibacterial properties (Mohanapriya et al. 2013). *Citrus* flavonoids function as free radical scavengers and show antioxidant properties.

Piper nigrum is commonly known as kali mirch. Berries of *Piper nigrum* have been part of traditional Ayurveda. Fruit of *Piper nigrum* contains ascorbic acid, β-carotene, lauric acid, myristic acid, palmitic acid, piperine, Insulin, and tannic acid. It is used as a spice in Indian foods and is full of antioxidant properties (Sharma et al. 2014). It is also used in the treatment of common cold, cough, parasitic infection, and has antidepressant, anti-inflammatory, anticancer, and antidiarrheal activity (Damanhouri and Ahmad 2014).

9.5 Components from Insect

Insects have been consumed by humans for thousands of years, in some cases as emergency food, in others as a mainstay, and in yet others as a delicacy (Bodenheimer 1951; DeFoliart 1995). Estimates of the number of bug species consumed by humans vary, but at least 2100 species have been reported as human food globally (Jongema 2017). In recent times, many communities have avoided entomophagy (the habit of eating insects) as ancient, unclean, or harmful. Nonetheless, insects are a vital and favored food source of protein, fat, minerals, and vitamins in many societies around the world (Belluco et al. 2013; Finke 2002; Melo et al. 2011). Protein values in crickets, grasshoppers, and locusts, for instance, often range between 60% and 80% on a dry weight basis (Rumpold and Schlüter 2013; Blásquez et al. 2012). Insect proteins are generally thought to be of high quality, being bioavailable and digestible (Belluco et al. 2013; Verkerk et al. 2007; Finke 2015). Essential amino acids derived from insects may be especially beneficial in areas where hunger is still a concern. Insects, fortunately, frequently include complementary necessary amino acids that are absent in staple-based diets dominated by grains (for example, maize), tubers, or legumes (Van Huis et al. 2013; Manditsera et al. 2019; Nadeau et al. 2015). In some areas, insects are a more affordable protein source than beef (Van Huis et al. 2013; Raksakantong et al. 2010). Harvesting, processing, shipping, and retailing edible forest insects provide an undetermined number of individuals across the world with exciting income and livelihood prospects. Traditionally, these operations were all local and largely unnoticed. However, more sophisticated and widespread marketing and commercialization of edible forest insects, including beautiful packaging and advertising, have recently advanced.

9.5.1 Diversity of Edible Forest Insect

The maximum number of insects that can be legally consumed worldwide ranges from 2000 to 3000, but the actual number may be much higher because most of the insects that indigenous cultures and other ethnic groups consume have not been systematically recognized (Hanboonsong et al. 2013). Therefore, despite the fact that incomplete data are available for some countries, the proportion of forest insects used in human nutrition and traditional medicine is still unknown (Jongema 2015; Mitsuhashi 2017). For instance, a total of 25 edible caterpillars were reported from the Bas-Congo province in the Democratic Republic of the Congo, with popular species including *Antheraea* spp., *Imbrasia* spp., *Cirina forda* Westwood, and *Bunaea alcinoe* (Stoll). Eight species (*alopia*, *anthina*, *ebilis*, *epimethea*, *melanops*, *ob- sura*, *petiveri*, and *swahlbergii*) have been identified in the one genus Imbrasia (Kelemu et al. 2015). In India, Manipur and Nagaland each have 41 species, Assam has 38 species, Meghalaya has 16 species, Kerala has five species, while Karnataka, Tamil Nadu, Odisha, and Madhya Pradesh each have one species of edible forest insect (Meyer-Rochow and Chakravorty 2013). Similar to prior surveys conducted in Nagaland, Meyer-Rochow and Changkija (1997) reported nine species of forest beetles belonging to seven genera as being eaten as food by Naga tribal people. Kakati and Chutia (2009) documented as many as 14 species of wild silkworms belonging to eight genera. Some edible insects are described in Table 9.1.

9.5.2 Advantages of Eating Insects

It is clear that both the prehistoric communities and the progenitors of *Homo sapiens* relied on insects for food and nourishment. As shown by coprolites, or fossilized human feces, insects were a significant element of human diets before they developed tools for food hunting and gathering (Ortiz et al. 2016; Hardy et al. 2017). For instance, coprolites from caves in the Ozark Plateau in the central United States contain ants, beetle larvae, lice, ticks, and mites. This region is located between Arkansas and Missouri (Mitsuhashi 2008). Most of the time, insects are known to be a readily available source of protein, fats, carbs, some vitamins, and minerals like calcium, iron, or zinc. Chitin, which makes up about 5–20% of the dry weight of insects, contains the majority of their carbohydrates (Chen et al. 2009; Payne et al. 2016). Stink bugs have a carbohydrate value of 6.71%, while cicadas have a carbohydrate content of 15.98% (Raksakantong et al. 2010). A significant number of polysaccharides found in them have been shown in studies to enhance human immunological functions. Chitin has minimal caloric values but is also recognized to have therapeutic benefits (Govorushko 2019).

If the primary objective of supporters of entomophagy is to reduce the environmental impact of food production, realistic goals that focus on systemic blame are vital. Given that insects are more attractive than animals due to their better conversion efficiency, perhaps the best course of action is to raise the latter by using the former (DeFoliart 1975; DeFoliart 1989). In addition to the ecological functions they offer, insects have long been associated with human civilization throughout history. This association dates back to antiquity. The following seven categories were created in the nineteenth century after extensive research on helpful insects: (1) insects that produce silk; (2) insects that produce honey, wax, etc.; (3) insects that produce dyes; (4) insects that produce manna (sap or juice released by a plant after being stung by an insect); (5) insects that are edible; (6) insects that are sources of medicine; and (7) insects that are used as ornaments. Since many helpful insects fall under more than one category, the aforementioned divisions are not mutually exclusive, but there is always a strong connection to ecological functions (Bodenheimer 1951).

The daily diets of rural communities sometimes include edible forest insects. This is especially evident in economically underdeveloped nations where family food insecurity and nutritional insecurity are linked not only to inadequate dietary intake of energy and nutrients but also to orthodox traditional food consumption patterns and socioeconomic position (Parappurathu et al. 2019). Major nutrients, including carbs (2.7–49.8 mg/kg, fresh weight), protein (20–76%, dry weight), and fat (2–50%, dry weight), are present in all edible insects. Some insects have more saturated than unsaturated fatty acids, as demonstrated by Sayed et al. (2019) for

Table 9.1 Diversity of insect species from the forest used for human consumption

S.no.	Insect sp.	Consuming stage	Country region	References
1	*Cirina forda* Westwood	Larva	Central African Republic, Democratic Republic of Congo, Nigeria	FAO (2004); Paiko et al. (2014)
2	*Imbrasia belina* Waterhouse	Larva	Central Africa, DRC, Zimbabwe	Kwiri et al. (2014); Nadeau et al. (2015)
3	*Macrotermes* spp.	Adult	East Africa, South Africa, Nigeria	Alemu et al. (2015); Netshifhefhe et al. (2018)
4	*Omphisa fuscidentalis* (Hamp.)	Larva	Thailand	Hanboonsong et al. (2013); Taylor and Wang (2018)
5	*Oryctes rhinoceros* (L.)	Larva	Thailand, Nigeria	Ratcliffe (2006); Okaraonye and Ikewuchi (2009)
6	*Oecophylla smaragdina* Fb.	Egg, adult	Thailand, India, Australia	Hanboonsong et al. (2013); Borgohain et al. (2014); Chakravorty et al. (2016)
7	*Ruspolia differens* (Serville)	Adult	Kenya, Uganda, Tanzania	Mmari et al. (2017); Fombong et al. (2017)
8	*Ruspolia nitidula* (Scopoli)	Adult	Kenya, Uganda	Ssepuuya et al. (2017)
9	*Rhynchophorus ferrugineus* Olivier	Larva	Egypt	Abdel-Moniem et al. (2017)
10	*Rhynchophorus* palmmarum (L.)	Larva	South America, Ivory Coast	Cerda et al. (2001); Gbogouri et al. (2013)
11	*Rhynchophorus phoenicis* (Fb.)	Larva	Nigeria, Cameroon	Ekpo (2010); Meutchieye and Niassy (2016)
12	*Phiosamia ricini Hutt.*	Pupa	India	Sarmah (2011); Longvah et al. (2011)
13	*Chortoicetes terminifera* Australian plague locust	Adult	Australia	Van Huis et al. (2013); Kouřimská and Adámková (2016)
14	*Tenebrio molitor* Yellow mealworm beetle	Larva	USA	Van Huis et al. (2013); Kouřimská and Adámková (2016)
15	*Atta mexicana* Mexican leafcutting ant	Adult	Mexico	Van Huis et al. (2013); Kouřimská and Adámková (2016)
16	*Gryllus bimaculatus* Two-spotted cricket	Adult	Thailand	Van Huis et al. (2013); Kouřimská and Adámková (2016)
17	*Oxya japonica* Japanese grasshopper	Adult	Thailand	Van Huis et al. (2013); Kouřimská and Adámková (2016)

(continued)

Table 9.1 (continued)

S.no.	Insect sp.	Consuming stage	Country region	References
18	*Cyrtacanthacris tatarica* Brown-spotted locust	Adult	Thailand	Van Huis et al. (2013); Kouřimská and Adámková (2016)
19	*Bombyx mori* Silkworm	Pupa	Thailand	Van Huis et al. (2013); Kouřimská and Adámková (2016)
20	*Locusta migratoria* African migratory locust	Adult	Netherlands	Van Huis et al. (2013); Kouřimská and Adámková (2016)
21	*Bunaea alcinoe*	Larva	West and central Africa	Adeoye et al. (2014)
22	*Oryctes* spp. *Oliver*	Larva	Africa	Adeoye et al. (2014)
23	*Analeptes trifasciata* Rhinocerus beetle	Larva	Africa	Adeoye et al. (2014)
24	*Anaphe venata* Caterpillar	Larva	Nigeria	Adeoye et al. (2014)
25	*Heteroligus meles* Billberger Yam beetle	Adult	Nigeria, Africa	Adeoye et al. (2014)
26	*Zonocerus Variegatus*, Grasshopper	Adult	West and Central Africa	Adeoye et al. (2014)
27	*Apis mellifera* Honeybee	Eggs, larvae, and pupae	Almost all over world	Adeoye et al. (2014)
28	*Macrotermes belliscosus* Termites	Winged adults, queen	Africa and Southest Asia	Adeoye et al. (2014)
29	*Brachytrupes* Cricket	Adult	Burkina Faso	Adeoye et al. (2014)
30	*Gryllotalpa Africana* Cricket	Adult	South Africa and Australia	Adeoye et al. (2014)

Bactrocera zonata Saunders and *Spodoptera littoralis* Boisduval. The overall unsaturated fatty acid concentration may be as high as 70% of the total fatty acids. Oleic, linoleic, and palmitic acids are the most prevalent unsaturated fatty acids, with essential amino acid levels typically ranging from 10 to 30%, covering 35 to 50% of all types of amino acids. This shows that a variety of bug species may contribute significantly to human nutrition. Generally speaking, amino acids can satisfy the FAO/WHO recommended daily requirement (Ayieko et al. 2012; Chakravorty et al. 2014; Chakravorty et al. 2016). Most insects include significant levels of the vitamins A, B, C, D, E, and K as well as the minerals P, K, Na, Cu, Fe, Zn, Ca, and Mg (Van Huis et al. 2013; Kouřimská and Adámková 2016; Ghosh et al. 2017). An insect's nutritional value can benefit from its intestinal composition as well (Mutungi et al. 2019). In Nigeria, 100 g of caterpillar supplies about 100% of an adult's vitamin needs and 76% of the daily necessary protein intake, respectively (Agbidye et al. 2009).

9.6 Forests Products as Source of Income

Forest products encompass a broad range of products with various biological origins, such as microbes (bacteria, fungi), plants, and animals (Nerfa et al. 2020). Thus, the materials collected from the forest ecosystem after further processing are a source of income when marketed with a proper marketing strategy (Hetemäki and Hurmekoski 2016). These forest products have been utilized as a source of income for the past decades (Arnold and Townson 1998). A few chief forest products with global recognition that include woods, paper, and nontimber products such as mushrooms, berries, nuts, medicinal plants, honey, broomsticks, roof materials, and extracted oils are also a source of rural income (Mukul et al. 2016; Lovrić et al. 2020; Talukdar et al. 2021). The population in rural areas is mainly dependent on forest products for their daily bread (Shrestha et al. 2020; Ushadevi and Vijaykumar 2022). A study from Patharia Hills Reserve Forest, South Assam, India investigated the area for nontimber forest products (Talukdar et al. 2021). The study reported the availability of food, construction, and roof materials. To earn money and support their daily lives, many households gather small goods to sell in their local marketplaces from the forest. Pegu et al. (2013) studied wild edible plants in the entire Jonai Subdivision, Dhemaji district, Assam, and observed 89 species, 52 families, and two fern species, *Cyclosorus extensa* and *Diplazium esculentum*. There are 26 species that are only used for food, whereas other species have multiple applications, like medicine and animal feed. Many species also provide livelihoods and sources of income. The majority of a plant's parts, including the leaves, stems, flowers, fruits, roots, and tubers, are edible and also provide income.

9.7 Environmental Services

Environmental services are another good source of poverty alleviation. It involves a direct and indirect role in poverty alleviation. Firstly, forest people directly benefit from a healthy forest ecosystem, for example, forests provide quantity and fresh quality of water supplies and enhance the fertility of soil by restoring soil and agroforestry systems (Sanchez et al. 1997). Moreover, forest biodiversity supplies various ecological benefits like germplasm for crop quality improvement. Off-site users typically pay forest people to maintain the ecological services of the forest. These payments can improve the income of forest people and help in reducing poverty (Lovrić et al. 2020).

9.8 Income from Nutri-Ayur Components of Forest

There are lots of nutritious products available in the forest which can be used in the diet (Nimbekar and Sanghi 2022). Medicinal plants from the forest are the main source of many medicines and most of the indigenous medicinal plants are used as food and spices by rural people. These medicinal plants are of extreme importance to the people and their health (Maes et al. 2011). Plant parts such as leaves, flowers, fruits, seeds, tubers, and roots are used for various medicinal purposes to cure many fatal diseases. Moreover, there are some secondary metabolites used for the treatment of a diverse group of diseases. Besides, a lot of physiological components associated with plants are exploited by traditional medicine practitioners in treating a diverse range of ailments (Ajibesin et al. 2011). So, we can say that forest is a storehouse of lots of medicinal plants used in Ayurveda. These medications are frequently a mainstay of the poor's access to healthcare, and many individuals take advantage of them. In actuality, 40–50% of individuals in Germany, 42% in the USA, 48% in Australia, and 49% in France use traditional medicines. Traditional medicines made from wild plant and animal sources are a significant export industry in both China and India (Pandey et al. 2016). In this way, Ayurveda completely depends on the forest product, and the whole income that comes from Ayurveda is a consequence of the forest product (Srivastava et al. 2022). Some forest products used as a source of income are given in Table 9.2. Bamboo, honey, spices, medicinal plants, fruits, and mushrooms are a few forest products that are frequently collected for income generation (Worku 2015; Ushadevi and Vijaykumar 2022). However, there are forest products which are directly utilized and not collected for sale purposes, such as medicinal plants, and are consumed directly as prescribed by the traditional practitioners (Beyene et al. 2020). In these cases, the additional step of processing the forest products is not required. Table 9.3 highlights the few forest products commonly collected for monetary reasons by humankind along with their uses.

The majority of the revenue from forest products is generated by timber-based forests, such as wood, furniture, and resins. Nutri-Ayur ingredients also originate from the forest, but knowledge of them is only available in the villages that rely on the forest for their survival. For future improvement, the knowledge of these components has to be expanded. Numerous ayurvedic medications originate in forests as well; however, research to discover the secret ingredients is ongoing.

9.9 Conclusions

Ayurvedic medicines, wholesome food, fruits, and many other necessities can be found in the forest. Our daily lives are made easier and more practical by the forest. Numerous nutrients are also obtained from plants and insects in the forest. Plant roots, stems, leaves, and bark are rich sources of several ingredients. Every part of a plant can be used to heal a variety of illnesses and provide energy. A nutrient-rich diet that includes proteins, minerals, nucleic acids, amino acids, vitamins, and a variety of electrolytes is one that includes insects that belong to the forest. The forest is a reliable source of income since it offers high-quality goods for daily use, medicines, and wood. This chapter highlights the utilization of forest products in ayurvedic treatment and nutrition, dietary management, and nutrition maintenance. Although it is simple to obtain nutri-ayur components from the forest, only those who live there are aware of its benefits. So, one needs to learn about these

Table 9.2 Forest products as a source of income

S.no.	Wild plants	Part used	Income information	References
1	*Amaranthus caudatus* L.	Tender leaves and shoots for vegetable	Weed, cash income	Mejía-Valvas et al. (2021)
2	*Anthocephalus chinensis* (Lamk.)	Mildly acidic fruit either eaten raw or cooked as a vegetable.	Ornamental; fuel wood; cash income	Rajalingam et al. (2017)
3	*Antidesma acidum* Retz.	Ripe fruit eaten; leaves prepared for curry.	Leaf preparation in headaches; stem to stimulate menstrual flow; fuel wood; cash income	Pegu et al. (2013)
4	*Baccuarea ramifolira*	Pulp of fruit is eaten by all community; tender shoots eaten cooked.	Bark for mouth ulcer in children. Fuel wood; cash income	Pegu et al. (2013)
5	*Bacopa monnieri (L.)*	Leaves cooked and taken as vegetable.	Whole plant for constipation, cough, fever, a clearing voice, and diabetes; nerve tonic. Cash income	Mohamed and Hamza (2022)
6	*Centella asiatica*	Aerial parts used as a vegetable with small fish. Prefers as chutney.	For stomach complaints and liver tonic, and for increasing memory. Leaf paste in wounds, cuts. Cash income	Puttarak et al. (2017)
7	*Cinnamomum tamala*	Mature leaves and bark are used to flavor curries, tea, polao, etc., for making yeast culture.	Antimicrobial and antioxidant; used to cure diarrhea and colic pain. Cash income	Kuna et al. (2020)
8	*Colocasia esculanta*	Tender leaves, runners, and corms eaten cooked with fruits of *Dillenia indica* and dried fish. Leaves grinded with dried fish and kept in the bamboo tube for future use	Whole plant is used as medicine to purify blood, coagulant; pig feed. Cash income	Talwana et al. (2009)
9	*Dillenia indica L.*	Misings and Bodos prefer to cook the fruit with fish and pork.	Fresh fruit for diabetes. Mucilage of fruit as hair washes. Cash income.	Tamang et al. (2020)

components. As such, lot of studies are being done in this area. There is a pressing need to study the importance and utilize the nutri-ayur components of forest products in a wise and sustainable manner.

Table 9.3 Common uses of forest products

S.no.	Forest product	Uses	References
1.	Bamboo *Dendrocalamus hamiltonii, D. longispathus, Melocanna baccifera, schizostachyum dullooa,*	House construction, furniture, cups, baskets, musical instruments such as flutes	Worku (2015); Talukdar et al. (2021)
2	Honey	Food/nutritional	Srećković et al. (2019)
3	*Calamus guruba, Calamus tenuis, Pinanga gracilis*	Roof material	Talukdar et al. (2021); Borah et al. (2020)
4	*Litsea khasyana, Artocarpus lakoocha, Vanilla planifolia, Garcinia gummigutta, Zanthoxylum rhetsa.*	Spices, food additives	Worku (2015); Hanumantha et al. (2019); Borah et al. (2020)
5	*Thunbergia grandiflora, Hoya verticillate, Alstonia scholaris, Aristolochia assamica, Aristolochia saccata Wall., Acmella paniculate, Chromolaena odorata, Mikania micrantha, Begonia silhetensis, Hodgsonia macrocarpa*	Medicinal plants	Borah et al. (2020)
6	*Solena heterophylla, Bauhinia variegate, Rhynchotechum ellipticum, Parabaena sagittate, Horsfieldia kingii, Lepionurus sylvestris, Artocarpus lacucha, Baccaurea ramiflora*	Consumable (raw/dried/cooked)	Borah et al. (2020)
7	*Cichorium intybus, Cirsium arvense, Matricaria chamomilla, Taraxacum officinale, Tussilago farfara, Betula* spp., *Vaccinium myrtillus.*	Beverage	Kolosova et al. (2020)

References

Abdel-Moniem ASH, El-Kholy MY, Elshekh WEA (2017) The red palm weevil, Rhynchophorus ferrugineus Olivier, as edible insects for food and feed a case study in Egypt. Res J Pharm Biol Chem Sci 8:1653–1658

Adeoye OT, Alebiosu BI, Akinyemi OD, Adeniran OA (2014) Socio economic analysis of forest edible insects species consumed and its role in the livelihood of people in Lagos State. Food Stud 3:104

Agbidye FS, Ofuya TI, Akindele SO (2009) Marketability and nutritional qualities of some edible forest insects in Benue State, Nigeria. Pak J Nutr 8(7):917–922

Aggarwal A, Brockington D (2020) Reducing or creating poverty? Analyzing livelihood impacts of forest carbon projects with evidence from India. Land Use Policy 95:104608

Ajibesin KK, Bala DN, Umoh UF (2011) The use of medicinal plants to treat sexually transmitted diseases in Nigeria: ethnomedicinal survey of Niger Delta Region. Int J Green Pharm 5(3):181

Alemu MH, Olsen SB, Vedel SE, Pambo KO, Owino VO (2015) Consumer acceptance and willingness to pay for edible insects as food in Kenya: the case of white winged termites IFRO working paper

Arnold M, Townson J (1998) Assessing the potential of forest product activities to contribute to rural incomes in Africa Natural Resources Perspectives 37. Overseas Development Institute, London, UK

Aronson JK (2001) Forbidden fruit. Nat Med 7(1):29–30

Atrayee B, Chowdhury M (2013) Forest degradation and livelihood of local communities in India: a human rights approach. J Hortic For 5(8):122–129

Ayieko MA, Kinyuru JN, Ndong'a MF, Kenji GM (2012) Nutritional value and consumption of black ants (Carebara vidua Smith) from the Lake Victoria region in Kenya. Adv J Food Sci Technol 4(1):39–45

Belluco S, Losasso C, Maggioletti M, Alonzi CC, Paoletti MG, Ricci A (2013) Edible insects in a food safety and nutritional perspective: a critical review. Compr Rev Food Sci Food Saf 12(3):296–313

Beyene AD, Mekonnen A, Hirons M, Robinson EJ, Gonfa T, Gole TW, Demissie S (2020) Contribution of non-timber forest products to the livelihood of farmers in coffee growing areas: evidence from Yayu Coffee Forest Biosphere Reserve. J Environ Plan Manag 63(9):1633–1654

Blásquez JRE, Moreno JMP, Camacho VHM (2012) Could grasshoppers be a nutritive meal. In Food Nutr Sci 3(2):164–175

Bodenheimer FS (1951) Insects as human food. In: A chapter of the ecology of man. The Hague

Borah D, Tangjang S, Das AP, Upadhaya A, Mipun P (2020) Assessment of non-timber forest products (NTFPs) in Behali Reserve Forest, Assam, Northeast India. Ethnobot Res Appl 19(43):1–15

Borgohain M, Borkotoki A, Mahanta R (2014) Total lipid, triglyceride and cholesterol contents in Oecophylla smaragdina, Fabricius consumed in Upper Assam of North East India. Int J Sci Res Publ 4(7):455

Cerda H, Martínez R, Briceño N, Pizzoferrato L, Manzi P, Ponzetta MT, Paoletti MG (2001) Palm worm:(Rhynchophorus palmarum) traditional food in Amazonas, Venezuela—nutritional composition, small scale production and tourist palatability. Ecol Food Nutr 40(1):13–32

Chakravorty J, Ghosh S, Jung C, Meyer-Rochow VB (2014) Nutritional composition of Chondacris rosea and Brachytrupes orientalis: two common insects used as food by tribes of Arunachal Pradesh, India. J Asia Pac Entomol 17(3):407–415

Chakravorty J, Ghosh S, Megu K, Jung C, Meyer-Rochow VB (2016) Nutritional and anti-nutritional composition of Oecophylla smaragdina (Hymenoptera: Formicidae) and Odontotermes sp.(Isoptera: Termitidae): two preferred edible insects of Arunachal Pradesh, India. J Asia Pac Entomol 19(3):711–720

Chen H, Zhu T, Krott M, Calvo JF, Ganesh SP, Makoto I (2013) Measurement and evaluation of livelihood assets in sustainable forest commons governance. Land Use Policy 30(1):908–914

Chen SY, Tengku RTM (2020) Effect of cooking methods on nutritional composition and antioxidant properties of lotus (Nelumbo nucifera) rhizome. Food Res 4(4):1207–1216

Chen X, Feng Y, Chen Z (2009) Common edible insects and their utilization in China. Entomol Res 39(5):299–303

Colfer CJP, Sheil D, Kishi M (2006) Forests and human health: assessing the evidence. CIFOR Occasional Paper No. 45; CIFOR: Bogor, Indonesia

Damanhouri ZA, Ahmad A (2014) A review on therapeutic potential of Piper nigrum L. (Black Pepper): the King of Spices. Med Aromat Plants 3(3):161

De Sherbinin A, VanWey LK, McSweeney K, Aggarwal R, Barbieri A, Henry S, Walker R (2008) Rural household demographics, livelihoods and the environment. Glob Environ Chang 18(1):38–53

DeFoliart GR (1975) Insects as a source of protein. Bull Entomol Soc Am 21(3):161e163

DeFoliart GR (1989) The human use of insects as food and as animal feed. Am Entomol 35(1):22–36

Defoliart GR (1995) Edible insects as minilivestock. Biodivers Conserv 4(3):306–321

Dinda S, Ghosh S, Chatterjee ND (2020) Understanding the commercialization patterns of non-timber forest products and their contribution to the enhancement of tribal livelihoods: an empirical study from Paschim Medinipur District, India. Small Scale For 19(3):371–397

Ekpo KE (2010) Nutrient composition, functional properties and anti-nutrient content of Rhynchophorus pheonicis (F) larva. Ann Biol Res 1(1):178–190

Falconer J, Arnold JEM (1989) Household Food Security and Forestry: an analysis of socio economic issues. Community Forestry Note 1, FAO, Rome, Italy

FAO (2004) Contribution des insects de la foret a la securite alimentaire: l'example des chenilles d'Afrique Central. NTFP working document no.1. FAO, Rome. http://www.fao.org/docrep/007/j3463f/j3463f3400.htm

Finke MD (2002) Complete nutrient composition of commercially raised invertebrates used as food for insectivores. Zoo Biol 21(3):269–285

Finke MD (2015) Complete nutrient content of four species of commercially available feeder insects fed enhanced diets during growth. Zoo Biol 34(6):554–564

Fombong FT, Van Der Borght M, Vanden Broeck J (2017) Influence of freeze-drying and oven-drying post blanching on the nutrient composition of the edible insect Ruspolia differens. Insects 8(3):102

Fransworth NR (1992) Ethnopharmacology and drug development. In: Chadwick DJ, Edt MU (eds) Ethnobotany and search for New drugs, Ciba Foundation Symposium, vol 183. Wiley, Chichester, p 42

Gbogouri GA, Beugre GAM, Brou K, Atchibri OA, Linder M (2013) Rhynchophorus palmarum L. larva, an edible insect in Côte D'ivoire: nutritional value and characterization of the lipid fraction. Int J Chem Sci 11:1692–1704

Ghosh S, Lee SM, Jung C, Meyer-Rochow VB (2017) Nutritional composition of five commercial edible insects in South Korea. J Asia Pac Entomol 20(2):686–694

Govorushko S (2019) Global status of insects as food and feed source: a review. Trends Food Sci Technol 91:436–445

Guha A (2006) Ayurvedic concept of food and nutrition. School Med Articles 25:4–7

Häkkinen SH, Kärenlampi SO, Heinonen IM, Mykkänen HM, Törrönen AR (1999) Content of the flavonols quercetin, myricetin, and kaempferol in 25 edible berries. J Agric Food Chem 47(6):2274–2279

Hamm S, Bleton J, Connan J, Tchapla A (2005) A chemical investigation by headspace SPME and GC–MS of volatile and semi-volatile terpenes in various olibanum samples. Phytochemistry 66(12):1499–1514

Hanboonsong Y, Jamjanya T, Durst PB (2013) Six-legged livestock: edible insect farming, collection and marketing in Thailand. RAP Publ 3:8–21

Hanumantha M, Bisanalli SI, Patil RS, Manjunatha GO (2019) Utilization pattern of non-timber forest products (NTFPS) in Siddapura taluk of Uttara Kannada district of western Ghat region, Karnataka. J Pharmacogn Phytochem 8(3):901–905

Hardy K, Radini A, Buckley S, Blasco R, Copeland L, Burjachs F, Bermúdez de Castro JM (2017) Diet and environment 1.2 million years ago revealed through analysis of dental calculus from Europe's oldest hominin at Sima del Elefante, Spain. Sci Nat 104(1):1–5

Harmayani E, Kumalasari ID, Marsono Y (2011) Effect of arrowroot (Maranta arundinacea L.) diet on the selected bacterial population and chemical properties of caecal digesta of Sprague Dawley rats. Int Res J Microbiol 2(8):278–284

Hetemäki L, Hurmekoski E (2016) Forest products markets under change: review and research implications. Curr For Rep 2(3):177–188

Holmbom B, Willför S, Hemming J, Pietarinen S, Nisula S, Eklund P, Sjöholm R (2007) Knots in trees—a rich source of bioactive polyphenols. In: Argyropoulos DS (ed) Materials, chemicals and energy from forest biomass, ACS Symposium Series, vol 954. ACS, pp 350–362

Jain SK (1992) Ethnopharmacology and drug development. In: Chadwick DJ, March U (eds) Ethnobotany and search for New drugs, Ciba Foundation Symposium, vol 183. Wiley, Chichester, p 153

Jayakumar A, Suganthi A (2017) Biochemical and phytochemical analysis of Maranta arundinacea (L.) Rhizome. Int J Res Pharm Pharm Sci 2(3):26–30

Johns T, Maundu P (2006) Forest biodiversity, nutrition and population health in market-oriented food systems. Unasylva-FAO 57(2):34

Jongema Y (2015) List of edible insect species of the world. http://www. ent.wur.nl/UK/Edible (Insects Worldwide Species List)

Jongema Y (2017) List of edible insects of the world. www.wageningenur.nl/en/Expertise-Services/Chair-groups/Plant-Sciences/Laboratory-of-Entomology/Edible-insects/Worldwide-species-list.htm. Accessed 18 September 2018

Kacprzak KM (2013) Chemistry and biology of Cinchona alkaloids. Nat Prod 1:605–641

Kakati LN, Chutia BC (2009) Diversity and ecology of wild sericigenous insects in Nagaland, India. Trop Ecol 50(1):137–146

Kathirvel A, Rai AK, Maurya GS, Sujatha V (2014) Dryopteris cochleata rhizome: a nutritional source of essential elements, phytochemicals, antioxidants and antimicrobials. Int J Pharm Pharm Sci 6:179–188

Kelemu S, Niassy S, Torto B, Fiaboe K, Affognon H, Tonnang H, Ekesi S (2015) African edible insects for food and feed: inventory, diversity, commonalities and contribution to food security. J Insects Food Feed 1(2):103–119

Kolosova V, Belichenko O, Rodionova A, Melnikov D, Sõukand R (2020) Foraging in Boreal Forest: wild food plants of the republic of Karelia, NW Russia. Foods 9(8):1015

Kouřimská L, Adámková A (2016) Nutritional and sensory quality of edible insects. NFS J 4:22–26

Kris-Etherton PM, Hecker KD, Bonanome A, Coval SM, Binkoski AE, Hilpert KF, Etherton TD (2002) Bioactive compounds in foods: their role in the prevention of cardiovascular disease and cancer. Am J Med 113(9):71–88

Kuna A, Sahoo MR, Mandarapu S, Mayengbam PD, Dasgupta M, Mulinti S (2020) Nutrient, antioxidant and anti nutrient composition of value added products made with underutilized forest produce bay leaf (Cinnamomum tamala). Agric Eng Int CIGR J 22(2):226–234

Kwiri R, Winini C, Muredzi P, Tongonya J, Gwala W, Mujuru F, Gwala ST (2014) Mopane worm (Gonimbrasia belina) utilisation, a potential source of protein in fortified blended foods in Zimbabwe: a review. Glob J Sci Front Res D Agric Vet 14:55–66

Longvah T, Mangthya K, Ramulu PJFC (2011) Nutrient composition and protein quality evaluation of eri silkworm (Samia ricinii) prepupae and pupae. Food Chem 128(2):400–403

Lovrić M, Da Re R, Vidale E, Prokofieva I, Wong J, Pettenella D, Mavsar R (2020) Non-wood forest products in Europe–A quantitative overview. Forest Policy Econ 116:102175

Maes J, Paracchini ML, Zulian G (2011) A European assessment of the provision of ecosystem services. Towards and atlas of ecosystem services. Ispra: Joint Research Centre, IES (EUR 24750 EN – 2011)

Manditsera FA, Luning PA, Fogliano V, Lakemond CM (2019) The contribution of wild harvested edible insects (Eulepida mashona and Henicus whellani) to nutrition security in Zimbabwe. J Food Compos Anal 75:17–25

Mejía-Valvas RL, Gómez-Pando L, Pinedo-Taco R (2021) Characterization of the productive units of kiwicha (Amaranthus caudatus) cropping in the provinces of Yungay, Huaylas and Carhuaz, department of Ancash, Peru. Cienc Tecnol Agropecuaria 22(1):1440

Melo V, Garcia M, Sandoval H, Jiménez HD, Calvo C (2011) Quality proteins from edible indigenous insect food of Latin America and Asia. Emir J Food Agric 23(3):283

Meutchieye F, Niassy S (2016) Preliminary observations on the commercialisation of Rynchophorus phoenicis larvae at Mvog-Mbi market in Yaoundé, Cameroon. J Insects Food Feed 2(3):199–202

Meyer-Rochow VB, Chakravorty J (2013) Notes on entomophagy and entomotherapy generally and information on the situation in India in particular. Appl Entomol Zool 48(2):105–112

Meyer-Rochow VB, Changkija S (1997) Uses of insects as human food in Papua New Guinea, Australia, and North-East India: cross-cultural considerations and cautious conclusions. Ecol Food Nutr 36(2–4):159–185

Mitsuhashi J (2008) Entomophagy: human consumption of insects. In: Capinera JL (ed) Encyclopedia of entomology 3. Springer, Heidelberg, pp 1341–1134

Mitsuhashi J (2017) Edible insects of the world. CRC Press, Boca Raton, FL, p 296

Mmari MW, Kinyuru JN, Laswai HS, Okoth JK (2017) Traditions, beliefs and indigenous technologies in connection with the edible longhorn grasshopper Ruspolia differens (Serville 1838) in Tanzania. J Ethnobiol Ethnomed 13(1):1–11

Mohamed MF, Hamza EM (2022) Mass propagation, Cultivation, Phytochemical and Fingerprint of Bacopa monnieri L. in Egypt. Egypt J Hortic 49(2):199–213

Mohanapriya M, Ramaswamy L, Rajendran R (2013) Health and medicinal properties of lemon (Citrus limonum). Int J Ayurvedic Herb Med 3(1):1095–1100

Moutsatsou P (2007) The spectrum of phytoestrogens in nature: our knowledge is expanding. Hormones (Athens) 6(3):173

Mukul SA, Rashid AM, Uddin MB, Khan NA (2016) Role of non-timber forest products in sustaining forest-based livelihoods and rural households' resilience capacity in and around protected area: a Bangladesh study. J Environ Plan Manag 59(4):628–642

Mutungi C, Irungu FG, Nduko J, Mutua F, Affognon H, Nakimbugwe D, Fiaboe KKM (2019) Postharvest processes of edible insects in Africa: a review of processing methods, and the implications for nutrition, safety and new products development. Crit Rev Food Sci Nutr 59(2):276–298

Nadeau L, Nadeau I, Franklin F, Dunkel F (2015) The potential for entomophagy to address undernutrition. Ecol Food Nutr 54(3):200–208

Nerfa L, Rhemtulla JM, Zerriffi H (2020) Forest dependence is more than forest income: development of a new index of forest product collection and livelihood resources. World Dev 125:104689

Netshifhefhe SR, Kunjeku EC, Duncan FD (2018) Human uses and indigenous knowledge of edible termites in Vhembe District, Limpopo Province, South Africa. S Afr J Sci 114(1–2):1–10

Nimbekar T, Sanghi D (2022) Wild edible vegetables used for health benefit by rural people of Gondia District in Maharashtra State, India. Tradit Med 3(1):1–9

Nishaa S, Vishnupriya M, Gopalkrishnan VK (2013) Qualitative assessment of ethanolic extract of Maranta arundinacea L. rhizome using HPLC. Int Res J Pharm 4(2):76–83

Ogbuewu IP, Jiwuba PD, Ezeokeke CT, Uchegbu MC, Okoli IC, Iloeje MU (2014) Evaluation of phytochemical and nutritional composition of ginger rhizome powder. Int J Agric Rural Dev 17(1):1663–1670

Okaraonye CC, Ikewuchi JC (2009) Nutritional potential of Oryctes rhinoceros larva. Pak J Nutr 8(1):35–38

Ortiz JC, Ruiz AT, Morales-Ramos JA, Thomas M, Rojas MG, Tomberlin JK, Yi L, Han R, Giroud L, Jullien RL (2016) Insect mass production technologies. In: Dossey AT, Morales-Ramos JA, Guadalupe Rojas M (eds) Insects as sustainable food ingredients. Production, processing and food applications. Academic Press, London, pp 153–201

Paiko YB, Jacob JO, Salihu SO, Dauda BE, Suleiman MA, Akanya HO (2014) Fatty acid and amino acid profile of emperor moth caterpillar (Cirina forda) in Paikoro Local Government Area of Niger State, Nigeria. Am J Biochem 4(2):29–34

Pandey AK, Tripathi YC, Kumar A (2016) Non timber forest products (NTFPs) for sustained livelihood: challenges and strategies. Res J For 10(1):1–7

Pandey MM, Rastogi S, Rawat AKS (2013) Indian traditional ayurvedic system of medicine and nutritional supplementation. Evid Based Complement Alternat Med 2013:376327

Parappurathu S, Kumar A, Bantilan MCS, Joshi PK (2019) Household-level food and nutrition insecurity and its determinants in eastern India. Curr Sci 117(1):71–79

Payne CL, Scarborough P, Rayner M, Nonaka K (2016) A systematic review of nutrient composition data available for twelve commercially available edible insects, and comparison with reference values. Trends Food Sci Technol 47:69–77

Pegu R, Gogoi J, Tamuli AK, Teron R (2013) Ethnobotanical study of wild edible plants in Poba Reserved Forest, Assam, India: multiple functions and implications for conservation. Res J Agric For Sci 2320:6063

Peterson CT, Denniston K, Chopra D (2017) Therapeutic uses of triphala in ayurvedic medicine. J Altern Complement Med 23(8):607–614

Porro R, Lopez-Feldman A, Vela-Alvarado JW (2015) Forest use and agriculture in Ucayali, Peru: livelihood strategies, poverty and wealth in an Amazon frontier. Forest Policy Econ 51:47–56

Pradeepkumar T, Pradeep K (2008) Management of horticultural crops, Horticulture Science Series, vol 11. New India Publishing Agency, New Delhi, pp 81–84

Puttarak P, Dilokthornsakul P, Saokaew S, Dhippayom T, Kongkaew C, Sruamsiri R, Chaiyakunapruk N (2017) Effects of Centella asiatica (L.) Urb. on cognitive function and mood-related outcomes: a systematic review and meta-analysis. Sci Rep 7(1):1–12

Rajalingam GV, Parthiban KT, Sivakumar K, Divya MP (2017) Growth and productivity of vegetables under Anthocephalus cadamba-based silvihorticultural system. Indian J Agrofor 19(1):79–82

Raksakantong P, Meeso N, Kubola J, Siriamornpun S (2010) Fatty acids and proximate composition of eight Thai edible terricolous insects. Food Res Int 43(1):350–355

Rao AV (2002) Mind in ayurveda. Indian J Psychiatry 44(3):201

Rasmussen LV, Watkins C, Agrawal A (2017) Forest contributions to livelihoods in changing agriculture-forest landscapes. Forest Policy Econ 84:1–8

Ratcliffe BC (2006) Scarab beetles in human culture. Coleopt Bull 60(5):85–101

Reen RK, Karan M, Singh K, Karan V, Johri RK, Singh J (2001) Screening of various Swertia species extracts in primary monolayer cultures of rat hepatocytes against carbon tetrachloride-and paracetamol-induced toxicity. J Ethnopharmacol 75(2–3):239–247

Rumpold BA, Schlüter OK (2013) Nutritional composition and safety aspects of edible insects. Mol Nutr Food Res 57(5):802–823

Sanchez PA, Shepherd KD, Soule MJ, Place FM, Buresh RJ, Izac AMN, Woomer PL (1997) Soil fertility replenishment in Africa: an investment in natural resource capital. Replenishing soil fertility in Africa 51, pp 1–46

Sarmah MC (2011) Eri pupa: a delectable dish of North East India. Curr Sci 100(3):279

Sayed WA, Ibrahim NS, Hatab MH, Zhu F, Rumpold BA (2019) Comparative study of the use of insect meal from Spodoptera littoralis and Bactrocera zonata for feeding japanese quail chicks. Animals 9(4):136

Sen S, Chakraborty R (2017) Revival, modernization and integration of Indian traditional herbal medicine in clinical practice: importance, challenges and future. J Tradit Complement Med 7(2):234–244

Shackleton CM, Shackleton SE, Buiten E, Bird N (2007) The importance of dry woodlands and forests in rural livelihoods and poverty alleviation in South Africa. Forest Policy Econ 9(5):558–577

Sharma A, Shinde YB, Sirigoud LS, Shirke U, Yadav J (2022) A novel approach of ayurveda towards the understanding of Shookdhanya Varga (Cereals) and their fundamental characteristics and health benefits: a critical study. Int J Ayurveda Pharma Res 10(3):119–125

Sharma AK, Kumar S, Chashoo G, Saxena AK, Pandey AK (2014) Cell cycle inhibitory activity of Piper longum against A549 cell line and its protective effect against metal-induced toxicity in rats. Indian J Biochem Biophys 51:358–364

Shrestha S, Shrestha J, Shah KK (2020) Non-timber Forest products and their role in the livelihoods of people of Nepal: a critical review. Grassroots J Nat Resour 3(2):42–56

Shukla G, Chakravarty S (2012) Ethnobotanical plant use of Chilapatta reserved forest in West Bengal. Indian Forester 138(12):1116

Singh A, Kumar S, Bajpai V, Kumar B (2017) Simultaneous determination of pyrroquinazoline alkaloids and flavonoids in Adhatoda beddomei and Adhatoda vasica and their marketed herbal formulations using ultra-high-performance liquid chromatography coupled with triple quadrupole linear ion trap mass spectrometry. Biomed Chromatogr 31(3):e3827

Srećković NZ, Mihailović VB, Katanić-Stanković JS (2019) Physico-chemical, antioxidant and antimicrobial properties of three different types of honey from central Serbia. Kragujevac J Sci 41:53–68

Srivastava S, Li C, Lingelbach M, Martín-Martín R, Xia F, Vainio KE, Fei-Fei L (2022) Behavior: benchmark for everyday household activities in virtual, interactive, and ecological environments. In: Conference on Robot Learning ser. Proceedings of Machine Learning Research, vol 164. PMLR, pp 477–490

Ssepuuya G, Mukisa IM, Nakimbugwe D (2017) Nutritional composition, quality, and shelf stability of processed Ruspolia nitidula (edible grasshoppers). Food Sci Nutr 5(1):103–112

Subrat N, Iyer M, Prasad R (2002) The ayurvedic medicine industry: current status and sustainability. Ecotech Services (India) Pvt. Ltd. and International Institute for Environment and Development, New Delhi, pp 1–176

Sunderlin WD, Angelsen A, Belcher B, Burgers P, Nasi R, Santoso L, Wunder S (2005) Livelihoods, forests, and conservation in developing countries: an overview. World dev, 33(9):1383–1402

Talukdar NR, Choudhury P, Barbhuiya RA, Singh B (2021) Importance of non-timber forest products (NTFPs) in rural livelihood: a study in Patharia Hills Reserve Forest, northeast India. Trees For People 3:100042

Talwana HAL, Serem AK, Ndabikunze BK, Nandi JOM, Tumuhimbise R, Kaweesi T, Palapala VA (2009) Production status and prospects of Cocoyam (Colocasia esculenta L. Schott.) in East Africa. J Root Crops 35:98–107

Tamang A, Kuchi VS, Das BC, Ray S (2020) Identification of superior genotypes of Chalta (Dillenia indica) through germplasm characterization. J Pharmacogn Phytochem 9(3):1579–1584

Taylor G, Wang N (2018) Entomophagy and allergies: a study of the prevalence of entomophagy and related allergies in a population living in North-Eastern Thailand. Biosci Horiz 11:hzy003

Ting Z, Haiyun C, Shivakoti GP, Cochard R, Homcha-aim K (2011) Revisit to community forest in northeast of Thailand: changes in status and utilization. Environ Dev Sustain 13(2):385–402

Urso V, Signorini MA, Tonini M, Bruschi P (2016) Wild medicinal and food plants used by communities living in Mopane woodlands of southern Angola: results of an ethnobotanical field investigation. J Ethnopharmacol 177:126–139

Ushadevi KN, Vijaykumar N (2022) Problems faced by tribals in collection and marketing of Non-timber Forest Products (NTFPs) in Kerala, India. Asian J Agric Ext Econ Sociol 40(11):251–258

Van Huis A, Van Itterbeeck J, Klunder H, Mertens E, Halloran A, Muir G, Vantomme P (2013) Edible insects: future prospects for food and feed security. Food and agriculture organization of the United Nations, Rome

Venkateshappa SM, Sreenath KP (2013) Potential medicinal plants of Lamiaceae. Am Int J Res Formal Appl Nat Sci 3(1):82–87

Verkerk MC, Tramper J, Van Trijp JCM, Martens DE (2007) Insect cells for human food. Biotechnol Adv 25(2):198–202

Vincenti B, Eyzaguirre P, Johns T (2008) The nutritional role of forest plant foods for rural communities. In: Colfer C (ed) Human health and forests. A global overview of issues, ractice and policy. People and plants international. Conservation series. London, UK, Earthscan, pp 63–96

Wakdikar S (2004) Global health care challenge: Indian experiences and new prescriptions. Electron J Biotechnol 7(3):02–03

Williamson EM (2002) Major herbs of Ayurveda. Churchill Livingstone. Elsevier, Edimburgh

Worku M (2015) Traditional uses of non-timber forest products in southwest Ethiopia: opportunities and challenges for sustainable forest management. J Agric Environ Sci 1(1):42–63

Zada M, Shah SJ, Yukun C, Rauf T, Khan N, Shah SAA (2019) Impact of small-to-medium size forest enterprises on rural livelihood: evidence from Khyber-Pakhtunkhwa, Pakistan. Sustainability 11(10):2989

Zenteno M, Zuidema PA, de Jong W, Boot RG (2013) Livelihood strategies and forest dependence: new insights from Bolivian forest communities. Forest Policy Econ 26:12–21

Indian Traditional Medicine: A Medical Inheritance

10

Dinesh Kumar and Rishabh Kaundal

Abstract

Indian Traditional Medicines are in practice from centuries for the local and global health care. They are also one of the cornerstones for treatment of new and chronic disorders and practiced throughout the world, particularly in West Asia (India, Pakistan, Tibet), East Asia (China, Korea, Japan, Vietnam), Africa, and the Americas. India's wealth of biodiversity and cultural heritage has been always fascinated for its unparalleled natural qualities and values. India is a botanical treasure trove with over 18,000 plant species that spread across the 15 diverse agroclimatic zones. These zones are rich in medicinal plants that provides raw material for traditional medicines and further serve significantly for ancient medical systems like Ayurveda, Unani, Siddha, Homoeopathy, Naturopathy, etc. The Vedic scripts are so rich in information that it led to explore bioactive metabolites and discovery of modern drugs. These natural products are diverse, with applications in human, veterinary, and agricultural sectors. The current information insights the medical inheritance of Indian traditional medicines with global impact.

Keywords

Inheritance · Vedic · Medicine · Ayuveda · Naturopathy

D. Kumar (✉) · R. Kaundal
Chemical Technology Division, CSIR-Institute of Himalayan Bioresource Technology, Palampur, Himachal Pradesh, India

Academy of Scientific and Innovative Research, (AcSIR), Ghaziabad, Uttar Pradesh, India
e-mail: dineshkumar@ihbt.res.in

A. Kumar et al. (eds.), *Innovations in Ayurvedic Nutrition*,
https://doi.org/10.1007/978-981-95-1213-3_10

10.1 Introduction

India's rich cultural legacy and diverse biodiversity have always captivated people, exhibiting unmatched natural qualities and ideals. India is a botanical treasure trove, home to over 18,000 plant species spread across 15 diverse agroclimatic zones, of which 6000–7000 are known for their medicinal qualities (Bhanot et al. 2011). These therapeutic plants are essential to Indian society in many ways, as they are used as main elements in ancient medical systems including Ayurveda, Unani, Siddha, Homoeopathy, and Sowa-Rigpa. They are also used by companies that make plant-based pharmaceuticals in their formulations.

With a predicted value of Rs. 4.2 billion (US$ 56.6 million) in 2019, the Indian market for medicinal plants is expected to develop significantly at a compound annual growth rate (CAGR) of 38.5%, reaching Rs. 14 billion (US$ 188.6 million) by 2026. Notwithstanding this expansion, India's proportion of the world market for the export of herbs and herbal products is still small because of things like restricted captive production and complicated regulations pertaining to the commerce in medicinal plants. Nonetheless, throughout time, the export of value-added extracts and herbs that are used medicinally has gradually increased (Demain 2014). India exported US$ 330.18 million worth of herbs in the 2017–2018 fiscal year, a 14.22% increase over the previous year. Likewise, value-added extracts of medical herbs and herbal products saw a growth rate of 12.23% in exports, reaching US$ 456.12 million over the same time frame (WHO 2004). This increase is a sign of the growing demand, especially in outside markets like those in Europe and other developed nations, for herbal and value-added extracts of therapeutic plants (Katz and Baltz 2016).

Among the diverse array of medicinal plants, spices, and herbs, bioactive metabolites play a crucial role in providing health benefits. In Ayurveda, health is intricately linked to the balance of the sap dhatus and the three doshas (vatta, pitta, kapha). Similarly, traditional texts emphasize that health encompasses not just physical well-being but also mental and internal strength. The knowledge derived from traditional medicinal systems has led to the development of natural products (NPs) containing diversified secondary metabolites with a wide range of biological activities (Katz and Baltz 2016). These NPs continue to find applications in human, veterinary, and agricultural domains, showcasing the multifaceted benefits of harnessing nature's bounty (Ekor 2014). Some of the important medicinal plants and their uses in traditional practices are discussed in Table 10.1 and Fig. 10.1 (Wah et al. 2014; Dev 1999; Pandey et al. 2013; Prasad 2002).

Traditional medicine in India encompasses the utilization of drugs with Indian origins or those that have been adopted into Indian culture from other countries (Barnes & Heinrich (2004)). This rich tradition is depicted in Fig. 10.2, showcasing the diverse range of medicinal practices and treatments. India boasts a deep-rooted history of traditional medicine, revolving around six primary systems: Ayurveda, Unani, Siddha, Naturopathy, Yoga, and Homeopathy. Each of these systems contributes unique perspectives, principles, and methodologies to the holistic approach to healthcare in India (Ravishankar and Shukla 2007). Figure 10.3 illustrates the extent to which plants are used in different systems of medicine.

Table 10.1 Some common medicinal plants used in traditional medicine

Scientific name	Sanskrit/Hindi name	Uses
Adhatoda vasica Nees	Adusa/Vasaka	Cough, asthma, bronchitis
Ananas comosus	Ananas	Sore throat, diabetes, heart disease, obesity
Acacia arabica Willd	Babool	Oral care, bleeding gums, wounds
Bacopa monnieri Pennell	Brahmi	Enhances memory, anxiety
Coriandrum sativum Linn	Dhaniya	Useful in indigestion, flatulence, controls spasmodic pain
Allium sativum	Lashun	Ringworm, dysentery, wounds
Cyperus rotundus Linn	Nagarmotha	Fever, diabetes, solar dermatitis
Ocimum sanctum Linn	Tulsi	Indigestion, heart health, respiratory diseases
Allium cepa Lin	Pyaj	Prostate health, digestive
Withania somnifera Dunal	Ashwgandha	Stress tolerance, immunity, joint pains, skin health
Aconitum ferox	Meetha Vish	Fever, diuretic action, arthritis
Cissampelos pareira Linn	Patha	Ulcers, sinuses, skin diseases, poisonous bites
Aconitum heterophyllum Wall	Atees	Fever, respiratory
Asparagus racemosus Willd	Shatavari	A strong Ayurvedic revitalization. It provides a variety of female hormones and is mostly advised for women who have undergone hysterectomies. In addition, it boosts immunity, cleanses blood, and supports urinary tract health.
Gymnema sylvestre R. Br.	Gurmarar	It has a glycolytic activity, lessens the strength of a glucose solution, and its Sanskrit name literally translates as "sugar destroyer." For millennia, Ayurveda has employed it to control the metabolism of sugar.
Melia azadirachta L.	Nimba, Neem	It is used as an astringent and tonic that aids in healing, and it has potent health-alleviating properties.

10.2 Ayurveda

Ayurveda stands as the ancient, most revered, practiced, and thriving native system of medicine in India. Its name is derived from the Sanskrit terms "ayur" (life) and "veda," meaning "The Science of Life" or "Knowledge of Life" (Ravishankar and Shukla 2007). In terms of mythology, the Ayurveda has two roots. The first is Dhanvantaridev, who gave Susruta access to this knowledge to relieve human suffering. Another is Brahma, who imparted this medicinal information to Prajapati Daha and is credited with creating the Agnivesha Treatise, an encyclopaedia of Ayurveda. It is thought that the creator of the universe gave philosophers a thorough

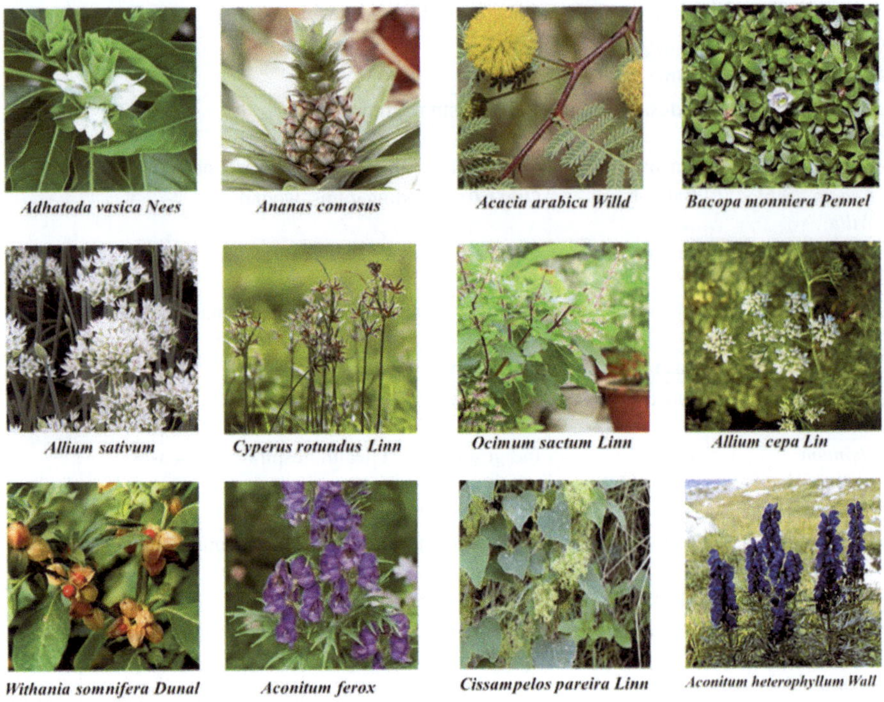

Fig. 10.1 Traditionally used Indian medicinal plants

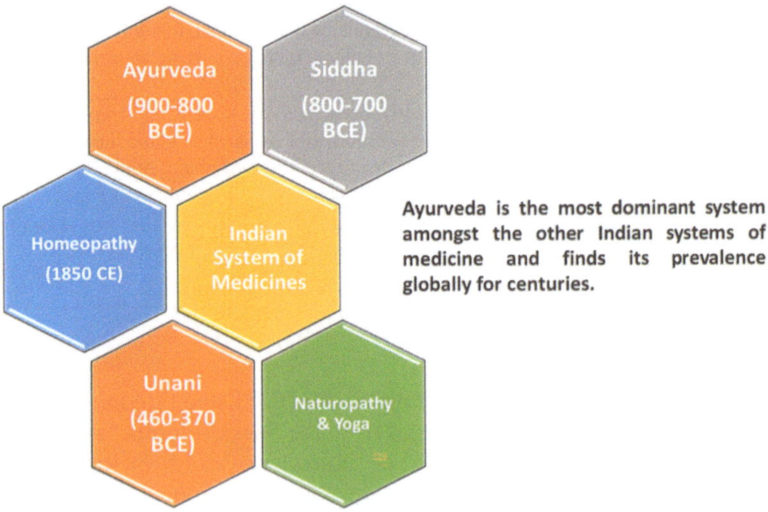

Fig. 10.2 Recognized systems of Indian medicinal practice

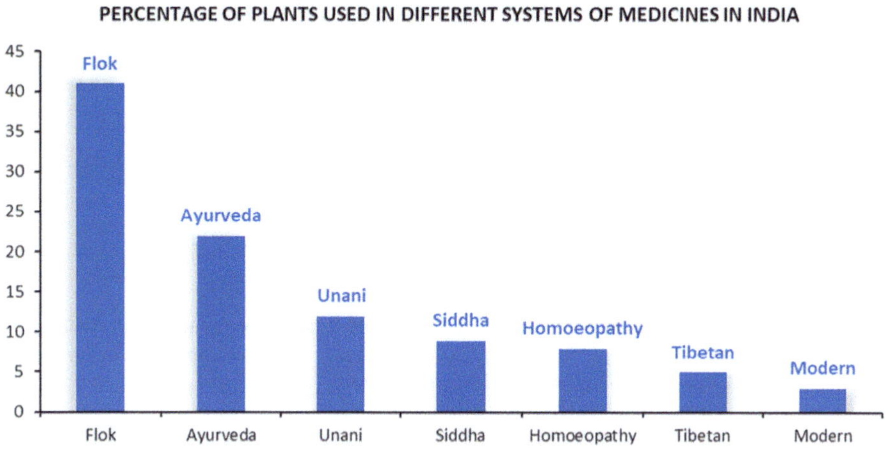

Fig. 10.3 Percentage of plants used in different systems of medicines

understanding of healing for the benefit of humanity. The sages then imparted this knowledge of conventional treatments to their pupils, who in turn disseminated it verbally and in writing to the broader public. The Yajur Veda, Rig Veda, Sam Veda, and Atharva Veda are revered as four prominent knowledge collections (Vedas) that form the cornerstone of the Hindu healing system. Among these Vedas, the Rig Veda stands out as the most renowned, containing 1028 Shlokas and references to 67 different plants with medicinal properties. Similarly, the Atharva Veda and Yajur Veda also provide valuable insights, describing 293 and 81 medicinally beneficial plants, respectively. The wisdom gleaned from these ancient texts serves as the foundational knowledge for the practice and principles of Ayurveda, a holistic system of medicine deeply rooted in the ancient traditions of India. Some of the important Ayurvedic formulations to treat diseases are discussed in Table 10.2 (Pandey et al. 2013).

Ayurveda has undergone a dramatic paradigm shift in recent decades, and scholars' perspectives on its uses have also changed significantly. Ayurvedic medicinal ideas emphasize prakriti and tridoshas, which explain that each person has a distinct constitution known as Prakriti. Prakriti ascertains how each person typically reacts to drugs, environmental circumstances, and nutritional considerations. Ayurveda has a long history, yet there have been shortcomings in techniques that have prevented it from advancing as much as the western medical system. The active ingredients of the herbal medications provided were unknown, and even now, many pharmaceuticals still require additional research to characterize their active constituents and explain how they work. Herbal medications still have several downsides even after decades of using cutting-edge analytical techniques for drug analysis. The complexity of studying the effects of various medications is increased by the administration of pharmacological combinations (Wah et al. 2014).

Table 10.2 Herbal remedies that are regularly utilized in India's ancient Ayurvedic system

Disease	*Formulation's ingredient*	Dose	Method of use
Anaemia	*Withania somnifera* (roots) 20% *Asparagus racemosus* (roots) 20% *Phyllanthus emblica* (fruits) 15% *Glycyrrhiza glabra* (roots) 15% *Tephrosia purpurea* (leaves) 10% *P. amarus* (leaves) 10% *Piper longum* (fruits) 5% *Plumbago zeylanica* (roots) 5%	Powder	4 g powder is given twice daily with water
Asthma/ bronchitis	*Solanum xanthocarpum* (whole plant) 25% *Adhatoda vasica* (leaves) 25% *Ocimum sanctum* (leaves) 10% *Curcuma zedoaria* (roots) 10% *Phyllanthus emblica* (fruits) 10% *Zingiber officinale* (roots) 10% Piper *longum* (fruits) 10%	Mixed powder water	4 g (one teaspoon full) twice a day (morning and at bedtime)
Blood circulation	*Zingiber officinale* (roots) 20% *Curcuma longa* (roots) 10% *Phyllanthus emblica* (fruits) 10% *Terminalia bellirica* (fruits) 10% *Withania somnifera* (roots) 10% *Tephrosia purpurea* (leaves) 10% *T. chebula* (fruits) 10% *Piper longum* (roots) 10% *Ocimum sanctum* (leaves) 10%	Mixed powder	4 g powder (twice daily with water)
Cough	*Phyllanthus emblica* (fruits) 25% *Glycyrrhiza glabra* (roots) 15% *Adhatoda vasica* (leaves) 20% *Solanum xanthocarpum* (whole plant) 10% *Piper longum* (fruits) 10% *Ocimum sanctum* (leaves) 10% *Zingiber officinale* (roots) 10%	Mixed powder	3 g powder mixed with honey and lukewarm water twice daily (in morning and night)
Diarrhoea	*Aegle marmelos* (fruits) 25% *Holarrhena antidysenterica* (bark) 25% *Terminalia chebula* (fruits) 10% *Phyllanthus emblica* (fruits) 10% *Cyperus rotundus* (roots) 10% *Zingiber officinale* (roots) 10% *Syzygium cumini* (seeds) 10%	Mixed powder	3 g powder mixed with curd (three times a day)
Hair problems	*Centella asiatica* (leaves) 15% *Phyllanthus emblica* (fruits) 15% *Glycyrrhiza glabra* (roots) 15% *Eclipta alba* (leaves) 15% *Tribulus terrestris* (fruits) 10% *Terminalia chebula* (fruits) 10% *T. bellirica* (fruits) 10% *Tinospora cordifolia* (stems) 10%	Mixed powder	4 g powder with honey (twice a day)

10.3 Siddha

The human body is made up of the five components (Fire, earth, space, water, air, Fig. 10.4) of the universe, or pancha mahabhootas, the Siddha system of medicine is founded on a similar theory to Ayurveda. The term "Siddha" means "holy harmony," "attaining excellence," or "known fact," and the "Siddhars" are thought to be supernatural creatures who acquire mental abilities via consistent use of this kind of medicine (Piet 1952). The Siddha system of medicine is attributed to the wisdom and contributions of the 18 Siddhars. These revered figures, including Thirumoolar, Bogar, Machchamuni, Konganar, Korakkar, Therayar, Karuvoorar, Nandi Devar, Idaikkadar, Iraamathevar, Sattamuni, Kuthampai, Paampaatti, Aluhanna, and Kahapusundar are believed to have laid the foundation for the Siddha system of medicines. Their collective knowledge and expertise have significantly influenced the principles, practices, and philosophies that define Siddha medicine (Sathasivampillai et al. 2017; Pillai 1998). In addition to five components, the Siddha system believes that 96 aspects influence a person's physical, moral, and physiological well-being. Among the 96 elements are voice, perception, and pulse reading. Perception is often used as a deciding factor for the psychosomatic system's therapy, with the help of minerals, metals, and to a lesser extent certain plant items. Several powdered preparations of plant and mineral origin that have undergone various preparation processes, such as calcinations, are used in the Siddha system.

Since most of the literature is not translated from the Tamil language, Siddha medications are less well-known in the west (Narayanaswami 1975). Siddha philosophy was developed from therapeutic, profound, and academic perspectives. It accords equal weight to the inner soul and the outer body and is particularly

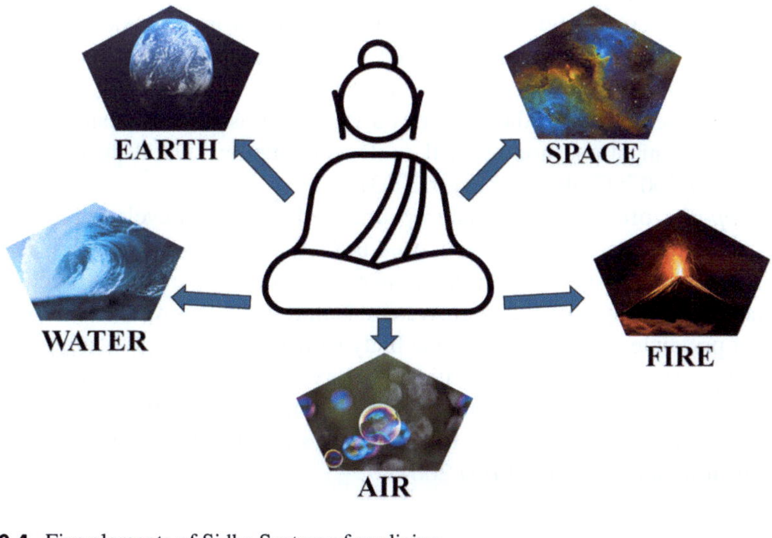

Fig. 10.4 Five elements of Sidha System of medicine

distinctive from ayurvedic medicine in that it uses alchemy (the transformation of base metals into gold), urine testing, and practise materia medica (Gordon 2013; Adhikari and Paul 2018). As of right present, all conditions except for emergencies can be effectively treated using Siddha remedies (Kalim et al. 2010).

10.4 Unani

Hippocrates, who lived from 460 BC to 366 BC, was a famous Greek physician and philosopher who is credited with founding the Unani medical system. The four humours that make up the human body blood, yellow bile, dark bile, and mucus have wet and dry properties (Chopra 2006). He developed the "humoral hypothesis" as a foundation for treating disorders. The foundation of Unani medicine is this fundamental idea. During the Mughal era, Unani medicine was incorporated into Indian culture and became well-known when a significant number of Indians adopted its practices. Following the Mongol invasion of Persia, Unani medicine which had its roots in Arab scholars and practitioners grew in popularity in India because of scholarly migration. Since that time, this medical system has established itself firmly in India and is approved by the Indian government for clinical use and research support (Alexander et al. 2013; Posadzki et al. 2011). Diet therapy, regimented treatment, and pharmacotherapy are the three categories of medications that the Unani system of medicine recommends. Oils, tinctures, powders, and ointments made from plants are utilized in treatment.

10.5 Yoga and Naturopathy

India is considered the historical birthplace of Yoga, a discipline that promotes introspective practices and lifestyle modification to promote peace of mind and improve well-being. Yoga combines treatments and diagnoses based on the Tridosha state analysis of a person's constitution as well as pulse analysis. Yoga is a form of physical and mental health that includes a variety of asanas, or positions, that are used in both clinical and non-clinical contexts to support overall health and well-being (Hoyez 2007; Grabia and Ernst 2003).

Naturopathy, often known as naturopathic medicine, was developed in Germany in the nineteenth century and is now used in several nations. Although it is not an old system of medicine, some practitioners of traditional medicine occasionally combine Naturopathy with the main system. Naturopathy is governed by an intriguing set of principles that recognizes the body's innate capacity for healing, places a strong emphasis on disease prevention, and exhorts individuals to take personal responsibility for their own welfare. According to naturopathic theory, the disease is viewed as a process of disruption to health and subsequent recovery in relation to natural healing mechanisms (Ernst 2004).

10.6 Homeopathy

Homoeopathy was first introduced by German physician Dr. Samuel Hahnemann in the middle of the seventeenth and early eighteenth centuries. The term "Homoeopathy" is derived from the Greek words "Homois," meaning similar, and "pathos," meaning suffering. The foundational principles of homeopathy revolve around concepts such as "immunological memory" and the "memory of water," as well as the correlations between a drug's pharmacological properties and the symptoms of the illness it treats. Homeopathy operates on the premise of treating a pathological condition by initially inducing or exacerbating similar symptoms, followed by administering drugs that cause symptoms resembling those of the disease. This treatment approach utilizes combinations of medicines whose effects on healthy individuals mirror the symptoms experienced by the specific patient, thereby aiming to stimulate the body's innate healing response (Ernst 1997; Linde et al. 1997). The technique is thought to operate on two key tenets (Baker et al. 2007)

1. "Like cures like"; a healthy person would experience the same symptom when taking the treatment, which means it treats the same ailment.
2. "Infinite dilution": Even when diluted beyond Avogadro's number, medicinal efficacy is increased by repeated dilution and succession.

To create formulations of very low potencies in homeopathy, aqueous extracts or the mother tinctures of the medications (plants, compounds of animal origin, venoms, and minerals) are diluted and succussed (a specific process of mixing or shaking).

10.7 Plant-Derived Drug Discovery

Plants serve as a rich source of diverse therapeutic properties, continually fuelling the development of innovative drugs. In modern pharmaceuticals, a significant portion of drugs is derived from natural products, particularly bioactive molecules. Through extensive research, numerous secondary metabolites with varied structures and pharmacological effects have been isolated from plants, microorganisms, and marine sources. The wealth of knowledge accumulated through traditional medicine systems has paved the way for exploring the potential of medicinal plants in drug development. One pivotal milestone in drug discovery was the identification of morphine, extracted from Papaver somniferum in 1803. This marked the beginning of a journey wherein medicinal plants became invaluable reservoirs of ethnobotanical compounds (Katiyar et al. 2012). Today, these compounds are extensively utilized in various drug discovery programs, contributing significantly to the pharmaceutical industry. The development of drugs from natural resources has led to the discovery of numerous therapeutic agents, as highlighted in Tables 10.3 and 10.4 and Fig. 10.5. Furthermore, advancements in genomics, proteomics, transcriptomics, and metabolomics have revolutionized the role of natural products in drug discovery. Metabolomic studies are increasingly utilized to identify novel drugs and drug targets, elucidate mechanisms of drug action, and document the therapeutic

Table 10.3 Plant derived drugs in the market

Plant species	Drug	Uses	Country
Salix spp	Salicilic acid-aspirin	Analgesic	Europe
Atropa belladonna	Atropine	Anti-cholinergic	Germany
Digitalis species	Digoxin, digitalin	Cardiotonic	UK-Europe
Cinchona species	Quinine	Antimalarial	Amazonia
Artemisia species	Artemisinin	Antimalarial	China
Rauwolfia serpentina	Reserpine	Antihypertensive	India
Dioscorea deltoidea	Diosgenin	Antifertility	India
Taxus species	Paclitaxel	Anticancer	Europe
Podophyllum spp.	Etoposide	Anticancer	Eastern USA
Colchicum autumnale	Colchicine	Antitumour	France
Catharanthus roseus	Vincristine, vinblastin	Anticancer	Madagascar
Mucuna deltoidea	(L)-dopa	Anti-Parkinson	Sweden
Papaver somniferum	Morphine	Analgesic	Mesopotamia
Colchicum autumnale	Colchicine	Antitumour	France
Physostigma venenosum	Physostigmine	Memory enhancement	West Africa
Chondrodendron spp.	Tubocurarine	Muscle relaxant	Amazonia
Calophyllum teysmannii	Calanolide B	Anti-HIV	America
Camptotheca acuminata	Topotecan	Anti-cancer	China
Cephalotaxus harringtonia	Homoharringtonine	Anti-cancer	China
Combretum caffrum	Combretastatins	Anti-cancer	S. Africa

Table 10.4 Medicinal plants in Indian sphere with major phytochemicals and therapeutic properties

Plant name	Major constituents	Major therapeutic activity	References
Abutilon indicum	Gallic acid and quercetin	It is used as febrifuge, anthelmintic, antiemetic, anti-inflammatory, and in the treatment of urinary and uterine discharges problems, piles, lumbago	Hussain et al. (2012b)
Averrhoa bilimbi L.	Ascorbic acid & tannic acid	Used to cure scurvy, fever, skin conditions, and to treat diarrhoea, hepatitis, and inflammatory conditions.	Patil et al. (2013)
Averrhoa bilimbi L. & *Averrhoa carambola*	Tannic acid	Often used to treat inflammatory conditions, diarrhoea, hepatitis, fever, scurvy, and skin disorders	Patil et al. (2011)
Averrhoa bilimbi L. & *Averrhoa carambola*	Ascorbic acid	Used to cure scurvy, fever, skin conditions, and to treat diarrhoea, hepatitis, and inflammatory conditions.	Patil et al. (2011)

(continued)

Table 10.4 (continued)

Plant name	Major constituents	Major therapeutic activity	References
Berberis aristata	Berberine	Its uses include anti-inflammatory, antimicrobial, antiprotozoal, hypotensive, immune stimulating, febrifugal, anticholinergic, and antiarrhythmic effects.	Gurme et al. (2022)
Bergenia ciliata and Bergenia ligulata	Bergenin, catechin, gallic acid	Antioxidant	Dhalwal et al. (2008)
Cassia fistula	Epicatechin, procyanidin B2, rhein, sennoside A & B, chrysophanol,	Antifertility, antifungal, antipyretic, antitumour, antitussive, Clastogenic effect, CNS activities, laxative, sedative, Hepatoprotective, antianxiety effect, and wound healing activity	Patidar et al. (2012); Thirumal et al. (2012)
Curcuma longa	Curcumin	Antitumour, antioxidant, hepatoprotective, anti-inflammatory etc.	Ashraf et al. (2012)
Naringi crenulata (Rutaceae)	Crenulatine, Sitosterol, xanthotoxin, limonin	It is used in the treatment of body pain, fever, vomiting, dysentery, and have antiaging property	Subramanian and Ramakrishnan (2011)
Withania somnifera (Ashwagandha)	Withanolides, omniferinin, anaferine, anahygrine	Adaptogenic, immune modulatory, antioxidant, analgesic, hypnotic, antipyretic, sedative anti-inflammatory, tonic, anticonvulsant, diuretic, and abortifacient properties	Alam et al. (2012)
Rauwolfia tetraphylla	Reserpiline yohimbine, soreserpiline, 10-methoxy tetrahydroalstonine	It has anti-tumour, antimalarial, antimicrobial, antihypertensive properties and used in the disorders of central nervous system	Gupta et al. (2012)
Gmelina arborea	6-*O*-(2″,3″-dibenzoyl)-α-L-rhamnopyranosylcatalpol	It is used as a diuretic, appetite stimulant, several gynaecological disorders and also in ayurvedic preparations e.g. *Dashmularishta*	Yadav et al. (2008)
Solanum xanthocarpum	Solasonine, solamargine and khasianine	It is used in the treatment of allergic bronchitis, asthma, cold, fever, and inflammations, etc.	Shanker et al. (2011)

(continued)

Table 10.4 (continued)

Plant name	Major constituents	Major therapeutic activity	References
Stevia rebaudiana	Steviolbioside, sativoside, rebaudioside-A	It is used as a natural sweetener, antioxidant. And helpful in the treatment of used as hypotensive and hypoglycemic	Jaitak et al. (2008)
Tephrosia purpurea (leaves)	Qurecetin and rutin	It is used for the treatment of asthma, diarrhoea, gonorrhoea, rheumatism, ulcers, and urinary disorders, etc.	Jain et al. (2009)
Tecomella undulata (bark)	Tecomin	It is used to treat leucorrhoea, enlarged spleen, jaundice, anaemia, intestinal worms, and urinary disorders.	Navneet et al. (2013)
Hygrophila auriculata	Lupeol and stigmasterol	It is used in jaundice, pain, fever, rheumatism, malaria, impotence and inflammation	Hussain et al. (2012a)
Ruellia tuberosa	RT-F2	It has been utilized in traditional medicine as an antipyretic, antidiabetic, diuretic, antidotal, thirst-quenching agent, analgesic, and anti-hypertensive.	Chothani et al. (2012)
Ricinus communis	Ferulic acid	It is used as stimulant cathartic, lactagogue, antirheumatic, antitumour and hepatoprotective, etc.	Verma et al. (2011)
Enicostemma littorale	Swertiamarin	It is used in diabetes, malaria, fever, etc.	Alam et al. (2012)
Lycopodium clavatum	Ferulic acid	It is used as antioxidant, hepatoprotective, and antitumour properties etc.	Srivastava et al. (2012)
Melaleuca alternifolia	Terpinen-4-ol	It is used in cosmetic as well as in perfumery industries, it has potential antimicrobial activity	Biju et al. (2005)
Valeriana wallichii	Hesperidin	Using valerian extract increases the quality of sleep and reduces sleep latency. Seen as beneficial for managing sleeplessness and anxiety	Sharma et al. (2012)

(continued)

Table 10.4 (continued)

Plant name	Major constituents	Major therapeutic activity	References
Ageratum conyzoides	Stigmasterol	They are employed as antimicrobials and to treat a variety of illnesses, including burns and wounds.	Kamboj and Saluja (2013)
Andrographis paniculata	Andrographolide	It is used in the treatment of diabetes, malaria, cholera dysentery, enteritis, gastritis, pneumonia, pyelonephritis, diarrhoea, even rabies etc.	Pawar et al. (2010)
Ganoderma lucidum	Total triterpenes	It is used as antioxidant, antitumour, mutagenic, antinociceptive, anti-inflammatory, anti-carcinogenic, and has cardio protective as well as nephroprotective effects	Smina et al. (2011)
Calotropis procera	Lupeol	It is used as antifungal, antipyretic and analgesic	Pathania et al. (2020)
Nyctanthes arbortristis	Lupeol	Ayurvedic doctors utilize it as a cholagogue, laxative, treatment for arthritis, stubborn sciatica, malaria, and as a tonic.	Pathania et al. (2020)
Cassia alata	Rhein and kaempferol	It is used as analgesic anti-inflammatory, antimutagenic and antimicrobial properties	Singh et al. (2012)
Semecarpus anacardium	Tetrahydroamentoflavone	It is used in neuritis, arthritis, leprosy, Helmintic infection, venereal disorders, etc.	Aravind et al. (2008)
Pueraria tuberosa	Puerarin	It is used in indigenous system of Indian medicine as tonic, aphrodisiac, diuretic antirheumatic and galactogogue. Ingredient of Chyawanprash (Ayurvedic medicine), Immunomodulator, etc.	Singh Chauhan and Kumar Dixit (2012)
Picrorhiza kurroa	Picroside-I, Picroside-II	It is used in the treatment of liver, kidney cardiac and respiratory disorders	Kumar et al. (2015)

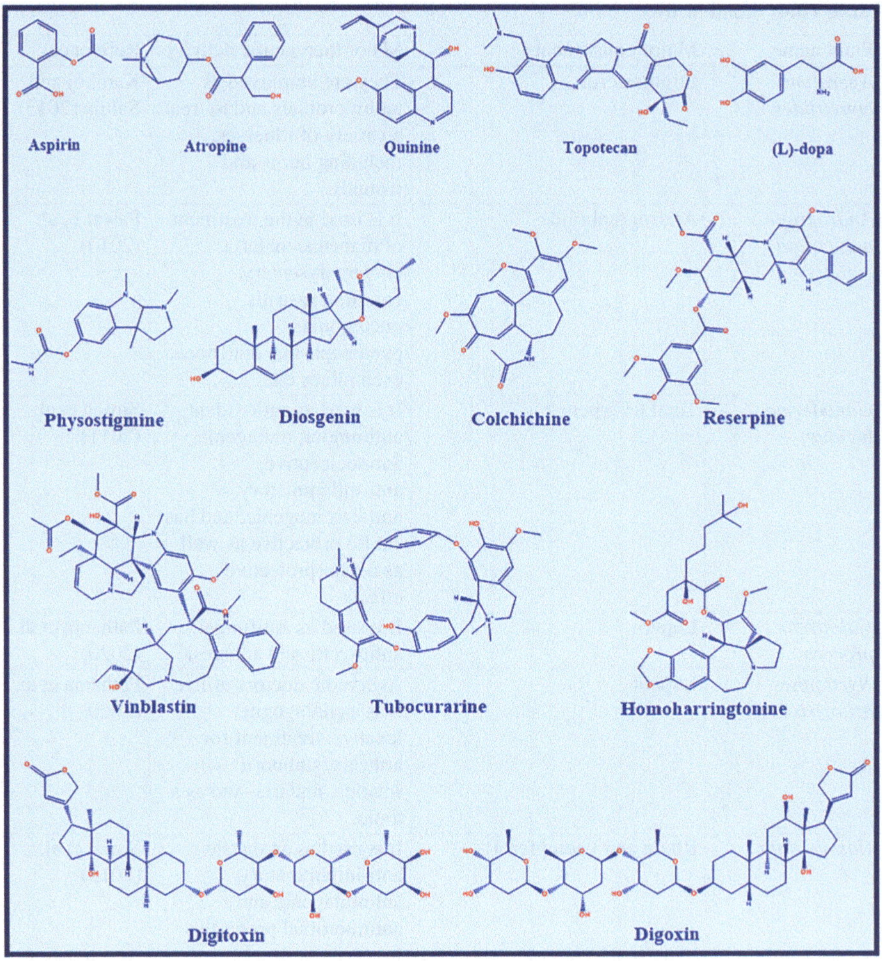

Fig. 10.5 Structure of plant-derived drug molecules (Newman and Cragg 2016)

effects of developed drugs. This multidisciplinary approach underscores the continued relevance and importance of natural products in the ever-evolving landscape of drug development.

10.8 Conclusion

NPs are the source of the majority of the bioactive compounds found in western medications. In the days before post-genomic medicine and high-throughput screening, more than 80% of pharmaceuticals came from natural products (NPs) or were modelled after natural substances. Although the term "ethno-pharmaceutical" may be used broadly to describe how people use plants as medicines, the most appropriate term for this practice is "ethno-botanic medicine"(Torri et al. 2011; Mukherjee et al. 2010).

As part of India's sociocultural tradition, Ayurveda and plant-based medical treatments have advanced thanks to everyday interactions. Additionally, according to the WHO, between 80% and 85% of the population in underdeveloped nations relies on complementary or alternative medicine for basic therapeutic needs Samal (2014). Medicinal plants are thought to be the mainstay and significant impact on all traditional medical systems. It is difficult to estimate the total number of medicinal plants in existence, but according to some estimates, between 35,000 and 70,000 plant species are utilized in human health care services globally, and the Indian pharmacopeia alone contains more than 3000 medications from natural sources.

However, there is a persistent argument between those who use NP treatments for various illnesses and disorders and others who rely on contemporary, modern medicine for treatment. People who favour current medical treatments argue that using NP for treatment is large "smoke and mirrors" and that nothing can be understood through its use. They believe that people who have received dishonest education typically choose bogus natural remedies. But nowadays many modern medical professionals are realizing this and beginning to suggest alternative (natural) treatments to their patients when modern medications do not work. This is also because natural treatments have fewer side effects, if any, and are less dangerous for prolonged use than allopathic synthetic medications, which often have fatal side effects.

Indian System of medicines has long history, yet there have been shortcomings in techniques that have prevented it from advancing just as the western system of medicine. The active ingredients of the herbal medications provided were unknown, and even now, many pharmaceuticals still require additional research to characterize their active constituents and explain how they work. Herbal medications still have several downsides even after decades of using cutting-edge analytical techniques for drug analysis. The complexity of studying the effects of various medications is increased by the administration of pharmacological combinations. As was previously mentioned, one advantage of traditional medical systems is that they prioritize the treatment of the patient rather than the sickness. However, this aspect also poses a barrier to the general population's ability to apply drugs. A comparison of the medications used in traditional system of medicines (TSM) is desperately needed because of a number of issues, such as species-based variations in potency, a lack of integrated coding for all species commonly used in traditional system of medicines (TSM), geographical variations in drug growth locations, inaccurate identification, adulteration of medications, inconsistent quality control standards, and variations in processing techniques.

References

Adhikari P, Paul SB (2018) History of Indian traditional medicine: a medical inheritance. History 11(1):421

Alam P, Gupta J, Firdouse S, Sultana A, Fathima N, Ummara U (2012) HPTLC method for qualitative estimation of withania somnifera linn in polyherbal formulation. Pharmacie Globale 3(11):1

Alexander GK, Innes KE, Selfe TK, Brown CJ (2013) "More than I expected": perceived benefits of yoga practice among older adults at risk for cardiovascular disease. Complement Ther Med 21(1):14–28

Aravind SG, Arimboor R, Rangan M, Madhavan SN, Arumughan C (2008) Semi-preparative HPLC preparation and HPTLC quantification of tetrahydroamentoflavone as marker in Semecarpus anacardium and its polyherbal formulations. J Pharm Biomed Anal 48(3):808–813

Ashraf K, Mujeeb M, Ahmad A, Amir M, Mallick MN, Sharma D (2012) Validated HPTLC analysis method for quantification of variability in content of curcumin in Curcuma longa L (turmeric) collected from different geographical region of India. Asian Pac J Trop Biomed 2(2):S584–S588

Baker DD, Chu M, Oza U, Rajgarhia V (2007) The value of natural products to future pharmaceutical discovery. Nat Prod Rep 24(6):1225–1244

Barnes J, Heinrich M (2004) Fundamentals of pharmacognosy and phytotherapy. Churchill Livingstone

Bhanot A, Sharma R, Noolvi MN (2011) Natural sources as potential anti-cancer agents: a review. Int J Phytomed 3(1):9–26

Biju SS, Ahuja A, Khar RK (2005) Tea tree oil concentration in follicular casts after topical delivery: Determination by high-performance thin layer chromatography using a perfused bovine udder model. J pharm sciences 94(2):240–5

Chopra D (2006) The seven spiritual laws of yoga. Wiley

Chothani DL, Patel MB, Mishra SH (2012) HPTLC fingerprint profile and isolation of marker compound of Ruellia tuberosa. Chromatogr Res Int 2012:1

Demain AL (2014) Importance of microbial natural products and the need to revitalize their discovery. J Ind Microbiol Biotechnol 41(2):185–201

Dev S (1999) Ancient-modern concordance in Ayurvedic plants: some examples. Environ Health Perspect 107(10):783–789

Dhalwal K, Shinde VM, Biradar YS, Mahadik KR (2008) Simultaneous quantification of bergenin, catechin, and gallic acid from Bergenia ciliata and Bergenia ligulata by using thin-layer chromatography. J Food Compos Anal 21(6):496–500

Ekor M (2014) The growing use of herbal medicines: issues relating to adverse reactions and challenges in monitoring safety. Front Pharmacol 4:66193

Ernst E (1997) Homoeopathy: past, present and future. Br J Clin Pharmacol 44(5):435

Ernst E (2004) Anthroposophical medicine: a systematic review of randomised clinical trials. Wien Klin Wochenschr 116(4)

Gordon T (2013) Theorizing yoga as a mindfulness skill. Procedia Soc Behav Sci 84:1224–1227

Grabia S, Ernst E (2003) Homeopathic aggravations: a systematic review of randomised, placebo-controlled clinical trials. Homeopathy 92(02):92–98

Gupta S, Shanker K, Srivastava SK (2012) HPTLC method for the simultaneous determination of four indole alkaloids in Rauwolfia tetraphylla: a study of organic/green solvent and continuous/pulse sonication. J Pharm Biomed Anal 66:33–39

Gurme ST, Patil DN, Jadhav SV, Ahire ML, Mundada PS (2022) Azadirachta indica (Neem) and Berberis aristata (Indian Barberry). Herbs, Shrubs, and Trees of Potential Medicinal Benefits 365–376. CRC Press

Hoyez AC (2007) The 'world of yoga': the production and reproduction of therapeutic landscapes. Soc Sci Med 65(1):112–124

Hussain MS, Fareed S, Ali M (2012a) Simultaneous HPTLC-UV530 nm analysis and validation of bioactive lupeol and stigmasterol in Hygrophila auriculata (K. Schum) Heine. Asian Pac J Trop Biomed 2(2):S612–S617

Hussain MS, Fareed S, Ali M, Rahman MA (2012b) Validation of the method for the simultaneous estimation of bioactive marker gallic acid and quercetin in *Abutilon indicum* by HPTLC. Asian Pac J Trop Dis 2:S76–S83
Jain A, Lodhi S, Singhai AK (2009) Simultaneous estimation of quercetin and rutin in Tephrosia purpurea Pers by high performance thin layer chromatography. Asian J Tradit Med 4(3):104–109
Jaitak V, Gupta AP, Kaul VK, Ahuja PS (2008) Validated high-performance thin-layer chromatography method for steviol glycosides in Stevia rebaudiana. J Pharm Biomed Anal 47(4–5):790–794
Kalim MD, Bhattacharyya D, Banerjee A, Chattopadhyay S (2010) Oxidative DNA damage preventive activity and antioxidant potential of plants used in Unani system of medicine. BMC Complement Altern Med 10:1–11
Kamboj K, Saluja AK (2013) HPTLC estimation of stigmasterol from petroleum ether extract of dried leaf, stem and flower of Ageratum conyzoides L. Int J Pharm Sci Rev Res 19:60–65
Katiyar C, Gupta A, Kanjilal S, Katiyar S (2012) Drug discovery from plant sources: an integrated approach. AYU 33(1):10–19
Katz L, Baltz RH (2016) Natural product discovery: past, present, and future. J Ind Microbiol Biotechnol 43(2–3):155–176
Kumar D, Kumar R, Singh B, Ahuja PS (2015) Reproducible reversed-phase high-performance thin-layer chromatography-based quality-control method for the endangered medicinal plant Picrorhiza kurroa Royle ex Benth. J Planar Chromatogr Mod TLC 28(3):256–261
Linde K, Clausius N, Ramirez G, Melchart D, Eitel F, Hedges LV, Jonas WB (1997) Are the clinical effects of homoeopathy placebo effects? A meta-analysis of placebo-controlled trials. Lancet 350(9081):834–843
Mukherjee PK, Venkatesh P, Ponnusankar S (2010) Ethnopharmacology and integrative medicine–let the history tell the future. J Ayurveda Integr Med 1(2):100
Narayanaswami V (1975) Introduction to the siddha system of medicine. A. Anandakumar, Pandit SS Anandam Research Institute of Siddha medicine
Navneet N, Manisha A, Sandeep R, Gaurav S, Reni K (2013) Quantitative estimation of tecomin in Tecomella undulata bark using HPTLC method. J Biomed Pharm Res 2(1)
Newman DJ, Cragg GM (2016) Natural products as sources of new drugs from 1981 to 2014. J Nat Prod 79(3):629–661
Pandey MM, Rastogi S, Rawat AKS (2013) Indian traditional ayurvedic system of medicine and nutritional supplementation. Evid Based Complement Alternat Med 2013:1
Pathania S, Bansal P, Gupta P, Rawal RK (2020) Genus Calotropis: a hub of medicinally active phytoconstituents. Current Traditional Medicine, 6(4):312–331
Patidar P, Dubey D, Dashora K (2012) Quantification of (−) epicatechin by HPTLC method in Cassia fistula crude drug, lab extract and commercial extract. Asian J Pharm Clin Res 5:140–143
Patil AG, Koli SP, Patil DA (2013) Pharmcognostical standardization and HPTLC fingerprint of *Averrhoa bilimbi* (L.) fruits. J Pharm Res 6(1):145–150
Patil AG, Patil DA, Sharma AJ, Naresh Chandra NC (2011) Comparative in vitro antioxidant activity and HPTLC fingerprint of Averrhoa bilimbi Linn. and Averrhoa carambola Linn. fruit extracts
Pawar RK, Sharma S, Singh KC, Sharma KR (2010) Development and validation of HPTLC method for the determination of andrographolide from Andrographis paniculata (whole plant). Int J Chem Res:15–19
Piet JH (1952) A logical presentation of the Saiva Siddhanta philosophy
Pillai NK (1998) History of siddha medicine. Department of Indian Medicine and Homeopathy, Chennai, India, pp 33–35
Posadzki P, Ernst E, Terry R, Lee MS (2011) Is yoga effective for pain? A systematic review of randomized clinical trials. Complement Ther Med 19(5):281–287
Prasad LV (2002) Indian system of medicine and homoeopathy traditional medicine in Asia. WHO-Regional Office for Southeast Asia-New Delhi, pp 283–286
Ravishankar B, Shukla VJ (2007) Indian systems of medicine: a brief profile. Afr J Tradit Complement Altern Med 4(3):319–337

Samal J (2014) Indian public health standards for Ayurveda, Yoga and Naturopathy, Unani, Siddha and Homoeopathy facilities: an assessment. Int J Med Public Health 4(4):331

Sathasivampillai SV, Rajamanoharan PR, Munday M, Heinrich M (2017) Plants used to treat diabetes in Sri Lankan Siddha Medicine–an ethnopharmacological review of historical and modern sources. J Ethnopharmacol 198:531–599

Shanker K, Gupta S, Srivastava P, Srivastava SK, Singh SC, Gupta MM (2011) Simultaneous determination of three steroidal glycoalkaloids in Solanum xanthocarpum by high performance thin layer chromatography. J Pharm Biomed Anal 54(3):497–502

Sharma P, Kirar V, Meena DK, Suryakumar G, Misra K (2012) Adaptogenic activity of Valeriana wallichii using cold, hypoxia and restraint multiple stress animal model. Biomed Aging Pathol 2(4):198–205

Singh B, Nadkarni JR, Vishwakarma RA, Bharate SB, Nivsarkar M, Anandjiwala S (2012) The hydroalcoholic extract of Cassia alata (Linn.) leaves and its major compound rhein exhibits antiallergic activity via mast cell stabilization and lipoxygenase inhibition. J Ethnopharmacol 141(1):469–473

Singh Chauhan N, Kumar Dixit V (2012) Development of HPTLC Method for Puerarin Estimation in Pueraria tuberosa (Roxb. ex Willd.) DC. Pharmaceutical. Crops 3(1)

Smina TP, Mathew J, Janardhanan KK, Devasagayam TPA (2011) Antioxidant activity and toxicity profile of total triterpenes isolated from Ganoderma lucidum (Fr.) P. Karst occurring in South India. Environ Toxicol Pharmacol 32(3):438–446

Srivastava S, Singh AP, Rawat AKS (2012) A HPTLC method for the identification of ferulic acid from Lycopodium clavatum. Asian Pac J Trop Biomed 2(1):S12–S14

Subramanian S, Ramakrishnan N (2011) Chromatographic finger print analysis of Naringi crenulata by HPTLC technique. Asian Pac J Trop Biomed 1(2):S195–S198

Thirumal M, Srimanthula S, Kishore G (2012) Cassia fistula Linn-Pharmacognostical, phytochemical and pharmacological review. Crit Rev Pharm Sci 1(1):43–65

Torri MC, Herrmann TM, Torri MC, Herrmann TM (2011) Traditional ethnobiological knowledge and bioprospecting. In: Bridges between tradition and innovation in ethnomedicine: fostering local development through community-based enterprises in India, pp 43–84

Verma SC, Rachana R, Pramila P, Padhi M, Jain CL, Ramesh B (2011) Quantitative determination of ferulic acid in Ricinus communis Linn. leaves and its geographical variation using HPTLC fingerprint

Wah HLK, Ramchurn K, Alladin SB (2014) Metal levels in traditional Chinese and Ayurvedic medicines. In: Chemistry: the key to our sustainable future. Springer, Netherlands, pp 321–337

World Health Organization (2004) WHO guidelines on safety monitoring of herbal medicines in pharmacovigilance systems. World Health Organization

Yadav AK, Tiwari N, Srivastava P, Singh SC, Shanker K, Verma RK, Gupta MM (2008) Iridoid glycoside-based quantitative chromatographic fingerprint analysis: a rational approach for quality assessment of Indian medicinal plant Gambhari (Gmelina arborea). J Pharm Biomed Anal 47(4–5):841–846

Ayurvedic Biology for Holistic Healing

11

Sandeep Kumar Jhade, Poonam Verma,
Poonam Kumari Pathak, Karthik Kalidoss,
Manoj Kumar Tripathi, and Rahul Shrivastava

Abstract

Ayurvedic biology is an ancient system of medicine rooted in the Indian subcontinent that offers a holistic and integrative approach to health and well-being. Ayurveda's foundational principles revolve around three doshas—Vata, Pitta, and Kapha, each representing a combination of the five basic elements and governing various physiological and psychological functions. By understanding the unique constitution (Prakriti) of individuals, Ayurveda emphasizes personalized healthcare, focusing on preventing disease by maintaining balance within these doshas. Ayurveda offers a comprehensive framework for achieving optimal health through personalized diagnostics and treatments, including diet, herbal remedies, and lifestyle adjustments. This chapter explores foundational concepts of ayurvedic biology, highlighting its relevance and application in modern holistic healing practices, and discusses the scientific validation of ayurvedic principles, highlighting the convergence of traditional wisdom with modern biomedical research. Future directions emphasize collaborative research, interdisciplinary education, and sustainable practices. The holistic and integrative nature of ayurveda makes it a valuable addition to modern healthcare, offering insights into personalized and preventive medicine.

S. K. Jhade · P. K. Pathak · K. Kalidoss · R. Shrivastava (✉)
Department of Biological Science and Engineering, Maulana Azad National Institute of Technology, Bhopal, Madhya Pradesh, India

P. Verma
Department of Biotechnology and Microbiology, ISBM University, Gariyaband, Chhattisgarh, India

M. K. Tripathi
ICAR- Central Institute of Agricultural Engineering, Bhopal, Madhya Pradesh, India

A. Kumar et al. (eds.), *Innovations in Ayurvedic Nutrition*,
https://doi.org/10.1007/978-981-95-1213-3_11

Keywords

Ayurveda · Doshas · Holistic healing · Personalized medicine · Traditional medicine

11.1 Introduction

Ayurvedic biology, an ancient yet evolving science, offers a profound understanding of health and healing by integrating the physical, mental, and spiritual dimensions of human existence. Rooted in ancient vedic texts, ayurveda views health as a harmonious balance of three doshas—Vata, Pitta, and Kapha. These doshas govern various physiological and psychological functions, and their balance is crucial for overall well-being. Unlike conventional medicine, which often focuses on treating symptoms, ayurveda emphasizes preventing illness by maintaining doshic equilibrium (Steer 2019). This ancient science has been practiced for thousands of years and continues to evolve, incorporating modern scientific research to validate its methods. Today, Ayurveda's principles resonate with contemporary holistic health trends, emphasizing natural remedies, personalized care, and lifestyle adjustments. By understanding the interplay of doshas and adopting ayurvedic practices, individuals can achieve a balanced state of health that encompasses physical, mental, and spiritual dimensions (Sharma 2016; Jaiswal and Williams 2017).

11.2 The Foundation of Ayurvedic Biology

Ayurvedic biology is grounded in the ancient Vedic philosophy of India, which perceives health as a state of dynamic equilibrium between the body, mind, and spirit. This holistic system is based on the concept of the three doshas—Vata, Pitta, and Kapha, which are fundamental bioenergetic forces present in all living beings (Hankey 2005). These doshas derive from the five basic elements: ether, air, fire, water, and earth. The unique combination of these elements in varying proportions gives rise to the individual constitution, or "Prakriti," which influences a person's physical characteristics, mental tendencies, and susceptibility to certain health conditions (Sharma 2016) (Fig. 11.1).

11.2.1 Vata (Air and Ether)

Vata is the principle of movement and is associated with qualities like lightness, coldness, dryness, and mobility. It governs bodily functions such as circulation, respiration, and nerve impulses. Vata's imbalance can lead to symptoms such as anxiety, dry skin, and irregular digestion. Those with a dominant Vata constitution are often creative, quick-thinking, and energetic, but may also experience restlessness and fatigue (Majumder and Ray 2022).

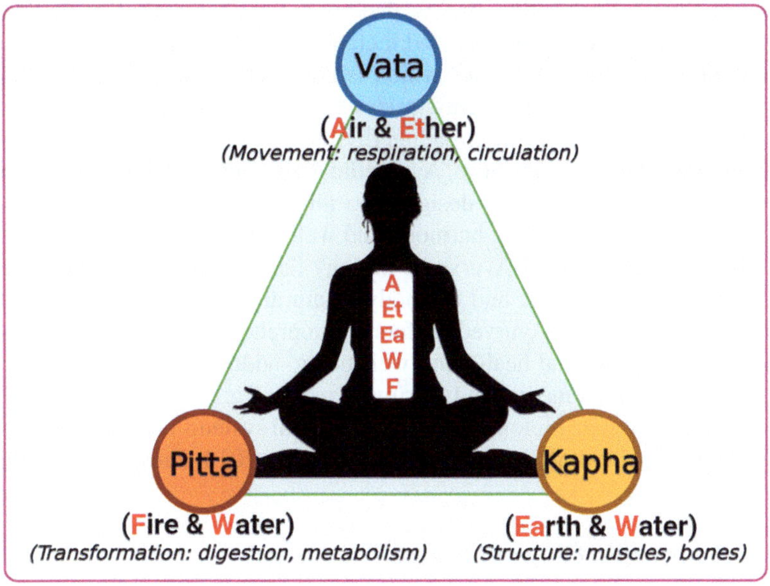

Fig. 11.1 Integration of doshas with biological functions in holistic healing: This image illustrates the fundamental principles of Ayurveda, showing the connection between the three doshas and their corresponding biological functions, reflecting a holistic approach to health and healing

11.2.2 Pitta (Fire and Water)

Pitta represents the energy of transformation and metabolism. It is linked with heat, sharpness, and fluidity, and controls digestion, metabolism, and body temperature. Pitta imbalance can manifest as inflammation, ulcers, and irritability. Individuals with a predominant Pitta constitution are typically intelligent, ambitious, and articulate, yet may also be prone to anger and impatience (Sharma 2016; Jaiswal and Williams 2017).

11.2.3 Kapha (Water and Earth)

Kapha embodies the principles of structure and cohesion, associated with heaviness, stability, and moisture. It governs the physical structure of the body, including bones, muscles, and fat, and is responsible for the lubrication and protection of tissues. An excess of Kapha can lead to lethargy, weight gain, and respiratory issues. Those with a Kapha-predominant constitution tend to be calm, strong, and nurturing but may struggle with complacency and resistance to change (Patel et al. 2020) (Fig. 11.1).

Ayurvedic biology posits that health is maintained by balancing these doshas according to one's unique prakriti. This balance can be influenced by various factors, including diet, lifestyle, climate, and emotional states (Patwardhan 2014). The concept of "agni," or digestive fire, is also crucial in Ayurveda. It is believed that strong agni leads to good digestion and metabolism, while weak agni can cause the accumulation of toxins, or "ama," which is considered the root cause of disease (Sharma 2016). Ayurveda also emphasizes the importance of the body's natural cycles and rhythms, such as the circadian rhythm, seasonal changes, and life stages, in maintaining health. For instance, Ayurvedic daily routines "dinacharya" and seasonal routines "ritucharya" are designed to align the body's internal clock with these natural cycles, promoting harmony and well-being (Shrivastava et al. 2020).

Briefly, the foundation of Ayurvedic biology lies in understanding the interplay of the doshas, the elements, and the body's natural rhythms. By recognizing and maintaining this balance, Ayurveda offers a comprehensive framework for achieving and sustaining optimal health and well-being, addressing not just physical ailments but also health's mental and spiritual aspects. This holistic approach is what distinguishes Ayurvedic biology from other medical systems and continues to make it relevant in contemporary health practices (Rastogi 2010; Patwardhan 2014).

11.3 Ayurvedic Diagnosis and Treatment

Ayurvedic diagnosis and treatment are grounded in a holistic understanding of the individual's physical, mental, and spiritual states. Unlike conventional medicine, which often focuses on treating specific symptoms or conditions, ayurveda seeks to identify and address the root causes of imbalance within the body and mind. This comprehensive approach involves a detailed assessment of the individual's constitution (Prakriti), the current state of doshas (Vikriti), and the presence of toxins (Ama). The goal is to restore balance and promote overall well-being.

11.3.1 Ayurvedic Diagnosis

Ayurvedic diagnosis is a multifaceted process that includes the following key components (Thakar 1982):

3.1.1 Pulse Diagnosis (Nadi Pariksha): One of the most critical aspects of Ayurvedic diagnosis, pulse diagnosis involves feeling the radial pulse at the wrist to assess the balance of the doshas. An experienced Ayurvedic practitioner can discern subtle qualities in the pulse that indicate imbalances in Vata, Pitta, and Kapha and specific organ systems (Joshi et al. 2007).

3.1.2 Observation (Darshanam): This involves the visual examination of the patient's body, including the skin, eyes, tongue, and nails. For instance, the color, coating, and texture of the tongue can reveal digestive issues, while the quality of the skin and eyes can provide insights into the body's internal state (Kurande et al. 2013).

3.1.3 Questioning (Prashnam): A thorough case history is taken to understand the patient's lifestyle, dietary habits, emotional state, and medical history. This helps in identifying factors that may be contributing to the imbalance of doshas (Kurande et al. 2013).

3.1.4 Touch (Sparshanam): This involves palpation and physical examination of the body, including checking the body's temperature, texture, and the presence of any abnormalities or discomfort (Thakar 1982; Kurande et al. 2013).
3.1.5 Urine, Stool, and Other Bodily Fluids Examination: Analysis of these can provide additional clues about the state of digestion, metabolism, and overall health.

11.3.2 Ayurvedic Treatment

The treatment approach in Ayurveda identifies and considers the individual's prakriti, the nature and severity of the imbalance, and the individual's environment and lifestyle (Patwardhan 2014). Key components of Ayurvedic treatment include:

Dietary Modifications: Ayurveda places great emphasis on the role of diet in maintaining health. Foods are categorized based on their taste (rasa), energy (virya), and post-digestive effect (vipaka). A tailored diet is prescribed to balance the doshas, considering factors like the individual's constitution, current doshic imbalance, and the season. For example, a Pitta-pacifying diet may include cooling, non-spicy foods, while a Vata-pacifying diet emphasizes warm, moist, and grounding foods (Tachaparamban 2014).

Herbal Medicine (Dravyaguna Vijnana): Ayurveda utilizes a vast pharmacopoeia of herbs, minerals, and other natural substances. These are selected based on their specific properties and actions on the doshas and body tissues. Commonly used herbs include ashwagandha for stress and vitality, turmeric for inflammation, and Triphala for digestive health (Kumar et al. 2011; Patibandla et al. 2024).

Panchakarma: This is a five-step detoxification and rejuvenation process designed to cleanse the body of accumulated toxins (ama) and restore doshic balance. Panchakarma includes therapies such as:

- Vamana (therapeutic vomiting).
- Virechana (purgation).
- Basti (medicated enemas).
- Nasya (nasal administration of medicated oils).
- Raktamokshana (bloodletting).

These therapies are often preceded by preparatory procedures like snehana (oleation) and swedana (sudation), which help loosen and mobilize toxins (Conboy et al. 2009; Vinjamury et al. 2012; Yadav et al. 2019).

Lifestyle and Behavioral Adjustments (Dinacharya and Ritucharya): Ayurveda prescribes daily and seasonal routines to align the individual's lifestyle with natural rhythms. Dinacharya includes practices like waking up early, tongue scraping, oil pulling, and self-massage (abhyanga). Ritucharya provides guidelines for dietary and lifestyle adjustments according to seasonal changes, helping to prevent seasonal illnesses and maintain doshic balance (Shrivastava et al. 2020).

Yoga and Meditation: These practices are integral to Ayurveda and are used to balance the mind, improve physical flexibility and strength, and promote mental clarity and emotional stability. Specific yoga postures (asanas) and breathing exercises (pranayama) are recommended based on the individual's constitution and current health status (Rioux and Howerter 2019).

Rasayana Therapy: This rejuvenation therapy involves the use of specific herbs, dietary regimens, and lifestyle practices to promote longevity, enhance immunity, and slow the ageing process. Rasayana is particularly beneficial in restoring vitality and preventing disease in those who are recovering from illness or experiencing age-related decline (Patibandla et al. 2024).

Mantra and Spiritual Practices: Recognizing the mind-body connection, ayurveda often incorporates spiritual practices like chanting mantras, meditation, and prayer to promote mental peace and spiritual well-being.

11.4 Ayurveda and Modern Science

The integration of Ayurveda with modern science represents an exciting convergence of ancient wisdom and contemporary research methodologies. As the world increasingly seeks holistic and personalized approaches to health care, Ayurveda's principles have garnered interest for their potential to complement and enhance modern medical practices (Patwardhan et al. 2008; Rastogi 2010; Patwardhan 2014). This section explores the scientific validation of ayurvedic concepts, the growing body of research on Ayurvedic treatments, and the synergistic possibilities between Ayurveda and modern medicine.

11.4.1 Scientific Validation of Ayurvedic Principles

11.4.1.1 Doshas and Biological Correlates

One of the central tenets of ayurveda is the concept of the three doshas—Vata, Pitta, and Kapha, which are believed to govern various physiological and psychological processes. Modern research has begun to explore the biological underpinnings of these doshas. For example, studies have suggested that Vata may correspond to the nervous system, Pitta to metabolic processes, and Kapha to structural and immune functions. This mapping offers a framework for understanding how doshic imbalances manifest as specific health conditions, providing a bridge between Ayurvedic theory and biomedical science (Morandi et al. 2011).

11.4.1.2 Prakriti and Genomics

Prakriti, the unique constitution of an individual, is a fundamental concept in Ayurveda that influences susceptibility to diseases and responses to treatment. Modern genetics and genomics research has begun to explore the correlation between prakriti types and genetic markers. Preliminary studies have shown that certain genetic polymorphisms correlate with specific prakriti types, indicating a genetic basis for the individual variations described in ayurveda. This research is paving the way for a deeper understanding of personalized medicine, aligning with the personalized approach ayurveda has advocated for millennia (Rotti et al. 2014; Prasher et al. 2016).

11.4.1.3 Agni and Metabolism

Agni, or digestive fire, is crucial in ayurveda, representing the body's ability to digest food and assimilate nutrients (Agrawal et al. 2010). Modern research on gut health, microbiota, and metabolism has provided insights into how digestive efficiency and microbiome composition can impact overall health (Shreiner et al. 2015), echoing ayurvedic emphasis on maintaining a strong agni for good health.

11.5 Research on Ayurvedic Treatments

11.5.1 Herbal Medicine and Phytochemistry

Ayurveda's extensive use of herbs has attracted significant scientific interest. Many Ayurvedic herbs are now studied for their pharmacological properties. For instance, turmeric (*Curcuma longa*), with its active compound curcumin, has been extensively researched for its anti-inflammatory and antioxidant effects (Sharifi-Rad et al. 2020; El-Saadony et al. 2022). Ashwagandha (*Withania somnifera*) is known for its adaptogenic properties, helping the body manage stress (Singh et al. 2011; Mikulska et al. 2023). Scientific research is uncovering the bioactive compounds in these herbs and elucidating their mechanisms of action, supporting their traditional uses.

11.5.2 Panchakarma and Detoxification

Panchakarma, Ayurveda's detoxification and rejuvenation therapy, is being studied for its effects on metabolic health, immune function, and chronic diseases. Research indicates that Panchakarma can influence biochemical markers of inflammation and oxidative stress, suggesting its potential benefits in managing chronic inflammatory conditions (Conboy et al. 2009; Vinjamury et al. 2012).

11.5.3 Mind-Body Practices

The inclusion of yoga and meditation in Ayurvedic treatment protocols has also been supported by modern research. Studies have demonstrated the benefits of these practices in reducing stress, improving mental health, and enhancing physical well-being. Research into the neurobiological effects of meditation and pranayama (breath control) aligns with Ayurvedic concepts of prana (life force) and mental balance (Field 2011).

11.6 Synergistic Possibilities Between Ayurveda and Modern Medicine

11.6.1 Integrative Health Care

The holistic and personalized approach of Ayurveda complements modern medicine's focus on disease diagnosis and acute treatment. Integrative health care models that combine Ayurvedic and allopathic approaches offer comprehensive care, addressing not only physical symptoms but also mental and emotional well-being. For example, ayurvedic dietary recommendations and herbal supplements can be used alongside conventional treatments for chronic conditions like diabetes (Thomas 2023), hypertension (Menon and Shukla 2018), and autoimmune diseases (Shingadiya et al. 2017) to enhance overall treatment efficacy.

11.6.2 Preventive Health

Ayurveda's emphasis on preventive health, including lifestyle and dietary guidelines, aligns well with modern preventive medicine's goals. Incorporating ayurveda into diseases and public health strategies can promote healthier lifestyles, reduce the prevalence of chronic diseases, and improve quality of life (Sharma et al. 2019).

11.6.3 Personalized Medicine

The concept of prakriti in Ayurveda provides a framework for personalized medicine, a rapidly growing field in modern healthcare. By considering individual differences in constitution, metabolism, and genetics, Ayurveda offers insights into personalized treatment plans. Modern tools like genetic testing can further refine these approaches, making Ayurveda's ancient wisdom even more relevant today (Joshi 2004).

11.7 Challenges and Future Directions

While ayurveda offers a rich and holistic approach to health and wellness, its integration with modern healthcare systems and scientific research presents several challenges. These challenges range from standardization and quality control to acceptance and understanding within the broader medical community (Gupta 2024). This section explores the key challenges faced by Ayurveda today and explores potential future directions to address these issues and enhance the practice's integration with modern science.

11.8 Challenges

11.8.1 Standardization and Quality Control

One of the primary challenges in the practice of ayurveda is the lack of standardization in formulations and treatments. Ayurvedic medicines often consist of complex mixtures of herbs and minerals, and the quality and potency of these ingredients can vary significantly. Ensuring consistent quality and efficacy requires stringent quality control measures, standardized processing methods, and accurate labelling. Contamination, adulteration, and variation in the concentration of active compounds are significant concerns that need to be addressed to build credibility and safety in ayurvedic products (Sahoo and Manchikanti 2013).

11.8.2 Scientific Validation and Evidence-Based Practice

While Ayurveda has a vast repository of knowledge based on traditional wisdom, there is a need for rigorous scientific research to validate its principles and practices. The current body of evidence is often seen as insufficient or lacking in the methodological rigor required by modern medical standards (Patwardhan 2014). Conducting well-designed clinical trials and pharmacological studies to investigate the efficacy, safety, and mechanisms of ayurvedic treatments is crucial for wider acceptance and integration into mainstream healthcare.

11.8.3 Regulatory Challenges

The regulatory landscape for ayurvedic products and practices varies widely across different countries. In some regions, ayurvedic products are classified as dietary supplements, which may not require the same level of regulatory scrutiny as pharmaceuticals. This can lead to variations in quality and safety standards. Establishing clear regulatory guidelines and standards that ensure the safety and efficacy of ayurvedic products while respecting traditional knowledge is a significant challenge (Parasuraman et al. 2014).

11.8.4 Intellectual Property and Traditional Knowledge

The global interest in ayurveda has raised issues regarding the protection of traditional knowledge and intellectual property rights. Ensuring that the benefits of ayurvedic practices are shared equitably and that traditional knowledge holders are recognized and compensated is an important challenge.

11.9 Future Directions

11.9.1 Standardization and Quality Assurance

Future efforts in ayurveda should focus on developing standardized protocols for the cultivation, harvesting, and processing of medicinal plants. Implementing good manufacturing practices and establishing pharmacopeial standards for ayurvedic products can enhance quality control and safety. Additionally, developing analytical methods to ensure the consistency and purity of herbal formulations will help build trust among consumers and healthcare providers.

11.9.2 Collaborative Research and Evidence Building

Collaborative research between ayurvedic practitioners and modern scientists can lead to a better understanding of the mechanisms behind ayurvedic treatments. Large-scale clinical trials, observational studies, and case series can provide robust evidence for the efficacy and safety of ayurvedic interventions. Research into the pharmacokinetics and pharmacodynamics of ayurvedic herbs and formulations will also help in understanding their actions and interactions with modern drugs.

11.9.3 Educational Integration and Interdisciplinary Training

Promoting interdisciplinary education and training programs that include ayurveda and modern medical sciences can bridge the knowledge gap between the two fields. Integrative medicine courses, workshops, and conferences can provide platforms for dialogue and collaboration, among practitioners.

11.9.4 Protecting Traditional Knowledge and Promoting Sustainable Practices

It is crucial to protect the intellectual property rights of traditional knowledge holders and ensure that they benefit from the commercialization of ayurvedic products. Additionally, promoting sustainable practices in the cultivation and harvesting of medicinal plants is essential to preserve biodiversity and protect natural resources.

11.9.5 Public Awareness and Education

Increasing public awareness about the benefits and limitations of Ayurveda through educational campaigns and media can help demystify the practice and encourage informed choices. Providing reliable information about the safe use of ayurvedic products and treatments will empower consumers and build confidence in ayurveda as a complementary healthcare option.

11.10 Conclusion

Ayurvedic biology offers a rich and comprehensive framework for understanding health and disease. By focusing on the balance of doshas and personalized care, ayurveda offers a unique approach to preventing and treating diseases, emphasizing holistic well-being. The integration of ayurvedic principles with modern medicine can enhance individualized care and provide more comprehensive health solutions. Future efforts should focus on rigorous research, education, and sustainable practices to ensure Ayurveda's safe and effective integration into mainstream healthcare. As we move forward, embracing the synergies between Ayurveda and modern science will be crucial in advancing holistic healthcare. Overcoming challenges such as standardization, quality control, and broader acceptance will pave the way for Ayurveda's integration into mainstream medical practices, promoting a more inclusive approach to health.

References

Agrawal AK, Yadav CR, Meena MS (2010) Physiological aspects of Agni. Ayu 31(3):395–398. https://doi.org/10.4103/0974-8520.77159

Conboy L, Edshteyn I, Garivaltis H (2009) Ayurveda and Panchakarma: measuring the effects of a holistic health intervention. Sci World J 9:272–280. https://doi.org/10.1100/tsw.2009.35

El-Saadony MT, Yang T, Korma SA, Sitohy M, Abd El-Mageed TA, Selim S, Al Jaouni SK, Salem HM, Mahmmod Y, Soliman SM, SAA M'm, WFA M, El-Wafai NA, Abou-Aly HE, Sitohy B, Abd El-Hack ME, El-Tarabily KA, Saad AM (2022) Impacts of turmeric and its principal bioactive curcumin on human health: pharmaceutical, medicinal, and food applications: a comprehensive review. Front Nutr 9:1040259. https://doi.org/10.3389/fnut.2022.1040259

Field T (2011) Yoga clinical research review. Complement Ther Clin Pract 17(1):1–8. https://doi.org/10.1016/j.ctcp.2010.09.007

Gupta R (2024) Integrating Ayurveda with modern medicine for enhanced patient care: analysis of realities. The Physician 9(1):1–6. https://doi.org/10.38192/1.9.1.3

Hankey A (2005) The scientific value of Ayurveda. J Altern Complement Med 11(2):221–225. https://doi.org/10.1089/acm.2005.11.221

Jaiswal YS, Williams LL (2017) A glimpse of ayurveda – the forgotten history and principles of Indian traditional medicine. J Tradit Complement Med 7(1):50–53. https://doi.org/10.1016/j.jtcme.2016.02.002

Joshi RR (2004) A biostatistical approach to ayurveda: quantifying the tridosha. J Altern Complement Med 10(5):879–889. https://doi.org/10.1089/acm.2004.10.879

Joshi A, Kulkarni A, Chandran S, Jayaraman VK, Kulkarni BD (2007) Nadi Tarangini: a pulse based diagnostic system. Annu Int Conf IEEE Eng Med Biol Soc 2007:2207–2210. https://doi.org/10.1109/IEMBS.2007.4352762

Kumar A, Dubey SD, Prakas S, Singh P (2011) Principle of Dravyaguna (Ayurvedic pharmacology). Biomed Pharmacol J 4(1):147–152. http://biomedpharmajournal.org/?p=1785

Kurande V, Bilgrau AE, Waagepetersen R, Toft E, Prasad R (2013) Interrater reliability of diagnostic methods in traditional Indian ayurvedic medicine. Evid-Based Complement Altern Med 2013:658275. https://doi.org/10.1155/2013/658275

Majumder B, Ray S (2022) Studies on functions of Vata Dosha – a novel approach. Int J Ayurveda Pharma Res 10(S2):117–124. https://doi.org/10.47070/ijapr.v10iSuppl2.2542

Menon M, Shukla A (2018) Understanding hypertension in the light of Ayurveda. J Ayurveda Integr Med 9(4):302–307. https://doi.org/10.1016/j.jaim.2017.10.004

Mikulska P, Malinowska M, Ignacyk M, Szustowski P, Nowak J, Pesta K, Szeląg M, Szklanny D, Judasz E, Kaczmarek G, Ejiohuo OP, Paczkowska-Walendowska M, Gościniak A, Cielecka-Piontek J (2023) Ashwagandha (Withania somnifera)-current research on the health-promoting activities: a narrative review. Pharmaceutics 15(4):1057. https://doi.org/10.3390/pharmaceutics15041057

Morandi A, Tosto C, Sartori G, Roberti di Sarsina P (2011) Advent of a link between ayurveda and modern health science: the proceedings of the first international congress on ayurveda, "Ayurveda: the meaning of life-awareness, environment, and health" March 21–22, 2009, Milan, Italy. Evid-Based Complement Altern Med 2011:929083. https://doi.org/10.1155/2011/929083

Parasuraman S, Thing GS, Dhanaraj SA (2014) Polyherbal formulation: concept of ayurveda. Pharmacogn Rev 8(16):73–80. https://doi.org/10.4103/0973-7847.134229

Patel V, Sasmal G, Kumar A (2020) A critical review of kapha dosha in the modern perspective. Int Ayurvedic Med J 8(12):5315–5319. https://doi.org/10.46607/iamj1808122020

Patibandla S, Gallagher JJ, Patibandla L, Ansari AZ, Qazi S, Brown SF (2024) Ayurvedic herbal medicines: a literature review of their applications in female reproductive health. Cureus 16(2):e55240. https://doi.org/10.7759/cureus.55240

Patwardhan B (2014) Bridging Ayurveda with evidence-based scientific approaches in medicine. EPMA J 5(1):19. https://doi.org/10.1186/1878-5085-5-19

Patwardhan B, Vaidya A, Chorghade M, Joshi S (2008) Reverse pharmacology and systems approaches for drug discovery and development. Curr Bioact Compd 4(4):201–212. https://doi.org/10.2174/157340708786847870

Prasher B, Gibson G, Mukerji M (2016) Genomic insights into ayurvedic and western approaches to personalized medicine. J Genet 95(1):209–228. https://doi.org/10.1007/s12041-015-0607-9

Rastogi S (2010) Building bridges between Ayurveda and modern science. Int J Ayurveda Res 1(1):41–46. https://doi.org/10.4103/0974-7788.59943

Rioux J, Howerter A (2019) Outcomes from a whole-systems Ayurvedic medicine and yoga therapy treatment for obesity pilot study. J Altern Complement Med 25(S1):S124–S137. https://doi.org/10.1089/acm.2018.0448

Rotti H, Raval R, Anchan S, Bellampalli R, Bhale S, Bharadwaj R, Bhat BK, Dedge AP, Dhumal VR, Gangadharan GG, Girijakumari TK, Gopinath PM, Govindaraj P, Halder S, Joshi KS, Kabekkodu SP, Kamath A, Kondaiah P, Kukreja H, Kumar KLR, Nair S, Nair SNV, Nayak J, Prasanna BV, Rashmishree M, Sharanprasad K, Thangaraj K, Patwardhan B, Satyamoorthy K, Valiathan MVS (2014) Determinants of prakriti, the human constitution types of Indian traditional medicine and its correlation with contemporary science. J Ayurveda Integr Med 5(3):167–175. https://doi.org/10.4103/0975-9476.140478

Sahoo N, Manchikanti P (2013) Herbal drug regulation and commercialization: an Indian industry perspective. J Altern Complement Med 19(12):957–963. https://doi.org/10.1089/acm.2012.0275

Sharifi-Rad J, Rayess YE, Rizk AA, Sadaka C, Zgheib R, Zam W, Sestito S, Rapposelli S, Neffe-Skocińska K, Zielińska D, Salehi B, Setzer WN, Dosoky NS, Taheri Y, El Beyrouthy M, Martorell M, Ostrander EA, Suleria HAR, Cho WC, Maroyi A, Martins N (2020) Turmeric and its major compound curcumin on health: bioactive effects and safety profiles for food, pharmaceutical, biotechnological and medicinal applications. Front Pharmacol 11:01021. https://doi.org/10.3389/fphar.2020.01021

Sharma H (2016) Ayurveda: science of life, genetics, and epigenetics. Ayu 37(2):87–91. https://doi.org/10.4103/ayu.AYU_220_16

Sharma R, Shahi VK, Khanduri S, Goyal A, Chaudhary S, Rana RK, Singhal R, Srikanth N, Dhiman KS (2019) Effect of Ayurveda intervention, lifestyle modification and yoga in prediabetic and type 2 diabetes under the National Programme for Prevention and Control of Cancer, Diabetes, Cardiovascular Diseases and Stroke (NPCDCS)-AYUSH integration project. Ayu 40(1):8–15. https://doi.org/10.4103/ayu.AYU_105_19

Shingadiya RK, Sharma R, Bedarkar P, Prajapati PK (2017) Autoimmune bullous skin disease managed with ayurvedic treatment: a case report. Anc Sci Life 36(4):229–233. https://doi.org/10.4103/asl.ASL_91_16

Shreiner AB, Kao JY, Young VB (2015) The gut microbiome in health and in disease. Curr Opin Gastroenterol 31(1):69–75. https://doi.org/10.1097/MOG.0000000000000139

Shrivastava S, Soundararajan P, Agrawal A (2020) Ayurvedic approach in chronic disease management. In: Noland D, Drisko JA, Wagner L (eds) Integrative and functional medical nutrition therapy. Springer, Cham, pp 783–798. https://doi.org/10.1007/978-3-030-30730-1_45

Singh N, Bhalla M, de Jager P, Gilca M (2011) An overview on ashwagandha: a Rasayana (rejuvenator) of Ayurveda. Afr J Tradit Complement Altern Med 8(5 Suppl):208–213. https://doi.org/10.4314/ajtcam.v8i5S.9

Steer E (2019) A cross comparison between Ayurvedic etiology of major depressive disorder and bidirectional effect of gut dysregulation. J Ayurveda Integr Med 10(1):59–66. https://doi.org/10.1016/j.jaim.2017.08.002

Tachaparamban NA (2014) Unique features of ayurveda dietetics. EPMA J 5(S1):A165. https://doi.org/10.1186/1878-5085-5-S1-A165

Thakar VJ (1982) Diagnostic methods in ayurveda. Anc Sci Life 1(3):139–145. https://www.ncbi.nlm.nih.gov/pmc/articles/PMC3336683/

Thomas V (2023) Ayurveda approach in the treatment of type 2 diabetes mellitus – a case report. J Ayurveda Integr Med. 14(4):100744. https://doi.org/10.1016/j.jaim.2023.100744

Vinjamury SP, Vinjamury M, Sucharitakul S, Ziegler I (2012) Panchakarma: ayurvedic detoxification and allied therapies—is there any evidence? In: Rastogi S (ed) Evidence-based practice in complementary and alternative medicine. Springer Berlin Heidelberg, Berlin/Heidelberg, pp 113–137. https://doi.org/10.1007/978-3-642-24565-7_7

Yadav U, Solanki JS, Bansal N (2019) Various aspects of Panchakarma in ayurveda. Indian J Appl Res 9(11):29–32. https://www.worldwidejournals.com/indian-journal-of-applied-research-(IJAR)/article/various-aspects-of-panchakarma-in-ayurveda/MTkxNTc=/?is=1&b1=0&k=1

Basic principles of Ayurvedic Nutrition

12

Deepa Sharma, Manoj Kumar Tripathi, Anil Kumar,
and Chandrashekhar Y. Jagtap

Abstract

Ayurveda, an ancient system of medicine from India, places significant emphasis on nutrition as a key component of health and disease prevention. Unlike conventional approaches, ayurvedic nutrition focuses on the individual, recognizing that each person's body and mind operate uniquely based on their constitution, or *dosha—Vata, Pitta*, and *Kapha*. In this system, food is seen not just as fuel but as a vital tool for maintaining balance and harmony in the body. By understanding how different foods and eating practices interact with our physiology, ayurvedic principles offer personalized dietary recommendations aimed at supporting digestion, metabolism, and overall well-being. This chapter explores the scientific foundation of ayurvedic nutritional concepts in relevance to the dietary practices mentioned in various Ayurveda classics. The text discusses the importance of food in Ayurveda, different concepts related to the food such as types of food, basic principles of digestion, major primary attributes of food, relation of food with sense organs, bodily constitutions and seasons, daytime variation in food, etc. The chapter also encompasses various dietary rules mentioned in Ayurveda,

D. Sharma
Central Ayurveda Research Institute, Jhansi, Uttar Pradesh, India

M. K. Tripathi
ICAR- Central Institute of Agricultural Engineering, Bhopal, Madhya Pradesh, India

A. Kumar
Rani Lakshmi Bai Central Agricultural University, Jhansi, Uttar Pradesh, India

C. Y. Jagtap (✉)
Central Ayurveda Research Institute, Jhansi, Uttar Pradesh, India

Department of Rasashastra and Bhaishajya Kalpana, All India Institute of Ayurveda, New Delhi, India

A. Kumar et al. (eds.), *Innovations in Ayurvedic Nutrition*,
https://doi.org/10.1007/978-981-95-1213-3_12

sequence of consuming foods, key factors influencing the utility of food, food adjuvants, etc. A thorough exploration of Ayurveda offers valuable insights that can enhance our understanding of health and nutrition, potentially leading to more effective healthcare solutions. Ultimately, adherence to these dietary principles and practices is essential for fostering a healthy life, promoting overall wellness and preventing illness.

Keywords

Ayurveda *Ahara* · Dietary rules · *Jatharagni* · *Prakriti* · *Anupan*

12.1 Introduction

Ayurveda, an ancient system of medicine from India, places significant emphasis on nutrition as a key component of health and disease prevention. Unlike conventional approaches, ayurvedic nutrition focuses on the individual, recognizing that each person's body and mind operate uniquely based on their constitution, or *dosha*—*Vata, Pitta*, and *Kapha*. In this system, food is seen not just as fuel but as a vital tool for maintaining balance and harmony in the body. By understanding how different foods and eating practices interact with our physiology, ayurvedic principles offer personalized dietary recommendations aimed at supporting digestion, metabolism, and overall well-being. This chapter explores the scientific foundation of ayurvedic nutritional concepts and their relevance in contemporary health practices.

12.1.1 Understanding *Hita Ahara* (Wholesome Food)

The food which maintains the balance of *dhatus* (seven fundamental tissues that constitute the human body), brings normalcy and restores the equilibrium of malbalanced ones is considered as *hita ahara* or wholesome food (Charaka 2009a).

12.1.2 Importance of *Ahara* (Food) in Ayurveda

Ayurveda views food as not only nourishment but also a powerful healing tool. Foods are chosen based on their inherent qualities, seasonal availability, and how they interact with an individual's constitution. Proper digestion is considered key to good health, and foods are selected to support digestive fire (*Agni*) without causing imbalance. *Ahara* is one of the three pillars of life according to Ayurveda; the other two being sleep (*Nidra*) and regulated sexual life (*Brahmacharya*) (Charaka 2009b). Acharya Charaka emphasizes the fundamental importance of food, stating that it sustains the life of all living organisms, with the entire world depending on it for survival. Factors such as complexion, mental clarity, longevity, cognitive ability, emotional well-being, satisfaction, physical growth, strength, and intelligence are all directly influenced by the quality and consumption of food (Charaka 2009c, d). Moreover, the benefits of proper nutrition extend beyond the individual, contributing to the well-being of society and the environment on a universal scale. Food is mentioned as the *prana* (vital force of life) of living beings but if not used properly may lead to death. Acharya Charaka states that body and disease both are generated out of food (Charaka 2009e).

Acharya Kashyapa mentions *Ahara* as the only cause of presence of all living things in this world. He also emphasizes on the importance of food by calling it a "*Mahabhaishajya,*" which means the best medicine of all (Vriddhajivaka 2005a). Maharshi Sushruta emphasized the vital role of food in promoting cardiovascular health and enhancing overall physical strength. According to him, a proper diet supports cognitive function, improves appetite, boosts energy levels, and strengthens both the mind and body (Sushruta 2003a).

12.1.3 Types of *Ahara* (Food) in Ayurveda

In ayurvedic texts four types of *Ahara* are mentioned, namely, *Ashit* (eatable), *Khadit* (chewable), *Peet* (drinkable), and *Leedh* (lickable) (Charaka 2009h).[9] Acharya Charak has mentioned twelve groups of various food items, namely, *shuk dhanya* (awned grains), *shami dhanya* (legumes), *mansa* (meat), *shaka* (vegetables), *phala* (fruits), *harita* (salads/ chutney), *madya* (alcoholic drinks), *jala* (water), *gorus* (milk & its products), *ikshu vikar* (sugar cane & its products), *kritanna* (dietary preparations), and *aharopyogi* (spices and condiments) (Charaka 2009i).

Acharya Bhavamishra has done more detailed grouping of food items as follows:

1. *Dhanya varga—Shalidhanya, brihidhanya, shukdhanya, shimbi dhanya,* and *kshudra dhanya.* (Bhavamishra 2012a)
2. *Shaka varga—Patra, pushpa, phala, naal, kand,* and *sansvedaj.* These are heavy to digest in from first to last. (Bhavamishra 2012b)
3. *Mansa varga—Jangal* (meat of animals belonging to jungles) and *Anoop* (meat of aquatic animals or animals living near water). *Jangal mansa* is better than *Anoop mansa.* (Bhavamishra 2012c)
4. *Kritanna varga*—Food prepared after cooking different food items. (Bhavamishra 2012d)
5. *Vari varga*—Different sources of water and its properties are given. (Bhavamishra 2012e)
6. *Dugdha varga*—Different sources of milk and their features are mentioned here. (Bhavamishra 2012f)
7. *Dadhi varga*—Various types of dadhi (curd) are explained like *manda, svaadu, svaduamla, amla,* and *atyamla.* All of these vary in their properties. (Bhavamishra 2012g)
8. *Takra varga—Ghol, mathit, takra, udashvit,* and *chhachhika* are various types of buttermilks explained along with their properties. (Bhavamishra 2012h)

9. *Navneet varga*—In this group, properties of butter obtained from cow and buffalo are given. Along with this, properties of butter obtained by various process like butter extracted from milk, fresh butter, and old butter are also mentioned. (Bhavamishra 2012i)
10. *Ghrita varga*—This group has detailed properties of Ghee obtained from various sources like cow, buffalo, goat, camel, sheep, human, and mare. Ghee obtained by various process is also mentioned like ghee extracted from fresh milk, 1 day old milk, fresh ghee, and old ghee. (Bhavamishra 2012j)
11. *Taila varga*—Oils extracted from various sources like sesame, mustard, linseed, poppy seeds, castor, etc., are described with their properties. (Bhavamishra 2012k)
12. *Sandhan varga*—Fermented liquids like *kanjika, tushodak, sauvir, arnal, dhanyamla, shindaki, shukta*, alcohol, *arishta, sura,* etc., are described with their properties. (Bhavamishra 2012l)
13. *Madhu varga*—Honey of eight types is described in this group, namely, *makshik, Bhramar, kshaudra, pauttik, chhatra, ardhya, auddalak,* and *dalam*. Out of these *makshik* is the best honey and *kshaudra* is beneficial for diabetics. (Bhavamishra 2012m)
14. *Ikshu varga*—Types and properties of sugarcane and its products like *fanit, matsyandika, guda, khand,* and *sharkara* are mentioned here. (Bhavamishra 2012n)

12.2 Basic Principles of Digestion in Ayurveda

Ayurvedic nutrition, rooted in ancient Indian traditions, emphasizes balance, individual constitution, and harmony with nature. Its dietary guidelines are based on the concept of *Doshas—Vata, Pitta,* and *Kapha*—which represent distinct energies or functional principles governing the body and mind. Ayurvedic nutrition seeks to maintain or restore balance among these *Doshas* to promote health and well-being. The digestive fire, referred to as *Agni* in Ayurvedic terminology, plays a crucial role in the breakdown, absorption, and assimilation of nutrients from food. *Agni* is the root cause of lifespan, complexion, strength, health, enthusiasm, growth, luster, immunity, energy, metabolism, and *prana* (vital force of life) (Charaka 2009j). When digestive function (*Agni*) is operating optimally, it promotes strength (*Bala*), health (*Arogya*), longevity (*Ayu*), and supports life force (*Prana*) (Charaka 2009k). However, an imbalance in digestive activity is considered a primary factor contributing to the onset of many diseases. Maintaining proper digestive function is therefore essential for overall well-being and disease prevention.

Avasthapak (Stages of Digestion)—The ingested food comprising of six *rasa* (tastes) undergoes stages of *prapaka* (preliminary digestion). Due to predominance of *kapha* in initial stage, the food gets converted into frothy state (chyme) undergoing *Madhur avasthapak*. Thereafter, *pitta* is predominant and food undergoes *Amla Avasthapaka*. Finally, when the food reaches the pakvashaya, which is the seat of *vata*, it gets converted into solid mass undergoing *katu Avasthapak* (Charaka 2009j). The process of *avasthapak* can be understood in modern terms as when food is taken, it is chewed (mechanical digestion) in the mouth, it mixes with saliva having mucous and ptyalin enzyme, which breakup the food material into smaller parts making it smooth with frothy appearance and starts the digestion of starch. When the food reaches the stomach, gastric juices containing hydrochloric acid (HCl) and pepsin helps in digestion mainly protein. HCl and pepsin may damage the stomach lining so mucous and bicarbonates secreted by stomach wall protect it by providing a slimy layer (*kaphaj* attribute). After this partially digested food (chyme) undergoes *amla avasthapak,* it reaches the small intestine having pitta in the form of bile and other digestive enzymes, which digest the food and assimilation of nutrients start. Finally, it reaches the large intestine, where it undergoes *katu avasthapak*, where water and minerals are reabsorbed from the food, which reduces its water content bringing roughness and dryness to the *kitta bhag* (stool) and formation of *vayu* (flatus).

When *Jatharagni* functions optimally, it divides the food into *Ahar Rasa prasad* (nutrient portion) and *Kitta* (waste product) parts. After digestion of food in the gastrointestinal tract, the action of five types of *agni* pertaining to five *mahabhut* viz. *akash* (space*), vayu (air), jala (water), agni* (fire), and *Prithvi* (earth) act and digest the respective portions of the food and nourishes the respective *dhatus* as per the *panchbhautik* composition. The *ahar rasa prasad* part is transformed into seven *dhatus* (body components viz. *Rasa, Rakta, Mansa, Meda, Asthi, Majja, and Shukra*) and *updhatu* [*stanya* (breast milk), *asruja* (menstrual blood), *kandara* (tendons), blood vessels, *vasa* (subcutaneous fat, skin, ligaments, and joints) by the action of *dhatvagnis* (digestive fire of each dhatu)]. *Dhatu mala* (waste of *dhatu*) is also produced in this process. These mala are *kapha, pitta, kha mala* (dirt of external orifices), *sveda* (sweat), *kesh-loma* (hairs of head and body), *Sneha of Akshi, vit, and tvak* (smear of eyes, feces, and skin) for each *dhatu,* respectively, upto *majja.* The *kitta* portion formed after digestion by the action of *jatharagni* is transformed into the *mala* (excretory waste product viz. *mutra and purish*) (Charaka 2009l).

A well-functioning digestive system leads to the production of a biochemical substance known as *Ojas,* which is formed out of *sara* (purest form) of *shukra dhatu*, which is believed to nourish both the body and mind. The seat of *Ojas* is heart (*hridaya*), which is also the seat of *mana* (mind). *Ojas* is considered essential for maintaining homeostasis across various physiological systems and is thought to support vitality, enhance immune function, and sustain life (*prana*) throughout the body (Charaka 2009m).

12.2.1 Features of Proper Digestion

Desire to take meal, good appetite, happiness and lightness in body, stability and normal activities are symptoms of proper digestion (Vriddhajivaka 2005b).

12.2.2 Factors Deranging the *Agni*

Fasting, eating during indigestion, over eating, irregular eating, intake of *astamya* (unsuitable) heavy, cold, rough, contaminated food items, faulty administration of *vamana* (therapeutic emesis), and *virechan* (therapeutic purgation), faulty adaptation of place, time, and season and suppression of natural urges (Charaka 2009o).

12.2.3 Causes of Derangement of *Annavah srotas* (Digestive Channels) and Its Symptoms

If food is taken in excessive quantity, untimely, and which is unwholesome causes derangement of *annavaha srotas* (digestive channels) and *agni* (digestive fire). Loss of desire to take food, anorexia, indigestion, and vomiting are indicative of dysfunction within the *Annavaha Srotas* (Charaka 2009p).

12.3 Food and *Dosha*

Ayurveda is grounded in the concept of three *Doshas*: *Vata*, *Pitta*, and *Kapha*, which are dynamic forces with distinct characteristics influencing all entities in the universe. Each person is born with a unique constitution, known as Prakriti, which is defined by varying proportions of these three *Doshas*. According to Ayurvedic principles, imbalances between the *Doshas* lead to a state known as *Vikriti*, a deviation from one's natural constitution. This imbalance can contribute to various health issues. Ayurvedic texts emphasize that an individual's diet should be tailored to their *Prakriti* to maintain balance and health. Ayurveda identifies six essential tastes—sweet, sour, salty, pungent, bitter, and astringent—that should be incorporated into the daily diet (Charaka 2009q). Each taste exerts specific physiological effects. A diet lacking in one or more of these tastes can lead to health complications and may trigger cravings for unhealthy foods, further disrupting the body's balance.

In Ayurveda, each taste has distinct effects on the three *Doshas* (Charaka 2009q):

- Sweet taste (*Madhur*): Common in sugar, honey, rice, milk, cream, butter, wheat, and bread, the sweet taste pacifies *Vata* and *Pitta* but increases *Kapha*.
- Sour taste (*Amla*): Found in lemons, limes, vinegar, cheese, and plums, the sour taste increases *Kapha* and *Pitta*, while decreasing *Vata*.
- Salty taste (*Lavana*): Salty foods elevate both *Kapha* and *Pitta*, while pacifies *Vata*.
- Pungent taste (*Katu*): Present in red chili, ginger, black pepper, and various hot spices, the pungent taste stimulates digestion, decreases *Kapha*, while increasing *Pitta* and *Vata*.

- Bitter taste (*Tikta*): Found in foods like spinach, leafy greens, asparagus, tomatoes, coffee, unsweetened cocoa, and citrus peels, the bitter taste helps reduce both *Kapha* and *Pitta*, but it tends to increase *Vata*.
- Astringent taste (*Kashaya*): Legumes such as peanuts, beans, peas, and lentils exhibit astringent properties. This taste reduces *Kapha* and *Pitta*, but increases *Vata*.

For balanced nutrition, Ayurveda recommends incorporating all six tastes into meals, adjusted for one's *Dosha* constitution.

12.4 Major Primary Attributes of Food

- Heavy (*Guru*): The heavy quality decreases *vata* and *pitta*, but increases *kapha*. Heavy foods include butter, ghee, sugar, heavy vegetables, etc.
- Light (*Laghu*): The light quality decreases *kapha*, but increases *vata* and *pitta*. Light foods include millet, wheat, barley, corn, spinach, lettuce, pears, and apples.
- Oily (*Snigdha*): The oily quality decreases *vata* and *pitta*, but increases *kapha*. Oily foods include dairy products, fatty foods, and cooking oils.
- Dry (*Ruksha*): The dry quality decreases *kapha*, but increases *vata* and *pitta*. Dry foods include beans, potatoes, barley, and corn.
- Hot (*Ushna*): The hot quality decreases *vata* and *kapha*, but increases *pitta*. The hot quality describes hot beverages, warm, and spicy foods.
- Cold (*Sheeta*): The cold quality decreases *pitta*, but increases *kapha* and *vata*. The cold quality describes cold beverages and foods.

12.5 Food and *Panchendriya* (Five Sense Organs)

The sense organs are defined as *panchendriya* in Ayurveda classics, namely, *Chakshu indriya, Shrotra indriya. Ghrana indriya, Rasana indriya, and Sparsha indriya,* which have predominance of *tejas* (fire), *akash* (space), *prithvi* (earth), *apah* (water), *sparsh* (*vayu*), respectively. Ayurveda describe food as not only a fusion of all the basic ingredients like proteins, vitamins, fats, and carbohydrates, but when desired food is taken, it also serves as a source of energy for the body and the senses as well (Charaka 2009r). Food is the substance through which we bring nature's quality into our bodies. The food consumed not only serves as nutrition for body but also to our senses, which in turn stimulates and kindles *agni* that is the basis of proper digestion. The ears (*shrotra*) hear the sound either from biting or chewing or breaking the food items. So, the food must have the required *Shabda* (crunch) in it so as to please ears. The *sparsha* (touch) of the food stimulates the touch sense, so the food should be good to touch. The *roop* (visual appearance) of the food pleases the eyes (*chakshurendriya*). The aroma from the food satisfies the smell (*ghranendriya*), so it must have pleasant smell. The food should also have good taste to satisfy the tongue (*rasanendriya).*

12.6 Food and *Prakriti*

A basic concept in Ayurveda is *prakriti* or the constitutional type of all individuals. It suggests that *prakriti* is stable at origin and has three primary types—*vata, pitta, and kapha*. In traditional practice, the predominance of three *dosha* in *prakriti* is determined by the physician on the basis of physical, mental, and behavioral qualities which are listed in the classical texts such as Charaka Samhita. An individual's *prakriti* is another important cause of the influence of food on the biological system. The food should be taken to balance the *dosha,* which is dominant in *prakriti* of an individual (Charaka 2009s). In Ayurvedic medicine, individuals with a *Vata Prakriti*—characterized by a lean, dry body type and a tendency to feel cold—are advised to consume more grains, oils/unctuous food, salt, and mild spices in their diet. If *Vata*-dominant individuals do not receive adequate nourishment, they may be prone to conditions such as anxiety, constipation, and insomnia. These individuals require nutrient-dense foods. It is recommended that they limit the intake of salads, fruits, and legumes, instead opting for more grains, dairy products, and nuts. For individuals with a *Pitta Prakriti,* who tend to have a warm body temperature and a focused, intense nature, the consumption of raw vegetables and mildly spiced foods is encouraged. Excessive consumption of hot and spicy foods is believed to exacerbate issues such as skin rashes, liver disorders, and irritability.

Those with a *Kapha Prakriti,* who are typically heavier or stockier and have slower movement and speech patterns, benefit from lighter foods, including vegetables and salads, and thrive on hot, spicy meals. Overconsumption of sweet, heavy, or oily foods may lead to an increase in mucus production, weight gain, and a higher risk of conditions such as diabetes mellitus. *Kapha*-dominant individuals are advised to avoid sweets, dairy products, nuts, and most grains like wheat and rice, although they may consume lighter grains such as millets. By selecting foods that are appropriate for their unique *Prakriti,* individuals can maintain or restore the balance of their *Doshas*. This purpose is crucial for the practice of Ayurveda because prakriti determines an individual's predisposition to diseases and response to treatment.

12.7 Food and Season

Ayurveda emphasizes the importance of diet in alignment with natural rhythms and seasonal changes. If wholesome diet (*satmya ahara*) is taken according to different seasons it brings strength and complexion to one's body (Charaka 2009t).

12.7.1 Winter Season (*Hemant & Shishir*)

In this season, the digestive capacity increases due to enhanced internal circulation, supporting the digestion of heavier foods. Diet rich in fats, *amla* (sour), and *lavan* (salty) tastes, along with the *anup mansa* (meat of aquatic animals), *vileshaya* (meat of burrowing animals), and *prasaha* (meat of predatory birds such as hawks and crows) is beneficial. Honey, milk products, sugarcane products, fats (*vasa*), oils (*taila*), freshly harvested rice, and lukewarm water are also suitable for consumption. Although both *Hemanta* (early winter) and Shishira (late winter) seasons are similar, *Shishira* is characterized by a colder and drier climate. Therefore, foods that are light, cold, and predominantly bitter (*katu*), pungent (*tikta*), and astringent (*kashaya*) in taste should be avoided (Charaka 2009u).

12.7.2 Spring Season *(Vasant Ritu)*

According to Ayurvedic principles, the accumulated *Kapha* from the winter season liquefies under the influence of the sun's rays during spring. This process weakens digestive power. Therefore, it is advised to avoid frequent and excessive consumption of foods that are heavy (*guru*), sour (*amla*), oily (*snigdha*), and sweet (*madhur*). Additionally, daytime sleeping is discouraged during this season to maintain *doshik* balance in the body. During this season, barley, wheat, beverages like *Sidhu* and *Madhvika* are useful. Lighter food options are preferable, such as soups, *moong dal* (green gram), *patol* (pointed gourd), *sahajana* (drumstick), bitter gourd, honey (*Madhu*), and decoctions made from *Shunthi* (dry ginger). These choices help maintain digestive balance and promote overall well-being (Charaka 2009v).

12.7.3 Summer Season *(Grishma Ritu)*

In summer, the sun's rays deplete moisture from the environment, which results in reduced physical strength and may also impair digestive capacity. During this season, sweet, cold, liquid, and fatty foods are beneficial. It is recommended to consume meat broth, ghee and milk along with rice, cold, and sweet *mantha* (a liquid preparation made from coarsely powdered drug/grain and cold water). Conversely, alcohol, hot and spicy foods, sour foods, and excessive physical exertion should be avoided to prevent further strain on the body (Charaka 2009w).

12.7.4 Rainy Season *(Varsha Ritu)*

During the rainy season, atmospheric humidity increases significantly, which leads to a more weakening of both the body's digestive strength and overall vitality which is already weakened during summer. To support and maintain digestive function, it is recommended to consume sour, salted, and fatty foods which are helpful in pacifying *vata*. Food items such as honey, aged barley, wheat, rice, green gram, and lukewarm water, along with fermented herbal preparations like *Asava* and *Arishta* should be taken. Additionally, exposure to excessive sunlight, consumption of heavy meals, cold drinks, and strenuous physical activities should be avoided to prevent further depletion of digestive capacity (Charaka 2009w).

12.7.5 *Sharad Ritu* (Autumn)

During this season, sudden exposure to sunlight can lead to an accumulation of *pitta*, necessitating the consumption of easily digestible, light, sweet, cool, slightly bitter, and *pitta*-reducing foods and beverages. Regular dietary items may include rice, barley, wheat, bitter ghee (*tikta sarpi*), Indian gooseberry (*Emblica officinalis*), and pointed gourd (*Trichosanthes dioica*). It is recommended to avoid excessive intake of oily foods, curd, alkalis (*kshara*), alcoholic beverages, hot, or irritating foods that cause a burning sensation after digestion, highly spiced dishes, and the meat of aquatic or marsh-dwelling animals (Charaka 2009x).

12.8 Food and Daytime Variation

Adopting an Ayurvedic lifestyle involves making dietary choices that align with an individual's *Dosha* constitution, the quality of the food, seasonal variations, and geographical location. According to Ayurveda, the time of day also plays a crucial role in digestion. When Pitta is most dominant during afternoon, it is ideal for consuming the most complex meal, as the digestive fire (*Agni*) is strongest during this time. Additionally, the stages of life influence conscious eating practices, with Ayurveda offering guidelines on appropriate food and lifestyle choices to maintain optimal health and balance throughout life's cycles. Acharya Sushruta mentions that meals should be consumed in accordance with scheduled times, ensuring that portions are neither excessive nor insufficient. Failure to adhere to these guidelines can result in various gastrointestinal disorders, which may have serious health consequences. Acharya Charaka emphasized that a discerning individual, aware of the numerous health issues and discomforts associated with an unbalanced diet, should choose foods that are appropriate for their constitution and consumes them in the correct quantities. Additionally, it is essential to eat at appropriate times while maintaining self-discipline over one's desires (Charaka 2009y). Consistency in meal times, sleep patterns, and hydration, along with the consumption of freshly prepared, enjoyable meals, helps to support overall health.

12.9 Dietary Rules

An individual's diet and lifestyle should be tailored to counterbalance their innate constitution (*Prakriti*). This approach helps maintain physiological equilibrium and prevents imbalances that can lead to health issues. Dietary intake should be selected to counteract imbalances in the doshas *(dosha-viruddha)* while simultaneously supporting the nourishment and equilibrium of bodily tissues *(dhatu-samana).* This ensures that the diet helps maintain overall health by balancing both the *doshas* and the body's foundational tissues (Charaka 2009y).

12.9.1 Sequence of Consuming Food Items

The principle aligns with the classical teachings of Ayurveda regarding the sequence in which different food types should be consumed. This sequencing supports efficient digestion and helps in maintaining the balance of *doshas—Vata, Pitta,* and *Kapha*.

- *Snigdha* (unctuous) and *Madhura* (sweet) food items are recommended at the beginning of a meal. These foods are generally nourishing and grounding, which helps pacify *Vata* and *Pitta* doshas, aiding in the smooth functioning of digestive enzymes.
- *Ruksha* (dry) foods, being light and rough, and *Drava* (liquid) items are suggested to be consumed at the end. Dry foods help in balancing *Kapha* dosha, while liquids aid in digestion and assimilation of nutrients, helping to cleanse the digestive tract.
- Other food items that fall between these categories are taken in the middle of the meal. These foods are generally mixed in terms of their qualities and help to balance the transition between heavier and lighter foods.

This order promotes the natural flow of digestion, allowing the body to break down and assimilate food optimally, ensuring that the doshas remain balanced throughout the process (Charaka 2009z; Vriddhajivaka 2005c).

12.10 *Dashvidh Ahar Vidhi Vidhan* (Ten Types of Dietary Intake Rules)

Acharya Charak has mentioned ten rules for dietary intake (Charaka 2009aa):

Ushnam: The term *Ushna* (hot) refers to the temperature of the food rather than its inherent qualities. Foods with *Ushna guna* promotes *Vatanulomana* (proper bowel movement) and enhance *Pachakagni* (digestive fire), facilitating effective digestion of the consumed food. However, extremely hot food (*Ati Ushna*) is not recommended, nor should excessively cold food be consumed. Eating food that has been prepared a long time prior (*Chirasiddham*) can lead to various adverse effects, including *Stambhana* (stiffness), *Agnimandya* (reduced digestive power), *Aruchi* (loss of appetite), and *Hrillasa* (nausea). It is advised to consume freshly prepared warm food.

Snigdha: Foods should contain a moderate amount of unctuousness (*Snigdha*), as this helps to balance Vata dosha and supports digestive function (*Pachakagni*). However, excessively unctuous foods (*Atisnigdha*) should be avoided. Both dry foods (*Asnigdha*) and overly oily foods can disrupt digestion. Dryness (*Ruksha guna*) exacerbates *Vata*, impairing digestive power, while overly greasy foods (*Atisnigdha*) are heavy (*Guru*), requiring more time and energy to digest. This can lead to symptoms such as lethargy, loss of appetite, excessive salivation, and other digestive disturbances.

Matravat: According to Maharshi Charak, it is essential to consume food in moderation, with the appropriate amount determined by the strength of an individual's digestive fire (*Jatharagni*). He states that when food is consumed in proper measure, it can be digested efficiently without negatively affecting health. The food taken in proper amount provides strength, complexion, and health without disturbing *prakriti* (Charaka 2009ab).

Improper food quantity (*Amatra*) can be categorized into two types: insufficient (*Hina*) and excessive (*Adhika*). It is crucial to avoid both inadequate and excessive food intake.

Various types of dietary intake are mentioned as per the amount of and frequency of food taken viz. *Pramitashana, addhyashana, Vishamashana, Viruddhashana, and Samashana. Pramitashana* means when an individual takes food in a very small portion or after the suppression of hunger and thirst (Vriddhajivaka 2005e).

Adhyashana means excess intake of food, i.e., taking meal before proper digestion of previously ingested food (Charaka 2009ac).

Vishamashana means improper amount, routine, and pattern of eating.

Viruddhashana means taking food that are opposite in qualities such as their *guna* (property), *virya* (potency), and *vipak* (final bio-transformation of food after digestion).

Shamashana means taking *pathya* (beneficial) and apathy (non-beneficial) food in equal quantity and at same time (Charaka 2009ac). One should take food in proper quantity and this quantity depends on the digestive power (Charaka 2009ad). For this, the stomach's capacity can be conceptually divided into four parts for optimal digestion. It is recommended that two parts (or half of the stomach) be reserved for solid food, while one part should be filled with water or liquids. The final one part should remain empty to allow for proper movement of the body's physiological energies, or *doshas*, facilitating efficient digestion and preventing digestive discomfort (Vriddhajivaka 2005c). This approach is designed to promote balance and ensure smooth gastrointestinal function. The amount of food consumed should align with an individual's specific needs. Failing to adhere to this principle can result in a range of health issues.

Jirne Ashniyat: Refers to the principle that food should be consumed only after the complete digestion of the previous meal. It is essential to wait until earlier food is fully digested, which is indicated by several signs: cleared belching (*Udgara shuddhi*), enthusiasm (*Utsaha*), appropriate elimination of urges (*Yathochita vegotsarga*), hunger (*Kshut*), thirst (*Pipasa*), and a sense of lightness (*Laghuta*). If food is consumed without the presence of these indicators, it may remain undigested in the stomach, mixing with partially digested food and leading to the immediate aggravation of all *doshas*. This scenario is a significant contributor to many health issues arising from dietary irregularities. Conversely, if an individual delays eating even after the previous meal has been digested, this can also negatively impact health. Therefore, timely consumption of food (*Kala bhojana*), as emphasized by Acharya Charak, is essential for maintaining health and well-being.

Virya Aviruddha or dietary incompatibility, refers to the consumption of food items that are contradictory to the body's elemental composition, leading to potential disturbances within the system. Such foods are classified as *Viruddha Ahara* (incompatible foods). The frequent consumption of incompatible food items has become increasingly common in contemporary diets, contributing to various health issues attributed to *Viruddha Ahara.* Common examples of incompatible food combinations include the pairing of milk with salty foods (e.g., biscuits or bread) and mixing milk with fruits (smoothies/shakes), Additionally, preserved foods often contain excessive oil or salt to enhance shelf life, which can lead to incompatibility. Other problematic practices include consuming highly hot or cold beverages before or after meals, such as coffee, chilled water, carbonated drinks, and ice cream, as well as drinking water immediately before or after tea or coffee. These examples illustrate some common dietary practices that may disrupt digestive harmony, emphasizing the need for awareness of food compatibility in maintaining health.

Ishta Deshe and *Ishta Sarvopakarana* refer to the importance of consuming food in a favorable environment that meets all essential requirements for optimal psychological well-being during meals. A pleasant dining atmosphere positively influences both mental and physical functions, whereas an unpleasant setting can lead to mental distress, adversely affecting bodily functions. The dining space should be clean, hygienic, and free from disruptive emotions such as desire (*Kama*), anger (*Krodha*), excessive thinking (*Chinta*), fear (*Bhaya*), and sadness (*Vishada*). Creating an environment that fosters tranquility and focus enhances the overall dining experience, promoting better digestion and nutritional assimilation.

Na ati drutam emphasizes the importance of consuming food at a measured pace. Eating too quickly can disrupt the normal digestive process, potentially causing food to follow unintended pathways. Moreover, hastily consuming meals increases the risk of inadvertently swallowing foreign materials, such as hair or nails, which may go unnoticed. Taking time to eat mindfully helps ensure proper digestion and reduces the likelihood of such occurrences.

Na ati vilambitam refers to the importance of avoiding excessively delayed food consumption. Eating too slowly can lead to overeating without achieving a sense of satiety. Prolonged intervals between bites can cause the temperature of the food to change, with hot items cooling down over time. These factors can negatively impact *Agni* (digestive fire) and ultimately impair the proper digestion of food. Thus, maintaining a balanced pace while eating is essential for optimal digestive function.

Ajalpan, Ahasan, Tanmana bhunjita emphasizes the significance of consuming food with full concentration, without engaging in conversation or laughter. Eating in a calm and focused manner enhances digestion and enriches the overall dining experience. When meals are consumed with minimal distractions, it promotes mindful eating, allowing for better attention to the process of chewing and digestion, which can help mitigate the risk of digestive issues. Furthermore, this practice decreases the likelihood of unintentionally swallowing foreign materials such as hair or nails, which may occur when eating hurriedly. Mindful eating not only supports physical health but also cultivates a greater appreciation for the food being consumed.

Atmana Abhisamikshya Bhunjita highlights the importance of consuming food with self-awareness and respect for one's own needs. This entails recognizing one's abilities, understanding appropriate portion sizes, and discerning which foods are beneficial or harmful to health. By considering these factors, individuals can select the right type and amount of food for their unique circumstances. Conversely, consuming food without regard for personal health needs can lead to inappropriate dietary choices that may be detrimental to well-being. Mindful eating involves being attuned to the body's requirements, enabling informed dietary decisions. This practice ensures that the diet contributes positively to health, energy levels, and overall well-being.

12.11 *Ashta Ahara Vidhi Visheshayatana* (Eight Key Factors Influencing the Utility of Food)

Acharya Charaka identified eight key factors influencing the utility of food, referred to as "*Ashta Ahara Vidhi Visheshayatana*" (Charaka 2009ae). These factors are considered essential in the causative, preventive, and therapeutic aspects of disease management. They should be carefully assessed before, during, and after food consumption to ensure proper nutrition and health benefits. The first six factors, ranging from *Prakriti* (nature of the food) to *Kala* (timing of intake), pertain to the characteristics of the food itself. The seventh factor, *Upayoga Samstha*, deals with the method and context of eating and the last factor *Upyokta* relates with the person who is eating. All these eight factors are collectively known as *Ahara Vidhi Vidhana*, which governs appropriate eating practices. All eight factors hold equal significance in maintenance of health (Table 12.1).

12.12 Routine After Meal

After eating a meal, it is advised to rest for one *muhurta* (approximately 48 min). Following this rest period, a slow walk of 100 steps is recommended, after which additional rest should be taken. This routine is believed to support effective digestion by allowing the body to gradually process the food consumed (Vriddhajivaka 2005d).

12.13 *Anupana* (Food Adjuvants)

The drink taken after meal is called *anupana*. It should be contrary to the properties of food but not to *dhatus* (body components). It saturates, nourishes, provides energy, improve weight, brings satiety, settles down the food taken, helps in breaking food mass thereby producing softness, moistens the food, which facilitates

Table 12.1 Eight key factors influencing the utility of food

Sl. No.	*Ahara Vidhi Visheshayatana*	*Description*
1	*Prakriti* (nature)	It specifies the natural qualities of the food, i.e., the inherent qualities like *Guru* (heavy), *Laghu* (light), etc.
2	*Karana* (processing)	The process/preparation of food by water, fire, cleansing, churning, place, time, infusing, duration, utensil, etc., and thereby imparting other properties to it. This changes the natural quality of the food.
3	*Samyoga* (combination)	The grouping of two or more food items and the product exhibits different properties from the parent material.
4	*Rashi* (quantity)	It consists of *sarvagraha* (total amount) and *parigraha* (individual amount). This ascertains the results of the food as per the quantity consumed.
5	*Desha* (habitat)	It indicates the habitat which affect variations in the qualities due to geographic region, different soil, use, and their acclimatization to that particular region. Diet should be opposite qualities of area/*desha* and diseases.
6	*Kala* (time)	It specifies time factor and described in two ways, i.e., conditional (individuals' conditions of age and disease) and seasonal variations.
7	*Upayoga Samstha* (dietetic rules)	It consists of dietetic rules.
8	*Upayokta* (consumer)	The person who consumes food and develops suitability by practice (*oka-satmya*)

digestion, quick absorption, and assimilation of food promoting strength and life (Charaka 2009af). Water intake is necessary for life as well as for proper digestion and assimilation of food. Taking water before meal produces weight loss, if taken in during meal brings normalcy, and if taken after meal increases weight (Sushruta 2003b).

Taking water just after meal is like poison but if taken after digestion enhances strength. Excessive water intake causes indigestion but if taken in small amounts is beneficial. Intake of excessive amount of water after strenuous or prolonged exercise, thirst, and dehydration can produce electrolyte imbalance. During such type of conditions, level of ADH (antidiuretic hormones) is high preventing loss of water from body to maintain blood pressure. But when excessive amount of plain water is taken quickly, it lowers the sodium concentration in extracellular fluid (ECF) leading to movement of water from ECF into cells producing cell swelling. This may cause hyponatremia, headache, nausea, vomiting, confusion, muscle cramps, lethargy, breathing problems and can also be fatal. Therefore, in such conditions water should not be taken in excessive amount in one take instead it should always be taken in small amounts frequently along with some sort of food items/salts. Spices like ginger, cumin, and turmeric are often incorporated to stimulate Agni and enhance digestion.

12.14 Suppression of Hunger (*Kshudha*) and Thirst (*Trishna*)

The natural urge of hunger should not be suppressed as this may lead to emaciation, weakness, discoloration, body ache, anorexia, and giddiness. It should be managed with unuctuous, warm, and light diet. Suppression of thirst may lead to dryness of throat and mouth, deafness, fatigue, depression, and uneasiness. Cold and saturating drinks like *tarpan, manth, panak, coconut water, etc.*, can be taken (Charaka 2009f).

12.15 Consumption of Food Items

Nitya prayunjeet (Foods which can be used regularly) (Charaka 2009ab)	*Nitya Asevaneeya* (Food which should not be used regularly) (Charaka 2009al)
Shastik rice	Dried meat
Moong dal (Split green gram)	Dried vegetables
Saindhava (rock salt)	Lotus tubers and stem
Amalaki (*Emblica officinalis*)	Pork
Barley (*Yava*)	Beef
Cow milk	Buffalo meat
Meat from animals of *Jangal Pradesh* (forests of dry areas)	Fish
Cow ghee	Curd should be avoided at night unless combined with ghee, sugar, honey, moong dal (green gram), or Indian gooseberry (*Amalaki*) (Charaka 2009g)
Honey	Black gram (*udad*)
	Yavak

Pippali (*Piper longum* L.), *kshara* (alkali), and *lavana* (salts) should not be taken for long duration in excessive amount. *Pippali* is beneficial for digestion and produces quick benefits to the body but if used for long duration causes accumulation of doshas especially *kapha* and *pitta*. *Kshara* is used for digestion and acidity regulation but if used excessively it cause baldness, greying of hairs, blindness, impotency, and person becomes prone to cardiac disorders. *Lavana* promotes relish, digestion, moistening effect to food but its excessive use causes malaise, laxity, debility in body, untimely baldness, greying of hairs, and wrinkles (Charaka 2009n). The process of transitioning from unwholesome (*apathya*) to wholesome (*pathya*) foods, or vice versa, should be done gradually in a stepwise manner (*Padanshik Krama*) to allow the body to adjust smoothly (Charaka 2009t).

12.16 Conclusion

In conclusion, Ayurvedic nutrition emphasizes personalized dietary choices based on one's *Dosha* constitution, the balance of tastes, and the proper timing of meals. The approach views food as integral to physical, mental, and spiritual health, promoting harmony between the individual and their environment. The emphasis on diet and lifestyle to an individual's *prakriti*, age, and seasonal changes underscores the dynamic nature of wellness. Ayurveda asserts that food should nourish not only the physical body but also the intellectual and spiritual aspects of an individual. The sensory experiences associated with food, including aroma and the dining environment, are integral for enhancing digestion. Both *Ahara* (diet) and *Ahara Vidhi Vidhana* (dietetic rules) are essential for achieving optimal nutrition and health and preventing diseases with proper application being key to well-being. As healthcare costs are rising globally both in developed and developing countries, a focus on individual health management can significantly reduce expenses through a preventive approach. Ayurvedic principles can play a vital role in crafting integrated healthcare strategies. A thorough exploration of Ayurveda offers valuable insights that can enhance our understanding of health and nutrition, potentially leading to more effective healthcare solutions. Ultimately, adherence to these dietary principles and practices is essential for fostering a healthy life, promoting overall wellness and preventing illness.

References

Bhavprakash by Shri Bhavamishra with Vidyotini Hindi Commentary by Shri Brahmashankara Mishra and Shri Rupalalaji Vaishya Part I (2012a) Chaukhamba Sanskrit Bhawan, Varanasi, Dhanyvarga/1–90, pp 635–662

Bhavprakash by Shri Bhavamishra with Vidyotini Hindi Commentary by Shri Brahmashankara Mishra and Shri Rupalalaji Vaishya Part I (2012b) Chaukhamba Sanskrit Bhawan, Varanasi, Shakavarga/1–120, pp 663–704

Bhavprakash by Shri Bhavamishra with Vidyotini Hindi Commentary by Shri Brahmashankara Mishra and Shri Rupalalaji Vaishya Part I (2012c) Chaukhamba Sanskrit Bhawan, Varanasi, Mansavarga/1–129, pp 705–723

Bhavprakash by Shri Bhavamishra with Vidyotini Hindi Commentary by Shri Brahmashankara Mishra and Shri Rupalalaji Vaishya Part I (2012d) Chaukhamba Sanskrit Bhawan, Varanasi, Kritannavarga/1–184, pp 724–746

Bhavprakash by Shri Bhavamishra with Vidyotini Hindi Commentary by Shri Brahmashankara Mishra and Shri Rupalalaji Vaishya Part I (2012e) Chaukhamba Sanskrit Bhawan, Varanasi, Varivarga/1–86, pp 747–758

Bhavprakash by Shri Bhavamishra with Vidyotini Hindi Commentary by Shri Brahmashankara Mishra and Shri Rupalalaji Vaishya Part I (2012f) Chaukhamba Sanskrit Bhawan, Varanasi, Dugdhavarga/1–46, pp 759–766

Bhavprakash by Shri Bhavamishra with Vidyotini Hindi Commentary by Shri Brahmashankara Mishra and Shri Rupalalaji Vaishya Part I (2012g) Chaukhamba Sanskrit Bhawan, Varanasi, Dadhivarga/1–22, pp 767–770

Bhavprakash by Shri Bhavamishra with Vidyotini Hindi Commentary by Shri Brahmashankara Mishra and Shri Rupalalaji Vaishya Part I (2012h) Chaukhamba Sanskrit Bhawan, Varanasi, Takravarga/1–18, pp 771–773

Bhavprakash by Shri Bhavamishra with Vidyotini Hindi Commentary by Shri Brahmashankara Mishra and Shri Rupalalaji Vaishya Part I (2012i) Chaukhamba Sanskrit Bhawan, Varanasi, Navneetvarga/1–6, p 774

Bhavprakash by Shri Bhavamishra with Vidyotini Hindi Commentary by Shri Brahmashankara Mishra and Shri Rupalalaji Vaishya Part I (2012j) Chaukhamba Sanskrit Bhawan, Varanasi, Ghritavarga/1–20, pp 775–777

Bhavprakash by Shri Bhavamishra with Vidyotini Hindi Commentary by Shri Brahmashankara Mishra and Shri Rupalalaji Vaishya Part I (2012k) Chaukhamba Sanskrit Bhawan, Varanasi, Tailavarga/1–27, pp 779–782

Bhavprakash by Shri Bhavamishra with Vidyotini Hindi Commentary by Shri Brahmashankara Mishra and Shri Rupalalaji Vaishya Part I (2012l) Chaukhamba Sanskrit Bhawan, Varanasi, Sandhanvarga/1–35, pp 783–787

Bhavprakash by Shri Bhavamishra with Vidyotini Hindi Commentary by Shri Brahmashankara Mishra and Shri Rupalalaji Vaishya Part I (2012m) Chaukhamba Sanskrit Bhawan, Varanasi, Madhuvarga/1–30, pp 788–791

Bhavprakash by Shri Bhavamishra with Vidyotini Hindi Commentary by Shri Brahmashankara Mishra and Shri Rupalalaji Vaishya Part I (2012n) Chaukhamba Sanskrit Bhawan, Varanasi, Ikshuvarga/1–33, pp 792–797

Charaka Samhita of Agnivesha, Ayurved Dipika commentary by Chakrapanidutta, Edited by Acharya Jadavji Tikramji (2009a) Choukhamba Surabharati Prakashan Varanasi, Sutrasthana 6/3, p 44

Charaka Samhita of Agnivesha, Ayurved Dipika commentary by Chakrapanidutta, Edited by Acharya Jadavji Tikramji (2009b) Choukhamba Surabharati Prakashan Varanasi, Sutrasthana 11/35, p 74

Charaka Samhita of Agnivesha, Ayurved Dipika commentary by Chakrapanidutta, Edited by Acharya Jadavji Tikramji (2009c) Choukhamba Surabharati Prakashan Varanasi, Sutrasthana 27/3, p 152

Charaka Samhita of Agnivesha, Ayurved Dipika commentary by Chakrapanidutta, Edited by Acharya Jadavji Tikramji (2009d) Choukhamba Surabharati Prakashan Varanasi, Sutrasthana 27/349, p 174

Charaka Samhita of Agnivesha, Ayurved Dipika commentary by Chakrapanidutta, Edited by Acharya Jadavji Tikramji (2009e) Choukhamba Surabharati Prakashan Varanasi, Sutrasthana 28/45, p 181

Charaka Samhita of Agnivesha, Ayurved Dipika commentary by Chakrapanidutta, Edited by Acharya Jadavji Tikramji (2009f) Choukhamba Surabharati Prakashan Varanasi, Vimanasthana 2/15, p 240

Charaka Samhita of Agnivesha, Ayurved Dipika commentary by Chakrapanidutta, Edited by Acharya Jadavji Tikramji (2009g) Choukhamba Surabharati Prakashan Varanasi, Sutrasthana 27/6–7, p 153

Charaka Samhita of Agnivesha, Ayurved Dipika commentary by Chakrapanidutta, Edited by Acharya Jadavji Tikramji (2009h) Choukhamba Surabharati Prakashan Varanasi, Chikitsasthana 15/5, p 512

Charaka Samhita of Agnivesha, Ayurved Dipika commentary by Chakrapanidutta, Edited by Acharya Jadavji Tikramji (2009i) Choukhamba Surabharati Prakashan Varanasi, Chikitsasthana 15/3–4, p 512

Charaka Samhita of Agnivesha, Ayurved Dipika commentary by Chakrapanidutta, Edited by Acharya Jadavji Tikramji (2009j) Choukhamba Surabharati Prakashan Varanasi, Chikitsasthana 15/9-11, p 512

Charaka Samhita of Agnivesha, Ayurved Dipika commentary by Chakrapanidutta, Edited by Acharya Jadavji Tikramji (2009k) Choukhamba Surabharati Prakashan Varanasi, Chikitsasthana 15/9–11, p 512

Charaka Samhita of Agnivesha, Ayurved Dipika commentary by Chakrapanidutta, Edited by Acharya Jadavji Tikramji (2009l) Choukhamba Surabharati Prakashan Varanasi, Chikitsasthana 15/13–14, pp 513–514

Charaka Samhita of Agnivesha, Ayurved Dipika commentary by Chakrapanidutta, Edited by Acharya Jadavji Tikramji (2009m) Choukhamba Surabharati Prakashan Varanasi, Chikitsasthana 15/17–19, pp 514–515

Charaka Samhita of Agnivesha, Ayurved Dipika commentary by Chakrapanidutta, Edited by Acharya Jadavji Tikramji (2009n) Choukhamba Surabharati Prakashan Varanasi, Vimanasthana 1/18, p 234

Charaka Samhita of Agnivesha, Ayurved Dipika commentary by Chakrapanidutta, Edited by Acharya Jadavji Tikramji (2009o) Choukhamba Surabharati Prakashan Varanasi, Chikitsasthana 15/42–43, p 517
Charaka Samhita of Agnivesha, Ayurved Dipika commentary by Chakrapanidutta, Edited by Acharya Jadavji Tikramji (2009p) Choukhamba Surabharati Prakashan Varanasi, Vimanasthana 5/12, p 251
Charaka Samhita of Agnivesha, Ayurved Dipika commentary by Chakrapanidutta, Edited by Acharya Jadavji Tikramji (2009q) Choukhamba Surabharati Prakashan Varanasi, Vimanasthana 5/8, p 251
Charaka Samhita of Agnivesha, Ayurved Dipika commentary by Chakrapanidutta, Edited by Acharya Jadavji Tikramji (2009r) Choukhamba Surabharati Prakashan Varanasi, Sutrasthana 1/65, p 18
Charaka Samhita of Agnivesha, Ayurved Dipika commentary by Chakrapanidutta, Edited by Acharya Jadavji Tikramji (2009s) Choukhamba Surabharati Prakashan Varanasi, Sutrasthana 1/66, p 18
Charaka Samhita of Agnivesha, Ayurved Dipika commentary by Chakrapanidutta, Edited by Acharya Jadavji Tikramji (2009t) Choukhamba Surabharati Prakashan Varanasi, Sutrasthana 7/36-37, p 51
Charaka Samhita of Agnivesha, Ayurved Dipika commentary by Chakrapanidutta, Edited by Acharya Jadavji Tikramji (2009u) Choukhamba Surabharati Prakashan Varanasi, Sutrasthana 6/21, p 46
Charaka Samhita of Agnivesha, Ayurved Dipika commentary by Chakrapanidutta, Edited by Acharya Jadavji Tikramji (2009v) Choukhamba Surabharati Prakashan Varanasi, Sutrasthana 6/22-26, p 46-47
Charaka Samhita of Agnivesha, Ayurved Dipika commentary by Chakrapanidutta, Edited by Acharya Jadavji Tikramji (2009w) Choukhamba Surabharati Prakashan Varanasi, Sutrasthana 6/27-29, p 47
Charaka Samhita of Agnivesha, Ayurved Dipika commentary by Chakrapanidutta, Edited by Acharya Jadavji Tikramji (2009x) Choukhamba Surabharati Prakashan Varanasi, Sutrasthana 6/41-45, p 48
Charaka Samhita of Agnivesha, Ayurved Dipika commentary by Chakrapanidutta, Edited by Acharya Jadavji Tikramji (2009y) Choukhamba Surabharati Prakashan Varanasi, Nidanasthana 6/11, p 221
Charaka Samhita of Agnivesha, Ayurved Dipika commentary by Chakrapanidutta, Edited by Acharya Jadavji Tikramji (2009z) Choukhamba Surabharati Prakashan Varanasi, Sutrasthana 7/41, p 52
Charaka Samhita of Agnivesha, Ayurved Dipika commentary by Chakrapanidutta, Edited by Acharya Jadavji Tikramji (2009aa) Choukhamba Surabharati Prakashan Varanasi, Vimanasthana 1/24, p 106-108
Charaka Samhita of Agnivesha, Ayurved Dipika commentary by Chakrapanidutta, Edited by Acharya Jadavji Tikramji (2009ab) Choukhamba Surabharati Prakashan Varanasi, Sutrasthana 5/12, p 38
Charaka Samhita of Agnivesha, Ayurved Dipika commentary by Chakrapanidutta, Edited by Acharya Jadavji Tikramji (2009ac) Choukhamba Surabharati Prakashan Varanasi, Chikitsasthana 15/236, p 525
Charaka Samhita of Agnivesha, Ayurved Dipika commentary by Chakrapanidutta, Edited by Acharya Jadavji Tikramji (2009ad) Choukhamba Surabharati Prakashan Varanasi, Sutrasthana5/3, p 36
Charaka Samhita of Agnivesha, Ayurved Dipika commentary by Chakrapanidutta, Edited by Acharya Jadavji Tikramji (2009ae) Choukhamba Surabharati Prakashan Varanasi, Vimanasthana 1/21, p 305-306
Charaka Samhita of Agnivesha, Ayurved Dipika commentary by Chakrapanidutta, Edited by Acharya Jadavji Tikramji (2009af) Choukhamba Surabharati Prakashan Varanasi, Sutrasthana 6/50, p 8

Charaka Samhita of Agnivesha, Ayurved Dipika commentary by Chakrapanidutta, Edited by Acharya Jadavji Tikramji (2009ag) Choukhamba Surabharati Prakashan Varanasi, Sutrasthana 27/319, p 171
Charaka Samhita of Agnivesha, Ayurved Dipika commentary by Chakrapanidutta, Edited by Acharya Jadavji Tikramji (2009ah) Choukhamba Surabharati Prakashan Varanasi, Sutrasthana 7/325-326, p 172
Charaka Samhita of Agnivesha, Ayurved Dipika commentary by Chakrapanidutta, Edited by Acharya Jadavji Tikramji (2009ai) Choukhamba Surabharati Prakashan Varanasi, Sutrasthana 7/20, p 49
Charaka Samhita of Agnivesha, Ayurved Dipika commentary by Chakrapanidutta, Edited by Acharya Jadavji Tikramji (2009aj) Choukhamba Surabharati Prakashan Varanasi, Sutrasthana 7/21, p 49
Charaka Samhita of Agnivesha, Ayurved Dipika commentary by Chakrapanidutta, Edited by Acharya Jadavji Tikramji (2009ak) Choukhamba Surabharati Prakashan Varanasi, Sutrasthana 5/12, p 38
Charaka Samhita of Agnivesha, Ayurved Dipika commentary by Chakrapanidutta, Edited by Acharya Jadavji Tikramji (2009al) Choukhamba Surabharati Prakashan Varanasi, Sutrasthana 5/10-11, p 38
Charaka Samhita of Agnivesha, Ayurved Dipika commentary by Chakrapanidutta, Edited by Acharya Jadavji Tikramji (2009am) Choukhamba Surabharati Prakashan Varanasi, Sutrasthana 7/61, p 54
Charaka Samhita of Agnivesha, Ayurved Dipika commentary by Chakrapanidutta, Edited by Acharya Jadavji Tikramji (2009an) Choukhamba Surabharati Prakashan Varanasi, Vimanasthana 1/16, p 234
Charaka Samhita of Agnivesha, Ayurved Dipika commentary by Chakrapanidutta, Edited by Acharya Jadavji Tikramji (2009ao) Choukhamba Surabharati Prakashan Varanasi, Vimanasthana 1/17, p 234
Charaka Samhita of Agnivesha, Ayurved Dipika commentary by Chakrapanidutta, Edited by Acharya Jadavji Tikramji (2009ap) Choukhamba Surabharati Prakashan Varanasi, Vimanasthana 1/18, p 234
Charaka Samhita of Agnivesha, Ayurved Dipika commentary by Chakrapanidutta, Edited by Acharya Jadavji Tikramji (2009aq) Choukhamba Surabharati Prakashan Varanasi, Sutrasthana 7/36-37, p 51
Charaka Samhita of Agnivesha, Ayurved Dipika commentary by Chakrapanidutta, Edited by Acharya Jadavji Tikramji (2009ar) Choukhamba Surabharati Prakashan Varanasi, Sutrasthana, 5/10–11, p 38
Charaka Samhita of Agnivesha, Ayurved Dipika commentary by Chakrapanidutta, Edited by Acharya Jadavji Tikramji (2009as) Choukhamba Surabharati Prakashan Varanasi, Sutrasthana, 7/61, p 54
Charaka Samhita of Agnivesha, Ayurved Dipika commentary by Chakrapanidutta, Edited by Acharya Jadavji Tikramji (2009at) Choukhamba Surabharati Prakashan Varanasi, Vimanasthana, 1/16, p 234
Charaka Samhita of Agnivesha, Ayurved Dipika commentary by Chakrapanidutta, Edited by Acharya Jadavji Tikramji (2009au) Choukhamba Surabharati Prakashan Varanasi, Vimanasthana, 1/17, p 234
Charaka Samhita of Agnivesha, Ayurved Dipika commentary by Chakrapanidutta, Edited by Acharya Jadavji Tikramji (2009av) Choukhamba Surabharati Prakashan Varanasi, Vimanasthana, 1/18, p 234
Charaka Samhita of Agnivesha, Ayurved Dipika commentary by Chakrapanidutta, Edited by Acharya Jadavji Tikramji (2009aw) Choukhamba Surabharati Prakashan Varanasi, Sutrasthana, 7/36–37, p 51
Kashyap Samhita by Vriddhajivaka, revised by Pt. Hemaraja Sharma, Vidyotini Hindi Commentary by Shri Satyapala Bhishagacharya (2005a) Chaukhamba Sanskrit Sansthan, Varanasi, Khilasthana 4/4, p 249

Kashyap Samhita by Vriddhajivaka, revised by Pt. Hemaraja Sharma, Vidyotini Hindi Commentary by Shri Satyapala Bhishagacharya (2005b) Chaukhamba Sanskrit Sansthan, Varanasi, Sutrasthana Upakalpaneeyadhyaya 24, p 31

Kashyap Samhita by Vriddhajivaka, revised by Pt. Hemaraja Sharma, Vidyotini Hindi Commentary by Shri Satyapala Bhishagacharya (2005c) Chaukhamba Sanskrit Sansthan, Varanasi, Khilasthana 5/52-53, p 259

Kashyap Samhita by Vriddhajivaka, revised by Pt. Hemaraja Sharma, Vidyotini Hindi Commentary by Shri Satyapala Bhishagacharya (2005d) Chaukhamba Sanskrit Sansthan, Varanasi, Khilasthana 5/56, p 260

Kashyap Samhita by Vriddhajivaka, revised by Pt. Hemaraja Sharma, Vidyotini Hindi Commentary by Shri Satyapala Bhishagacharya (2005e) Chaukhamba Sanskrit Sansthan, Varanasi, Khilasthana 5/60, p 260

Sushruta Samhita edited with Ayurveda-tattva-sandipika hindi commentary by Kaviraja Ambikadutta Shastri, Part I (2003a) Chaukhamba Sanskrit Sansthan, Varanasi, Sutrasthan 24/68, p 109

Sushruta Samhita edited with Ayurveda-tattva-sandipika hindi commentary by Kaviraja Ambikadutta Shastri, Part I (2003b) Chaukhamba Sanskrit Sansthan, Varanasi, Sutrasthan 46/444

Ayurvedic Drugs: Pharmacological and Pharmaceutical Principles and Their Delivery Systems

13

Sandeep Kumar Jhade, Poonam Kumari Pathak, Karthik Kalidoss, Manoj Kumar Tripathi, and Rahul Shrivastava

Abstract

Ayurvedic drugs, originated from traditional knowledge, are gaining prominence in present healthcare systems worldwide. Pharmacologically, ayurvedic drugs exhibit diverse therapeutic actions and mechanisms, with recent research shedding light on their pharmacokinetics and pharmacodynamics. Furthermore, pharmaceutical principles guide the manufacturing, quality control, and formulation of ayurvedic medicines, ensuring safety and efficacy. This chapter provides a comprehensive overview of the pharmacological and pharmaceutical principles highlighting ayurvedic remedies and their delivery systems. Exploring the evolution of ayurvedic remedies from ancient texts to modern applications, we highlight their relevance in addressing global health challenges. Innovative delivery systems, including nanotechnology and novel drug delivery approaches, enhance the bioavailability and efficacy of ayurvedic formulations. Despite challenges in standardization and regulatory compliance, the future of ayurvedic pharmacology and pharmaceutical sciences is promising, with opportunities for interdisciplinary collaboration and personalized healthcare solutions. This chapter emphasizes the significance of integrating traditional ayurvedic wisdom with modern scientific insights to shape the future of medicine.

Keywords

Herbal Formulations · Ayurvedic Drug Repurposing · Nano-drug delivery

S. K. Jhade · P. K. Pathak · K. Kalidoss · R. Shrivastava (✉)
Department of Biological Science and Engineering, Maulana Azad National Institute of Technology, Bhopal, Madhya Pradesh, India

M. K. Tripathi
ICAR- Central Institute of Agricultural Engineering, Bhopal, Madhya Pradesh, India

A. Kumar et al. (eds.), *Innovations in Ayurvedic Nutrition*,
https://doi.org/10.1007/978-981-95-1213-3_13

13.1 Introduction

Ayurveda, an ancient holistic healing system originating from the Indian subcontinent, offers a treasure trove of natural remedies and therapeutic interventions deeply rooted in tradition and empirical evidence (Pandey et al. 2013). With a history spanning thousands of years, Aaurveda continues to captivate global attention due to its comprehensive approach to health and wellness, which emphasizes the harmony between mind, body, and spirit. Recent literature emphasizes the growing interest in ayurvedic drugs as complementary and alternative medicine options, driven by a surge in demand for holistic and personalized healthcare solutions (Chauhan et al. 2015). Moreover, the need for sustainable and nature-based therapies in the face of escalating healthcare challenges has further highlights the importance of ayurvedic interventions in promoting well-being and longevity (Nedungadi et al. 2023). By embracing Ayurvedic principles and practices, we not only honor a rich cultural heritage but also tap into a reservoir of therapeutic potential that resonates with the ethos of modern healthcare.

13.2 Evolution of Ayurvedic Remedies

The Evolution of Ayurvedic Remedies embodies a rich historical journey spanning millennia, reflecting the dynamic adaptation of ancient healing traditions to contemporary healthcare needs (Mishra et al. 2001). Originating from the Vedic period in ancient India, Ayurveda has traversed through various epochs, assimilating diverse influences and innovations along the way (Narayanaswamy 1981) (Fig. 13.1). From the classical formulations documented in ancient texts like Charaka Samhita and Sushruta Samhita to the modern resurgence of Ayurvedic practices, this evolutionary trajectory underscores the enduring relevance and adaptability of Ayurvedic remedies (Patwardhan 2013). Recent literature highlights the integration of Ayurveda into mainstream healthcare systems worldwide, fueled by growing recognition of its holistic approach and evidence-based efficacy (Buwanaka Jayakody and Buddhika Panditharathna 2023). Moreover, the evolution of Ayurvedic remedies reflects a synthesis of traditional wisdom with contemporary scientific advancements, ensuring their continued relevance in addressing global health challenges (Narayanaswamy 1981; Mukherjee et al. 2017).

13.3 Current Scenario of Ayurvedic Remedies

In the contemporary landscape, ayurvedic remedies have witnessed a remarkable resurgence, experiencing a renewed interest and acceptance in global healthcare systems. This revival is underpinned by a growing appreciation for holistic healing modalities and natural therapies, amidst concerns over the side effects and limitations of conventional medicine. Recent literature attests to the expanding role of ayurvedic remedies as complementary and alternative medicine options, with

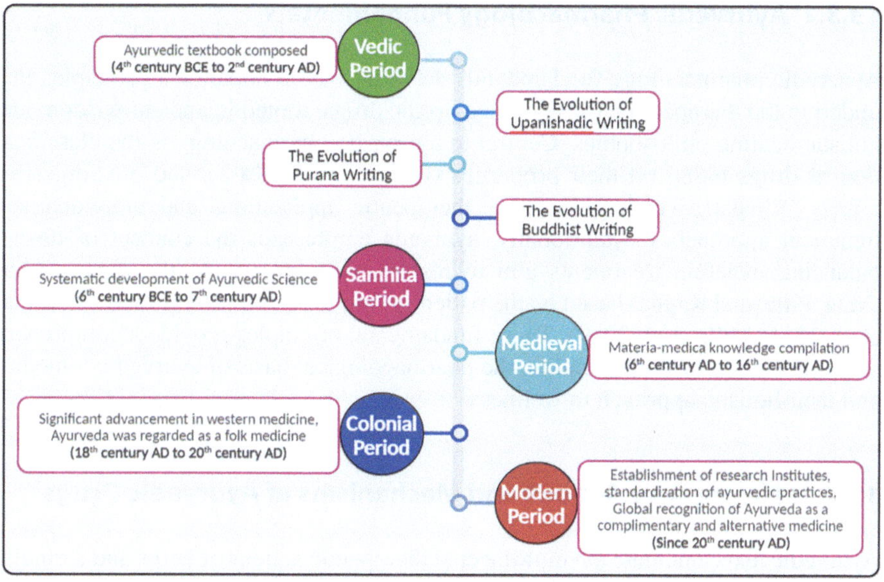

Fig. 13.1 Historical timeline for evolution of Ayurvedic Science

governments and regulatory bodies actively endorsing quality standards and research initiatives to enhance their credibility and safety (Chauhan et al. 2015). Furthermore, the integration of ayurvedic principles into mainstream healthcare reflects a paradigm shift towards personalized and patient-centric approaches to wellness (Patwardhan 2013; Nedungadi et al. 2023). This current scenario underlines the enduring relevance and adaptability of ayurvedic remedies in meeting the evolving healthcare needs of diverse populations worldwide.

13.3.1 Pharmacological Principles of Ayurvedic Drugs

The pharmacological principles of Ayurvedic drugs encompass a nuanced understanding of their therapeutic actions and mechanisms within the body. Rooted in ancient wisdom, ayurvedic pharmacology emphasizes individualized treatment approaches tailored to patient's unique constitutions and health conditions. Recent studies have elucidated the pharmacokinetic and pharmacodynamic profiles of ayurvedic drugs, highlight on their absorption, distribution, metabolism, and excretion pathways. Furthermore, research highlights the potential of ayurvedic herbs for repurposing in modern disease management, underscoring the relevance of traditional remedies in contemporary healthcare paradigms. Integrating traditional concepts with modern insights paves the way for evidence-based validation and innovative therapeutic interventions.

13.3.2 Ayurvedic Pharmacology Fundamentals

Ayurvedic pharmacology fundamentals delve into the foundational principles that underpin the therapeutic efficacy of ayurvedic drugs, rooted in ancient wisdom and holistic healing philosophies. Central to ayurvedic pharmacology is the classification of drugs based on their properties (Guna), tastes (Rasa), and post-digestive effects (Vipaka), which guide their therapeutic applications and individualized treatment approaches. Additionally, ayurveda emphasizes the concept of dosha-balancing, wherein treatments aim to restore harmony among the three doshas (Vata, Pitta, and Kapha) based on the patient's unique constitution (Prakriti) (Kumar et al. 2011; Mills et al. 2019). These fundamental principles provide a comprehensive framework for understanding the pharmacological basis of ayurvedic remedies and their holistic approach to wellness.

13.3.3 Therapeutic Actions and Mechanisms of Ayurvedic Drugs

Ayurvedic texts elucidate the multifaceted therapeutic actions of herbs and formulations, often attributing their efficacy to their ability to balance doshas, support organ function, and promote overall well-being. Moreover, modern research endeavors have unraveled the molecular mechanisms underlying the pharmacological effects of ayurvedic drugs, revealing interactions with various cellular signaling pathways and biochemical processes (Lele 2010; Kumar et al. 2017). This convergence of traditional wisdom with contemporary scientific insights enriches the understanding of Ayurvedic therapeutics and underscores their relevance in modern healthcare practices.

13.4 Pharmacokinetics and Pharmacodynamics of Ayurvedic Drugs

The pharmacokinetics and pharmacodynamics of ayurvedic drugs, delve into the dynamic interplay between ayurvedic remedies and the human body, unravelling their absorption, distribution, metabolism, and excretion profiles, along with their mechanisms of action. While ayurvedic pharmacokinetics traditionally accounts for factors like formulation type, route of administration, and individual constitution, modern research employs advanced techniques to assess the bioavailability and systemic effects of these drugs. Additionally, elucidating the pharmacodynamics of ayurvedic drugs involves understanding their interactions with biological targets, cellular pathways, and physiological processes, shedding light on their therapeutic mechanisms and potential adverse effects. Integrating traditional knowledge with contemporary pharmacological insights enhances the understanding of Ayurvedic pharmacokinetics and pharmacodynamics, facilitating evidence-based practice and personalized healthcare (Kaliappan et al. 2013).

13.5 Ayurvedic Drug Repurposing

Drug repurposing is the practice of identifying new therapeutic uses for existing drugs beyond their original intended purposes, often based on their known pharmacological properties. It offers a cost-effective and time-efficient strategy for discovering novel treatments for various diseases. (Khare et al. 2023) Ayurvedic drug repurposing signifies a promising avenue in modern pharmacology, leveraging the vast repository of traditional Ayurvedic remedies for novel therapeutic applications in contemporary medicine. This approach involves systematically exploring the potential of existing ayurvedic herbs and formulations for addressing modern diseases, backed by rigorous pharmacological research and clinical studies. Recent literature showcases compelling evidence supporting the repurposing of ayurvedic drugs for various health conditions, including metabolic disorders, neurodegenerative diseases, and immune-related disorders (Vaidya and Devasagayam 2007; Kumar Verma et al. 2021; Saggam et al. 2021; Krishnamurthy et al. 2022). Repurposing traditional remedies/drugs, not only harnesses their inherent therapeutic properties but also capitalize on their safety profile and cultural acceptance, offering cost-effective and accessible treatment options for diverse patient populations.

13.6 Traditional Concepts and Modern Insights in Ayurvedic Pharmacology

The synergy between tradition and modernity enables to validate the efficacy of traditional formulations through robust scientific research, employing pharmacological assays, clinical trials, and molecular studies (Patwardhan et al. 2008). Recent literature highlights the importance of integrating traditional ayurvedic concepts such as dosha-balancing and Rasayana therapy with modern pharmacological insights to develop evidence-based treatment strategies for chronic diseases and lifestyle disorders. Bridging the gap between tradition and modernity, fosters a holistic approach to healthcare that honors the legacy of Ayurveda while embracing the advancements of contemporary medicine (Gupta 2024).

13.7 Pharmaceutical Principles of Ayurvedic Drugs

Ayurveda, one of the oldest medical systems, provides a treasure trove of knowledge on the medicinal properties of herbs and minerals. The formulation, efficacy, and safety of ayurvedic medications are significantly influenced by pharmaceutical principles. These principles encompass various aspects aimed at optimizing formulation, safety, and therapeutic efficacy. Key considerations include drug formulation, extraction methods, dosage forms, and quality control measures (Pandey et al. 2013; Chauhan et al. 2015).

13.8 Manufacturing Processes and Standards in Ayurvedic Drug Production

Ayurvedic drug manufacturing is a complex and intricate process that begins with the selection of high-quality raw materials, followed by meticulous extraction, purification, and formulation. These processes are deeply ingrained in traditional ayurvedic texts such as Charaka Samhita and Sushruta Samhita, which serve as guiding principles for ayurvedic pharmacists. The integration of modern pharmaceutical techniques, including Good Manufacturing Practices (GMP), has revolutionized the industry, ensuring adherence to stringent quality and safety standards. Despite these advancements, Ayurvedic manufacturers remain committed to preserving the essence of traditional preparation methods, recognizing their significance in maintaining the authenticity and efficacy of Ayurvedic medicines (Manohar 2014; Mikulski et al. 2017).

13.9 Quality Control and Assurance in Ayurvedic Pharmaceuticals

Quality control is paramount in ayurvedic pharmaceuticals to ensure the safety, efficacy, and consistency of products. This process involves rigorous checks at every stage, from sourcing raw materials to the final product testing. Advanced analytical techniques such as chromatography and spectroscopy play a crucial role in standardizing herbal ingredients and finished products, thereby guaranteeing their potency and purity. The implementation of robust quality control measures not only meets regulatory requirements but also enhances consumer confidence in ayurvedic medicines (Jaishankar et al. 2014; Jan et al. 2015).

13.10 Formulation Techniques and Dosage Forms in Ayurvedic Medicine

Ayurvedic formulations are carefully crafted using a diverse array of herbs, minerals, and natural ingredients, each chosen for its specific therapeutic properties. These formulations are often tailored to individual constitutions or health conditions, drawing from classical recipes that have been passed down through generations. The flexibility of ayurvedic medicine is reflected in its wide range of dosage forms, including traditional churna (powder), kwatha (decoction), and taila (oil), as well as modern adaptations such as tablets, capsules, and syrups. This diversity ensures that patients have access to treatments that align with their preferences and lifestyles, further enhancing the holistic approach of ayurveda to healthcare (Manohar 2014; Rotti et al. 2014; Frattaruolo et al. 2019).

13.11 Delivery Systems of Ayurvedic Drugs

The delivery systems for ayurvedic drugs encompasses both traditional and modern approaches. Traditional methods include formulations such as churna (powder), kwatha (decoction), and taila (oil), which have been used for centuries to administer herbal remedies orally or topically (Bhatt and Deshpande 2020). In contrast, modern pharmaceutical advancements have introduced novel delivery systems like liposomes, nanoparticles, and microspheres tailored specifically for ayurvedic formulations. These modern approaches aim to enhance targeted delivery and sustained release, thereby improving the efficacy and bioavailability of ayurvedic drugs in line with contemporary pharmaceutical standards (Devi et al. 2010; Pandey et al. 2013; Bhatt and Deshpande 2020).

13.11.1 Traditional and Modern Drug Delivery Systems

Traditional ayurvedic medicines, rooted in natural sources like plants, animal products, and minerals, primarily utilize herbal formulations such as decoctions, powders, pills, and oils. These formulations rely on the body's inherent processes for metabolizing bioactive ingredients and absorption, with variability influenced by factors like raw materials and preparation methods. Unlike modern pharmaceutical formulations, which encompass a broad range of dosage forms including injections, patches, tablets, capsules, and inhalers, traditional ayurvedic drugs focus on promoting holistic health and balancing bodily energies (doshas) rather than complex drug delivery mechanisms (Katiyar 2019). While modern pharmaceuticals undergo rigorous testing to ensure the bioavailability of active ingredients, advancements such as nanoparticle technology, prodrug design, and micronization are employed to enhance absorption and therapeutic efficacy (Devi et al. 2010) (Fig. 13.2). Both traditional and modern drug delivery systems have witnessed significant advancements in targeted delivery and bioavailability, with nanotechnology emerging as a promising tool for improving drug delivery efficiency by overcoming biological barriers.

13.11.2 Nanotechnology in Ayurvedic Drug Delivery

Over the past two decades, nanotechnology has emerged as a cornerstone in the research and development of traditional herbal medicine. Its potential to revolutionize ayurvedic drug delivery holds promise for enhancing efficacy and precision. Nanoscale carriers and nanoparticles play a crucial role in this transformation, facilitating targeted delivery of bioactive compounds. Notably, bioactive compounds such as curcumin, berberine, and quercetin possess diverse biological activities against chronic diseases (Patel et al. 2024). Nanocarriers used in ayurvedic drug platforms, including polymeric nanoparticles and liposomes, serve as potent carriers that enhance bioavailability and protect active ingredients from degradation

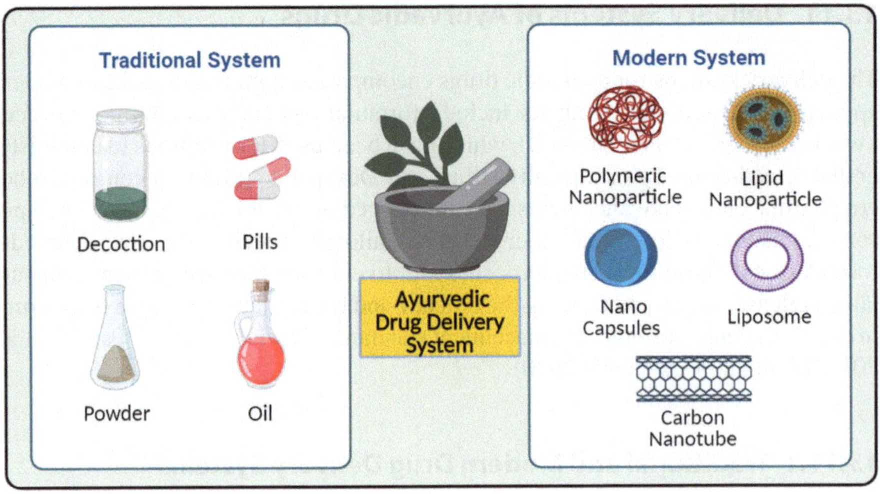

Fig. 13.2 Outline of traditional and modern drug delivery systems in Ayurveda

(Begines et al. 2020). These carriers encapsulate active ingredients from traditional ayurvedic formulations, thereby improving their bioavailability and therapeutic efficacy. Targeted delivery of nanoparticles ensures precise targeting of ayurvedic drugs towards specific tissues or cells, minimizing off-target effects and maximizing therapeutic outcomes (Abdelkawi et al. 2023). Surface modifications of nanoparticles facilitate their uptake by target cells or tissues, allowing for tailored drug delivery. By overcoming biological barriers, nanotechnology enhances the bioavailability of ayurvedic drugs, enabling lower doses, reduced side effects, and improved patient compliance.

13.12 Novel Drug Delivery Approaches for Ayurvedic Formulations

The exploration of novel drug delivery approaches holds substantial promise for enhancing the safety and efficacy of ayurvedic formulations. Contemporary drug delivery systems, including nanoparticles, liposomes, and microspheres, offer avenues to address challenges related to bioavailability, targeted delivery, and sustained release associated with traditional ayurvedic formulations (Sarangi and Padhi 2018). These advanced systems provide several advantages such as enhanced bioavailability, targeted delivery, sustained release, and protection of active ingredients (Singh and Sharma 2023). Nanotechnology-based delivery systems, for instance, enhance the solubility and absorption of active ingredients, thereby improving bioavailability (Bonifácio et al. 2014). Liposomes and nanoparticles enable precise delivery of ayurvedic formulations, minimizing off-target effects and enhancing therapeutic efficacy (Liu et al. 2022). Moreover, sustained-release systems like microspheres prolong the release of active ingredients, enhancing therapeutic effects and patient compliance (Ruan et al. 2022). Encapsulation of active ingredients in liposomes or nanoparticles protects them from degradation, ensuring stability and efficacy until reaching the target site. However, it is imperative to ensure compatibility between novel delivery systems and ayurvedic principles to preserve the holistic nature of ayurvedic medicine. Thorough preclinical and clinical studies are essential to evaluate the safety, efficacy, and pharmacokinetics of these advanced delivery systems tailored for ayurvedic formulations (Sarmukaddam et al. 2010). In conclusion, innovative drug delivery approaches have the potential to revolutionize herbal medicine, enabling personalized and targeted therapies.

13.13 Conclusion

The integration of ayurvedic principles with modern pharmacology and pharmaceutical sciences holds immense promise for advancing personalized healthcare paradigms. Through rigorous research and evidence-based validation, Ayurveda offers a holistic approach to wellness that complements conventional medical practices. However, this integration is not without its challenges. Standardization of herbal ingredients, regulatory compliance, and bridging the gap between traditional knowledge and contemporary scientific methodologies remain key hurdles to overcome. Nevertheless, the future of ayurvedic pharmacology and pharmaceutical sciences is bright, with emerging trends such as network pharmacology, personalized medicine, and nanotechnology poised to revolutionize drug discovery and delivery. Collaborative efforts between traditional healers, scientists, and healthcare professionals are essential for harnessing the full potential of ayurveda for addressing global health challenges and promoting well-being across diverse populations.

References

Abdelkawi A, Slim A, Zinoune Z, Pathak Y (2023) Surface modification of metallic nanoparticles for targeting drugs. Coatings 13(9):1660. https://doi.org/10.3390/coatings13091660

Begines B, Ortiz T, Pérez-Aranda M, Martínez G, Merinero M, Argüelles-Arias F, Alcudia A (2020) Polymeric nanoparticles for drug delivery: recent developments and future prospects. Nanomaterials 10(7):1403. https://doi.org/10.3390/nano10071403

Bhatt NS, Deshpande M (2020) A critical review and significance of Ayurvedic preparation Kwatha – herbal decoction. Int J Ayurvedic Med 11(2):155–164. https://doi.org/10.47552/ijam.v11i2.1495

Bonifácio BV, da Silva PB, Ramos MADS, Negri KMS, Bauab TM, Chorilli M (2014) Nanotechnology-based drug delivery systems and herbal medicines: a review. Int J Nanomedicine 9:1–15. https://doi.org/10.2147/IJN.S52634

Buwanaka Jayakody, Buddhika Panditharathna (2023) Integrating Ayurveda into mainstream healthcare systems: policy considerations. https://doi.org/10.13140/RG.2.2.17378.30403

Chauhan A, Semwal D, Mishra S, Semwal R (2015) Ayurvedic research and methodology: present status and future strategies. AYU Int Q J Res Ayurveda 36(4):364. https://doi.org/10.4103/0974-8520.190699

Devi VK, Jain N, Valli KS (2010) Importance of novel drug delivery systems in herbal medicines. Pharmacogn Rev 4(7):27–31. https://doi.org/10.4103/0973-7847.65322

Frattaruolo L, Carullo G, Brindisi M, Mazzotta S, Bellissimo L, Rago V, Curcio R, Dolce V, Aiello F, Cappello AR (2019) Antioxidant and anti-inflammatory activities of flavanones from Glycyrrhiza glabra L. (licorice) leaf phytocomplexes: identification of Licoflavanone as a modulator of NF-kB/MAPK pathway. Antioxid Basel Switz 8(6):186. https://doi.org/10.3390/antiox8060186

Gupta R (2024) Integrating Ayurveda with modern medicine for enhanced patient care: analysis of realities. Physician 9(1):1–6. https://doi.org/10.38192/1.9.1.3

Jaishankar M, Tseten T, Anbalagan N, Mathew BB, Beeregowda KN (2014) Toxicity, mechanism and health effects of some heavy metals. Interdiscip Toxicol 7(2):60–72. https://doi.org/10.2478/intox-2014-0009

Jan A, Azam M, Siddiqui K, Ali A, Choi I, Haq Q (2015) Heavy metals and human health: mechanistic insight into toxicity and counter defense system of antioxidants. Int J Mol Sci 16(12):29592–29630. https://doi.org/10.3390/ijms161226183

Kaliappan I, Kammalla AK, Ramasamy MK, Agrawal A, Dubey GP (2013) Emerging need of pharmacokinetics in ayurvedic system of medicine. Int J Res Ayurveda Pharm 4(5):647–651. https://doi.org/10.7897/2277-4343.04503

Katiyar CK (2019) Ayurvedic pharmaceutics, manufacturing processes and novel drug delivery systems in Ayurveda. In: Rastogi S (ed) Translational Ayurveda. Springer Singapore, Singapore, pp 33–52

Khare R, Jhade SK, Tripathi MK, Shrivastava R (2023) Drug repurposing: an approach for reducing multidrug resistance. In: Wani MY, Ahmad A (eds) Non-traditional approaches to combat antimicrobial drug resistance. Springer Nature, Singapore, pp 179–190

Krishnamurthy N, Grimshaw AA, Axson SA, Choe SH, Miller JE (2022) Drug repurposing: a systematic review on root causes, barriers and facilitators. BMC Health Serv Res 22(1):970. https://doi.org/10.1186/s12913-022-08272-z

Kumar A, Dubey SD, Prakas S, Singh P (2011) Principle of Dravyaguna (Ayurvedic pharmacology). Biomed Pharmacol J 4(1):147–152. https://doi.org/10.13005/bpj/273

Kumar S, Dobos GJ, Rampp T (2017) The significance of Ayurvedic medicinal plants. J Evid-Based Complement Altern Med 22(3):494–501. https://doi.org/10.1177/2156587216671392

Kumar Verma A, Kumar V, Singh S, Goswami BC, Camps I, Sekar A, Yoon S, Lee KW (2021) Repurposing potential of Ayurvedic medicinal plants derived active principles against SARS-CoV-2 associated target proteins revealed by molecular docking, molecular dynamics and MM-PBSA studies. Biomed Pharmacother 137:111356. https://doi.org/10.1016/j.biopha.2021.111356

Lele R (2010) Beyond reverse pharmacology: mechanism-based screening of Ayurvedic drugs. J Ayurveda Integr Med 1(4):257. https://doi.org/10.4103/0975-9476.74435

Liu P, Chen G, Zhang J (2022) A review of liposomes as a drug delivery system: current status of approved products, regulatory environments, and future perspectives. Molecules 27(4):1372. https://doi.org/10.3390/molecules27041372

Manohar PR (2014) Toxicity of Ayurveda medicines and safety concerns: the need to revive the branch of toxicology in Ayurveda. Anc Sci Life 34(1):1. https://doi.org/10.4103/0257-7941.150761

Mikulski MA, Wichman MD, Simmons DL, Pham AN, Clottey V, Fuortes LJ (2017) Toxic metals in ayurvedic preparations from a public health lead poisoning cluster investigation. Int J Occup Environ Health 23(3):187–192. https://doi.org/10.1080/10773525.2018.1447880

Mills PJ, Peterson CT, Wilson KL, Pung MA, Patel S, Weiss L, Kshirsagar SG, Tanzi RE, Chopra D (2019) Relationships among classifications of ayurvedic medicine diagnostics for imbalances and western measures of psychological states: an exploratory study. J Ayurveda Integr Med 10(3):198–202. https://doi.org/10.1016/j.jaim.2018.02.001

Mishra L, Singh BB, Dagenais S (2001) Ayurveda: a historical perspective and principles of the traditional healthcare system in India. Altern Ther Health Med 7(2):36–42

Mukherjee PK, Harwansh RK, Bahadur S, Banerjee S, Kar A, Chanda J, Biswas S, SkM A, Katiyar CK (2017) Development of Ayurveda – tradition to trend. J Ethnopharmacol 197:10–24. https://doi.org/10.1016/j.jep.2016.09.024

Narayanaswamy V (1981) Origin and development of Ayurveda: (a brief history). Anc Sci Life 1(1):1–7

Nedungadi P, Salethoor SN, Puthiyedath R, Nair VK, Kessler C, Raman R (2023) Ayurveda research: emerging trends and mapping to sustainable development goals. J Ayurveda Integr Med 14(6):100809. https://doi.org/10.1016/j.jaim.2023.100809

Pandey MM, Rastogi S, Rawat AKS (2013) Indian traditional Ayurvedic system of medicine and nutritional supplementation. Evid Based Complement Alternat Med 2013:1–12. https://doi.org/10.1155/2013/376327

Patel P, Garala K, Singh S, Prajapati BG, Chittasupho C (2024) Lipid-based nanoparticles in delivering bioactive compounds for improving therapeutic efficacy. Pharmaceuticals 17(3):329. https://doi.org/10.3390/ph17030329

Patwardhan B (2013) Historical future of Ayurveda. J Ayurveda Integr Med 4(4):189. https://doi.org/10.4103/0975-9476.123671

Patwardhan B, Vaidya A, Chorghade M, Joshi S (2008) Reverse pharmacology and systems approaches for drug discovery and development. Curr Bioact Compd 4(4):201–212. https://doi.org/10.2174/157340708786847870

Rotti H, Raval R, Anchan S, Bellampalli R, Bhale S, Bharadwaj R, Bhat BK, Dedge AP, Dhumal VR, Gangadharan GG, Girijakumari TK, Gopinath PM, Govindaraj P, Halder S, Joshi KS, Kabekkodu SP, Kamath A, Kondaiah P, Kukreja H, Kumar KLR, Nair S, Nair SNV, Nayak J, Prasanna BV, Rashmishree M, Sharanprasad K, Thangaraj K, Patwardhan B, Satyamoorthy K, Valiathan MVS (2014) Determinants of prakriti, the human constitution types of Indian traditional medicine and its correlation with contemporary science. J Ayurveda Integr Med 5(3):167–175. https://doi.org/10.4103/0975-9476.140478

Ruan L, Su M, Qin X, Ruan Q, Lang W, Wu M, Chen Y, Lv Q (2022) Progress in the application of sustained-release drug microspheres in tissue engineering. Mater Today Bio 16:100394. https://doi.org/10.1016/j.mtbio.2022.100394

Saggam A, Limgaokar K, Borse S, Chavan-Gautam P, Dixit S, Tillu G, Patwardhan B (2021) Withania somnifera (L.) Dunal: opportunity for clinical repurposing in COVID-19 management. Front Pharmacol 12:623795. https://doi.org/10.3389/fphar.2021.623795

Sarangi M, Padhi S (2018) Novel herbal drug delivery system: an overview. Arch Med Health Sci 6(1):171. https://doi.org/10.4103/amhs.amhs_88_17

Sarmukaddam S, Chopra A, Tillu G (2010) Efficacy and safety of Ayurvedic medicines: recommending equivalence trial design and proposing safety index. Int J Ayurveda Res 1(3):175–180. https://doi.org/10.4103/0974-7788.72491

Singh H, Sharma G (2023) Recent development of novel drug delivery of herbal drugs. RPS Pharm Pharmacol Rep 2:rqad028. https://doi.org/10.1093/rpsppr/rqad028

Vaidya ADB, Devasagayam TPA (2007) Current status of herbal drugs in India: an overview. J Clin Biochem Nutr 41(1):1–11. https://doi.org/10.3164/jcbn.2007001

Medicinal Plants and Sustainable Human Health

14

Ashwini Kumar Mishra, Divya Sharma, Rahul Maurya, Smita Jain, and Chandrashekhar Y. Jagtap

Abstract

The fact that medicinal plants (MPs) play a significant role in advancing sustained human health cannot be overstated. These plants exhibit medicinal properties in various parts of their structure. Their global utilization is increasing as they are utilized in diverse scenarios to support and prolong human well-being. MPs have played a pivotal role in sustainable human health management, fueling a growing interest in alternative medicines and the therapeutic use of plants. This is primarily attributed to their significantly lower cost in comparison to manufactured pharmaceutical alternatives. MPs are facing threats from human activities and unregulated wild harvesting. To ensure a steady supply of these plant species, intentional efforts to domesticate and cultivate them are strongly recommended. This chapter explores the correlation between MPs and human health and their utilization in various cultural contexts. The text discusses the progression of contemporary medicine from cures derived from plants, the difficulties in

A. K. Mishra
Department of Pharmaceutics, School of Pharmacy and Technology Management, SVKM's NMIMS Deemed-to-be University, Shirpur, Dhule, Maharashtra, India

D. Sharma
School of Pharmaceutical Sciences, Delhi Pharmaceutical Sciences and Research University, Delhi, India

R. Maurya
Central Ayurveda Research Institute, Jhansi, Uttar Pradesh, India

S. Jain
Department of Pharmacology, School of Pharmacy and Technology Management, SVKM's NMIMS Deemed-to-be University, Shirpur, Dhule, Maharashtra, India

C. Y. Jagtap (✉)
Department of Rasashastra and Bhaishajya Kalpana, All India Institute of Ayurveda, New Delhi, Delhi, India

A. Kumar et al. (eds.), *Innovations in Ayurvedic Nutrition*,
https://doi.org/10.1007/978-981-95-1213-3_14

safeguarding traditional knowledge of medicinal plants, sustainable methods to ensure their long-term availability, ways for collecting them in an environmentally friendly manner, and the advantages of producing medicinal plants in controlled settings. The chapter also examines the involvement of MPs in providing health benefits and promoting preventative healthcare. The challenges to the availability of MPs and conservation efforts are tackled through prospects for research and technologies.

Keywords

Herbal medicine · Sustainable harvesting · Sustainable health · Medicinal plants · Phytotherapy · Nutraceuticals

14.1 Introduction

Medicinal plants (MPs) have long been a vital source of novel pharmaceuticals. In Europe, more than 1300 MPs are utilized, with 90% sourced from wild resources. Approximately 118 of the top 150 prescription medications in the United States are derived from natural sources. Additionally, many people in underdeveloped countries depend entirely on herbal remedies for their primary healthcare needs. In contrast, over a quarter of prescribed medications in developed countries come from wild plant species. The global demand for herbal medicines, natural health products, and secondary metabolites of MPs continues to rise (Balunas and Kinghorn 2005; Mishra et al. 2024a; Pimm et al. 1995). Based on the International Union for Conservation of Nature and the World Wildlife Fund findings, there is a global count of around 50,000 to 80,000 flowering plant species utilized for their therapeutic properties. Around 15,000 species risk extinction due to excessive harvesting and losing their habitats. Additionally, 20% of their natural resources have already been depleted due to the growing human population and increased consumption of plants. The long-standing threat of extinction to MPs has been exacerbated by the rapid loss of species and degradation of habitats on a global scale. This risk is particularly high in Asia and East Africa (Chen et al. 2016). Extensive research has been conducted on the preservation and responsible utilization of MPs. Several recommendations have been made to protect plant species, including developing systems for species inventorying, status monitoring, and promoting coordinated conservation approaches that incorporate both in situ (on-site) and ex situ (off-site) techniques. The sustainable utilization of natural resources can serve as an effective conservation alternative for MPs facing dwindling supply. The situation in China and South Africa is particularly grave because of the substantial demands of their massive populations (Uprety et al. 2012; Hamilton 2004). Although there are several sets of guidelines for conserving and sustainably using MPs, only a limited number of them have successfully safeguarded medicinal plant resources through traditional conservation methods in natural reserves or botanic gardens. The pace of progress in attaining the United Nations' 2030 Agenda for Sustainable Development has been remarkably sluggish. There is a noticeable lack of action, and it is crucial that we adopt a new strategy to effectively achieve the interconnected Sustainable Development Goals (SDGs) and ensure health for everyone. The COVID-19 epidemic has highlighted the current disparities and inequalities at both local and global levels, which, although recognized, have not been given enough importance in our efforts to achieve the Sustainable Development Goals (SDGs) (Ottersen and Engebretsen 2020; Jha et al. 2024). The health of any individual is associated with every sector of society, ultimately leading to the formation of a healthy planet. Sustainable health involves recognizing the significance of these links and understanding how the current health improvements will impact future generations. To address health disparities, it is crucial to prioritize marginalized groups and people who are most vulnerable to the negative effects of global trends. Policies and interventions formulated and executed from this standpoint will guarantee fair and enduring health outcomes for individuals and the environment and will substantially influence other objectives of the 2030 Agenda for Development (Wanyenze et al. 2023). MPs for healing are an ancient therapy practice that dates back to the earliest days of human existence. The relationship between humans and their quest for medications in nature has existed since ancient times, with abundant evidence from many sources such as written records, surviving monuments, and even original plant remedies. The knowledge of the therapeutic use of plants has been acquired via prolonged efforts to combat illnesses, leading humans to seek medicinal substances in the bark, seeds, fruits, and other components of plants. Modern pharmacotherapy in contemporary research recognizes and considers the active effects of medications derived from plants, which were understood and utilized by ancient civilizations for thousands of years. Understanding the evolution of concepts about the utilization of MPs with consciousness has enhanced the capacity of chemists and physicians to address the emerging issues associated with expanding professional services in improving human well-being (Kumar Srivastava 2018; Sen and Samanta 2015). Drug delivery systems in pharmaceutical science can facilitate the administration of herbal or spice-based medicines synthesized from MPs. This herbal cure enhances the therapeutic efficacy of drugs by reducing their toxicity and adverse effects while improving their gastrointestinal absorption and metabolic effects (Rudrapal et al. 2022). This chapter delves into the relationship between MPs and human health and their use in different cultures. The evolution of modern medicine from plant-based remedies, challenges in preserving traditional knowledge of MPs, sustainable practices for long-term availability, sustainable harvesting techniques, and the benefits of cultivating MPs in controlled environments are also discussed. The chapter also discusses the role of MPs in health benefits and preventive healthcare. The threats to the availability of MPs and conservation efforts are addressed with future opportunities for research and innovations.

14.2 History of Medicinal Plants

14.2.1 Traditional Uses of Medicinal Plants in Different Cultures

MPs have been a cornerstone of traditional medicine across various cultures for centuries, with uses deeply rooted in local customs and beliefs.

Ayurveda: An ancient system of medicine from India, is based on the belief that health and wellness depend on a delicate balance between the mind, body, and spirit. It emphasizes the use of natural remedies, primarily MPs, to maintain this balance and treat various ailments (Jaiswal and Williams 2017). Here are some key aspects:

(a) *Tridosha Concept:* Ayurveda revolves around the concept of three doshas—*Vata* (air and ether), *Pitta* (fire and water), and *Kapha* (water and earth). Everyone has a unique combination of these doshas, and health is achieved by balancing them through diet, lifestyle, and herbal treatments.
(b) *Common Ayurvedic Plants:*
Turmeric (*Curcuma longa* L.): Known for its anti-inflammatory, antioxidant, and antimicrobial properties, turmeric is used in treating skin conditions and digestive disorders and as a general tonic (Fuloria et al. 2022).
Ashwagandha (*Withania somnifera* (L.) Dunal): This adaptogenic herb is used to reduce stress, boost energy levels, and enhance mental clarity (Mikulska et al. 2023).
Neem (*Azadirachta indica* A. Juss.): Neem is known for its detoxifying and purifying effects, commonly used in skin care, dental hygiene, and to manage blood sugar levels (Alzohairy 2016).
Tulsi (*Ocimum sanctum* L.): Also known as holy basil, *Tulsi* is revered for its ability to boost immunity, reduce respiratory issues, and promote overall health (Jamshidi and Cohen 2017).
(c) *Panchakarma*: Ayurveda includes a range of detoxification practices known as *Panchakarma*, which involves five therapies—*Vamana* (emesis), *Virechana* (purgation), *Basti* (enema), *Nasya* (nasal drops), and *Raktamokshana* (bloodletting). These are used to cleanse the body of toxins and restore *dosha* balance (Vinjamury et al. 2011).
(d) *Rasayana (Rejuvenation Therapy)*: This Ayurveda branch promotes longevity and vitality. It uses herbs like *Amalaki* (*Emblica officanalis* Gaertn.) and *Brahmi* (*Bacopa monnieri* (L.) Pennell) to rejuvenate the body, enhance cognitive function, and improve immunity (Singh et al. 2014).

Ayurveda is a holistic system that integrates physical, mental, and spiritual health, making it a comprehensive approach to well-being that has endured for over 5000 years.

14.2.2 Traditional Chinese Medicine (TCM)

It is a holistic medical system practiced in China for over 2000 years. It is based on balancing the body's energy, known as *Qi* (*Chi*), to maintain health and treat disease. TCM integrates various practices, including herbal medicine, acupuncture, massage (*Tui Na*), dietary therapy, and exercise (like *Tai Chi* and *Qigong*) (Marshall 2020). Here are the key components:

(a) *Yin and Yang:* TCM emphasizes the balance between *Yin* (the passive, cooling, and nurturing force) and *Yang* (the active, warming, and invigorating force) in the body. Health is seen as a state of harmony between these forces, and illness arises when there is an imbalance (Yin et al. 2024).

(b) *Five Elements Theory:* This theory links the body's functions and organs to five elements—Wood, Fire, Earth, Metal, and Water. Each element corresponds to specific organs, emotions, and seasons. TCM practitioners use this theory to diagnose and treat imbalances (Chung et al. 2017).

(c) *Meridians and Acupuncture:* The body is believed to have a network of meridians (energy channels) through which *Qi* flows. Acupuncture involves inserting fine needles into specific points along these meridians to unblock and regulate the flow of *Qi*, thereby restoring balance and health (Longhurst 2010).

(d) *Common Medicinal Herbs:*
   - *Ginseng* (*Panax ginseng* C.A.Mey.): Used to boost energy, improve mental clarity, and support immune function (Kang and Min 2012).
   - *Ginger* (*Zingiber officinale* Roscoe): Employed for its warming properties, it aids digestion, relieves nausea, and combats colds (Mao et al. 2019).
   - *Astragalus* (*Astragalus membranaceus* Fisch. ex Bunge): Known for its immune-boosting effects, it is often used to prevent illness and increase vitality (Fu et al. 2014).
   - *Liquorice Root* (*Glycyrrhiza glabra* L.): Commonly included in formulas to harmonize other herbs, it also soothes the throat, reduces inflammation, and boosts energy (Wahab et al. 2021; Bisht et al. 2021).

(e) *Herbal Formulae:* TCM often uses complex formulae of multiple herbs that work synergistically. These formulas are tailored to individual patients based on their specific symptoms and constitution, following the principle of balancing *Yin* and *Yang*, as well as the Five Elements (Eng et al. 2019).

(f) *Dietary Therapy:* Food is considered medicine in TCM, and dietary therapy is essential for treatment. Foods are categorized by their energy (e.g., hot, cold), flavor (e.g., sweet, bitter), and how they affect the body's organs and *Qi*. Practitioners recommend specific diets based on the patient's needs to restore balance (Eng et al. 2019).

(g) *Tui Na (Massage) and Qigong*: Tui Na is a form of therapeutic massage that manipulates the body's energy flow, while Qigong combines movement, meditation, and breathing exercises to strengthen and balance *Qi* (Garcia and Cohen 2020).

(h) *Diagnosis and Treatment:* TCM diagnosis involves observing the patient's physical appearance, tongue color, pulse, and overall energy. Treatments are highly individualized, focusing on correcting the underlying imbalance rather than just alleviating symptoms (Bai et al. 2022).

TCM remains an integral part of healthcare in China and has gained global recognition for its holistic approach, which combines ancient wisdom with modern health practices to promote overall well-being.

14.2.3 Native American Medicine

Native American medicine is a holistic approach to health and healing practiced by various Indigenous tribes in North America for centuries. It is deeply rooted in the spiritual, physical, and emotional aspects of life and often involves the use of natural remedies, rituals, and spiritual practices (Koithan and Farrell 2010).

Key components of Native American medicine include:

- *Herbal Medicine:* Using plants, herbs, and natural substances to treat illness and promote health. Each tribe has its own unique pharmacopeia, with plants like sage, tobacco, and sweetgrass being commonly used (Panduro et al. 2024; Jain et al. 2024).
- *Spiritual Healing:* Involves ceremonies, prayers, and rituals led by medicine men or women who are believed to have a special connection to the spiritual world. These practices often involve using sacred objects, songs, and dances.
- *Holistic Approach:* Health is viewed as a balance between the physical, mental, emotional, and spiritual aspects of life. Illness is often seen as a sign of imbalance, and treatment focuses on restoring harmony.
- *Ceremonies and Rituals:* Important ceremonies, such as the sweat lodge, vision quest, and sun dance, play a significant role in the healing process. These rituals are often community-centered and are meant to cleanse, purify, and connect individuals with the spiritual world (Panduro et al. 2024).
- *Community and Family Involvement:* Healing is often a communal effort, with family and community members supporting. The health of an individual is closely linked to the well-being of the community (Panduro et al. 2024).

Native American medicine emphasizes the interconnectedness of all living things and the importance of living in harmony with nature. It is often practiced alongside modern medicine today to promote healing and well-being.

14.2.4 African Traditional Medicine

African Traditional Medicine is a diverse and holistic system that varies widely across the continent but shares common principles of using natural resources, spiritual practices, and community involvement for healing (Ezekwesili-Ofili Josephine and Okaka Antoinette 2019) [23]. Here are the key elements:

(a) *Holistic Healing:* African traditional medicine views health as a balance between life's physical, spiritual, and social aspects. Illness is often seen as a disruption of this balance, and healing involves addressing all these dimensions.
(b) *Use of Medicinal Plants:*
   - *Baobab* (*Adansonia digitata* L.): Known as the "tree of life," its leaves, bark, and fruit are used for various purposes, including boosting immunity, treating digestive issues, and as a source of essential nutrients.
   - *Aloe Vera* (*Aloe vera* L.): Widely used for its healing properties, especially in treating skin conditions, wounds, and burns.
   - *Devil's Claw* (*Harpagophytum procumbens* DC. ex Meisn.): Traditionally used to treat pain, inflammation, and digestive problems.
   - *African Potato* (*Hypoxis hemerocallidea* Fisch.): Used for its immune-boosting properties and as a treatment for urinary infections and other ailments.
(c) *Spiritual Practices:* Traditional African healers, known as sangomas or herbalists, often incorporate spiritual practices into their healing methods. This may involve rituals, prayers, and communication with ancestors to diagnose and treat illness.
(d) *Divination:* Many African cultures use divination to understand the causes of illness and guide treatment. This might involve interpreting signs, casting bones, or using other methods to communicate with the spiritual world (Okpako 1999).
(e) *Rites and Rituals:* Healing rituals often involve music, dance, and offerings to ancestors or deities. These rituals are designed to appease spiritual forces, remove curses, or restore harmony within the community and the individual.
(f) *Community Involvement:* Healing is often a communal activity, with the community playing a crucial role in supporting the sick and participating in rituals and ceremonies. The collective effort is believed to enhance the effectiveness of the healing process.
(g) *Ancestral Worship:* Ancestors are revered in many African cultures, and their guidance is sought in healing practices. It is believed that the ancestors have the power to protect, heal, or cause illness, so maintaining a good relationship with them is essential for health.
(h) *Traditional Birth and Death Practices:* In African traditional medicine, special ceremonies and practices surround birth and death, emphasizing the continuity of life and the importance of respecting both the living and the dead.

African Traditional Medicine is deeply rooted in their respective cultures, emphasizing a harmonious relationship with nature, the importance of community, and the integration of spiritual practices in healing. These systems continue to be practiced and respected, often alongside modern medical approaches.

14.2.5 Amazonian Indigenous Medicine

Amazonian Indigenous Medicine is a deeply spiritual and holistic system of healing practiced by the indigenous tribes of the Amazon rainforest. It is characterized by its intimate connection with nature, particularly the rich biodiversity of the Amazon, which provides a vast array of MPs and natural remedies (Berlowitz et al. 2023). Here are the key aspects of Amazonian Indigenous Medicine:

(a) *Spiritual Healing and Shamanism:* Shamans, or traditional healers, are central figures in Amazonian medicine. They act as intermediaries between the physical and spiritual worlds, using their knowledge of plants, rituals, and spiritual practices to diagnose and treat illnesses. Healing is often seen as a journey that involves the mind, body, and spirit (Berlowitz et al. 2023).

(b) *Ayahuasca* (*Banisteriopsis caapi* (Spruce ex Griseb.)): One of the most well-known elements of Amazonian medicine is the use of ayahuasca, a powerful psychoactive brew made from the *Banisteriopsis caapi* (Spruce ex Griseb.) vine and other plants. Ayahuasca is used in ceremonial settings for spiritual cleansing, healing, and to gain insights. The visions induced by ayahuasca are believed to reveal the root causes of physical, emotional, or spiritual issues (Frecska et al. 2016).

(c) *Medicinal Plants:*
- *Cat's Claw* (*Uncaria tomentosa* DC.): Known for its anti-inflammatory, antioxidant, and immune-boosting properties, it is used to treat arthritis, digestive issues, and to enhance overall health.
- *Chuchuhuasi* (*Maytenus krukovii* A.C. Sm.): This bark is traditionally used for pain relief, particularly for joint and muscle pain, and as a general tonic to boost energy and stamina.
- *Camu Camu* (*Myrciaria dubia* (Kunth) McVaugh): A fruit high in vitamin C, used to boost the immune system and combat inflammation.
- *Sangre de Drago* (*Croton lechleri* Mull. Arg.): A red sap from the Croton tree, used for wound healing, as an antiseptic, and to treat gastrointestinal issues.

(d) *Plant Diets:* A key practice in Amazonian medicine is the "dieta," a period of isolation and fasting where the individual consumes specific MPs under the guidance of a shaman. This practice is believed to allow deeper communication with the plant spirits, leading to physical healing and spiritual insights (Frecska et al. 2016).

(e) *Purification Rituals:* Indigenous tribes often use plants such as tobacco, known as "mapacho," and other herbal smoke to cleanse the body and spirit. These rituals are believed to remove negative energies and prepare the individual for healing.

(f) *Connection with Nature:* Amazonian medicine emphasizes living harmoniously with nature. The forest is seen as a living entity with its own spirit, and the plants are respected as powerful allies in healing. This deep connection with the natural world is central to the healing practices and worldview of Amazonian tribes.

(g) *Community and Ancestral Wisdom:* Healing is often a communal activity, with the community coming together in ceremonies and rituals to support the sick. Knowledge of MPs and healing practices is passed down through generations, often orally, and is closely tied to ancestors' wisdom.
(h) *Ceremonial Healing:* Ceremonies often involve chants, music, and dance to invoke spiritual energies and guide healing. These ceremonies are deeply sacred and are believed to restore balance and harmony to the individual and the community.
(i) *Prevention and Holistic Health:* Amazonian medicine is not just about treating illness but also about maintaining health and preventing disease. This involves a holistic approach that includes a balanced diet, regular physical activity, and maintaining strong spiritual and social connections.

Amazonian Indigenous Medicine is a profound and complex system that embodies the deep connection between humans and the natural world. It is a testament to the rich cultural heritage and ecological knowledge of the indigenous peoples of the Amazon, who continue to practice and preserve these ancient healing traditions.

14.2.6 European Herbal Medicine

European Herbal Medicine has a rich history that spans thousands of years and is deeply rooted in the traditional practices of ancient civilizations such as the Greeks, Romans, and Celts. Over time, this knowledge evolved, blending with medieval and Renaissance medical practices to form the foundation of modern Western herbalism (Leonti and Verpoorte 2017). Here are key elements of European Herbal Medicine:

(a) *Historical Foundations:*
  - *Hippocrates and Galen:* Ancient Greek physicians like Hippocrates, often called the "Father of Medicine," laid the groundwork for European herbal medicine by advocating for the use of herbs in balancing the body's humor. Galen, another influential figure, expanded on this with his extensive writings on the medicinal properties of plants (Bennett 2007).
  - *Dioscorides:* A Greek physician in the Roman army, Dioscorides wrote "De Materia Medica," one of the most important herbal texts of the ancient world. This work catalogued hundreds of MPs and became a cornerstone of European herbal knowledge for centuries.

(b) *The Doctrine of Signatures:* This Renaissance-era theory suggested that a plant's shape, color, and other characteristics could indicate its medicinal uses. For example, the lung-shaped leaves of lungwort (Pulmonaria spp.) were believed to treat respiratory ailments, and the heart-shaped leaves of motherwort (*Leonurus cardiaca*) were used for heart conditions (Bennett 2007).
(c) *Monastic Medicine:* During the Middle Ages, monks preserved and expanded much of the knowledge of MPs in European monasteries. They cultivated herb gardens and compiled manuscripts like the "Hortulus" by St. Gall and the

"Physica" by Hildegard of Bingen, which detailed the medicinal uses of various plants (Will and Eisenmann-Tappe 2016).

(d) *Common Medicinal Herbs:*
  - *Chamomile* (*Matricaria chamomilla* L.): Used for its calming effects, chamomile is a popular remedy for anxiety, insomnia, and digestive issues (Srivastava et al. 2010).
  - *Peppermint* (*Mentha piperita* L.): Known for its soothing effect on the digestive system, peppermint is used to alleviate nausea, bloating, and headaches (Chumpitazi et al. 2018).
  - *St. John's Wort* (*Hypericum perforatum* L.): Traditionally used for treating mild depression and anxiety, as well as for its antiviral and anti-inflammatory properties (Klemow et al. 2011).
  - *Yarrow* (*Achillea millefolium* L.): Used to stop bleeding, heal wounds, and treat fevers, yarrow has been a staple in European herbal medicine for centuries (Thangavelu et al. 2011).
  - *Elderberry* (*Sambucus nigra* L.): Valued for its immune-boosting properties, elderberry is commonly used to prevent and treat colds and flu (Hawkins et al. 2019).

(e) *Culpeper's Herbal:* Nicholas Culpeper, a seventeenth-century English herbalist, made significant contributions to European herbal medicine with his book "The English Physician," also known as "Culpeper's Herbal." This work made herbal knowledge more accessible to the general public by translating Latin medical texts into English and advocating for the use of locally available herbs (Smith 2012).

(f) *Seasonal and Local Herbs:* European herbalists often emphasize using locally grown and seasonal plants, believing that herbs that grow in a particular environment best suit the people. This approach also reflects a deep connection to nature and the cycles of the seasons (Smith 2012).

(g) *Integration with Modern Medicine:* In recent times, European herbal medicine has seen a resurgence, with many people seeking natural remedies alongside conventional treatments. Herbalism is now integrated into modern health practices, with scientific research validating the efficacy of many traditional European herbs (Smith 2012; Rawat et al. 2024).

(h) *Traditional Herbal Practices:*
  - *Teas and Infusions:* Herbal teas are a common method of administering MPs, where leaves, flowers, or roots are steeped in hot water to extract their healing properties.
  - *Tinctures and Extracts:* Alcohol or glycerin-based extracts of herbs are used for their concentrated medicinal properties and longer shelf life.
  - *Poultices and Compresses:* Herbal poultices involve applying crushed or heated herbs directly to the skin to treat wounds, inflammations, and other localized conditions.

(i) *Folk Medicine:* Many regions in Europe have their own folk medicine traditions, which have been passed down through generations. These practices often involve using herbs, charms, and rituals to treat common ailments and maintain health. European Herbal Medicine is a dynamic and evolving tradition, grounded in ancient wisdom and continually enriched by scientific research. It remains a popular and respected approach to health and wellness, reflecting the enduring human connection to the healing power of plants (Grienke et al. 2014).

14.3 Evolution of Modern Medicine from Plant-Based Remedies

The evolution of modern medicine from plant-based remedies is a fascinating journey that spans millennia, reflecting humanity's deep connection with nature and the gradual development of scientific knowledge. Here is an overview of this evolution:

14.3.1 Ancient Times: The Roots of Herbal Medicine

(a) *Early Human Societies:* From the dawn of civilization, humans have relied on plants for healing. Ancient civilizations like the Sumerians, Egyptians, and Indigenous peoples across the globe documented the use of MPs for various ailments. These remedies were often discovered through trial and error, guided by observations of the natural world.
(b) *Traditional Medicine Systems:* In ancient China, India, and the Mediterranean, sophisticated medical systems like Traditional Chinese Medicine (TCM) and Ayurveda emerged, with extensive pharmacopeia of MPs. These systems not only used herbs for treating illnesses but also incorporated them into broader philosophies of health and wellness (Hassan 2015; Marshall 2020).

14.3.2 Classical Antiquity: The Foundation of Herbal Knowledge

(a) *Greek and Roman Medicine:* The works of Hippocrates and Galen laid the foundation for Western medicine, emphasizing the use of plants to balance the body's humor. Dioscorides, a Greek physician, compiled "De Materia Medica," a seminal text that catalogued hundreds of MPs and their uses.
(b) *Monastic Medicine:* During the Middle Ages, much of this knowledge was preserved and expanded upon in European monasteries, where monks cultivated medicinal herb gardens and compiled herbals that served as key references for centuries (Wagner et al. 2020).

14.3.3 Renaissance and Enlightenment: Transition to Modern Science

(a) *The Doctrine of Signatures:* In the Renaissance, the Doctrine of Signatures suggested that the appearance of plants indicated their therapeutic use (e.g., lungwort for lung ailments). While largely symbolic, this idea influenced the herbal practices of the time.

(b) *Paracelsus and Alchemy:* Paracelsus, a Swiss physician, challenged the traditional Galenic system and promoted using chemical substances derived from plants, laying early groundwork for pharmacology. He believed in extracting the active principles of plants, which foreshadowed modern drug development.
(c) *Development of Pharmacopeia:* The Enlightenment era saw the formalization of medical knowledge, with the publication of comprehensive pharmacopeia that standardized the use of MPs, Herbo-mineral medicines, and documented their preparation and dosages (Dal Cero et al. 2023; Jagtap et al. 2024).

14.3.4 Nineteenth Century: The Birth of Pharmacology

(a) *Isolation of Active Compounds:* The nineteenth century marked a turning point in isolating active compounds from plants. Morphine was extracted from opium poppies, quinine from cinchona bark, and salicin from willow bark. These discoveries demonstrated that specific chemical constituents were responsible for the medicinal effects of plants (Philippu and Seifert 2023; Deshmukh et al. 2024).
(b) *Rise of Synthetic Drugs:* The success of these isolated compounds led to the development of synthetic drugs, which could be produced in large quantities and with consistent potency Fig. 14.1. This period saw the emergence of pharmaceutical companies and the beginning of the modern pharmaceutical industry (Tainter and Marcelli 1959; Mishra et al. 2024b).

14.3.5 Twentieth Century: Integration and Innovation

(a) *Advances in Chemistry and Pharmacology:* The twentieth century brought rapid advancements in chemistry and pharmacology, leading to the synthesis of new drugs that were more effective than their natural counterparts. Aspirin, derived from salicin, became one of the first widely used synthetic drugs.

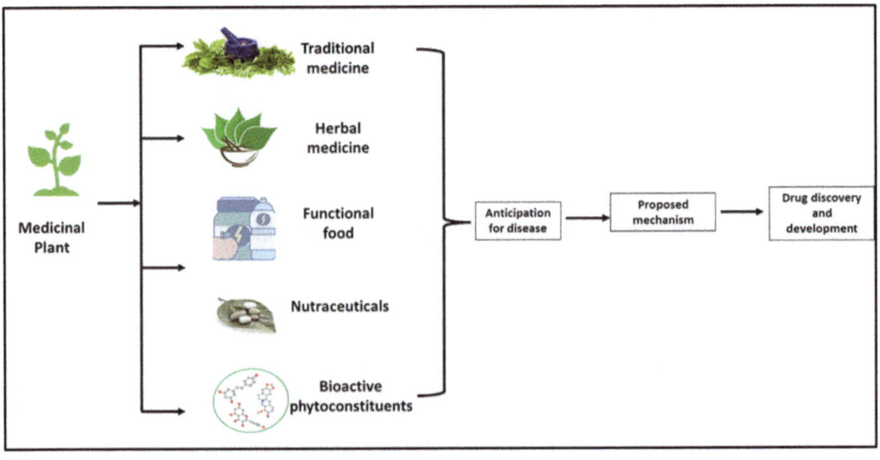

Fig. 14.1 The herbal plants for the Development of new drug

(b) *Antibiotics and Vaccines:* The discovery of penicillin, derived from a mold, revolutionized medicine by providing a powerful tool against bacterial infections. The development of vaccines further transformed public health, drastically reducing the incidence of many infectious diseases.
(c) *Shift from Plant-Based Remedies:* As synthetic drugs became more prevalent, the use of plant-based remedies declined, particularly in Western medicine. A multitude of liver illnesses with significant impact on the global population remain refractory to appropriate treatment. The primary obstacles or difficulties are inherent physiological barriers and non-specific pharmacological targeting, resulting in ineffective therapy. However, interest in herbal medicine persisted, especially in traditional and alternative medicine systems (Sulaiman et al. 2024; Mishra et al. 2022a).

14.3.6 Twenty-First Century: Return to Nature and Integration

(a) *Renewed Interest in Herbal Medicine:* The twenty-first century has seen a resurgence of interest in plant-based remedies, driven by a desire for natural and holistic approaches to health. Scientific research has validated the efficacy of many traditional herbs, leading to their integration into modern medicine.
(b) *Phytotherapy and Nutraceuticals:* Phytotherapy uses plant extracts for therapeutic purposes. It has gained popularity as a complementary approach to conventional medicine. Nutraceuticals—foods or supplements with medicinal properties—have also become important to health and wellness (Mishra et al. 2024c).
(c) *Bioprospecting and Conservation:* The search for new medicinal compounds in plants, known as bioprospecting, continues to be a major focus of pharmaceutical research. This has also raised awareness of the importance of biodiversity and the need to conserve MPs and traditional knowledge (Thomford et al. 2018).

14.3.7 Modern Drug Development: From Plants to Pills

(a) *Herbal Medicine in Clinical Practice:* Herbal medicine is recognized as a valuable complementary and alternative therapy. Many modern drugs, in combination with nanotechnological advances, are derived from plants or inspired by plant compounds, and herbal supplements are widely used for health and wellness (Veeresham 2012; Mishra and Sahoo 2022).
(b) *Integration with Evidence-Based Medicine:* While using plant-based remedies is increasingly supported by scientific evidence, the integration of herbal medicine with evidence-based practices remains a focus of ongoing research. This integration seeks to combine the best of traditional knowledge with modern scientific rigor (Chaachouay and Zidane 2024; Mishra et al. 2024a).

14.4 Challenges in Preserving Traditional Knowledge of MPs

Preserving traditional knowledge of MPs is critical for maintaining cultural heritage and supporting biodiversity, but several significant challenges threaten this valuable resource.

14.4.1 Loss of Language and Culture

Traditional knowledge of MPs is often transmitted orally within communities through languages and cultural practices. As languages die out and cultural practices diminish, this knowledge is at risk of being lost. Many indigenous languages, which carry detailed knowledge about local plants and their uses, are spoken by only a few remaining elders. As these speakers pass away without transferring their knowledge to younger generations, the traditional understanding of MPs also fades.

14.4.2 Environmental Changes

The rapid pace of environmental degradation directly threatens MPs. Deforestation, urbanization, and agricultural expansion destroy natural habitats, losing plant species crucial for traditional medicine. Additionally, climate change alters growing conditions, affecting plant availability and medicinal properties. The resultant decline in plant populations jeopardizes not only the plants themselves but also the traditional knowledge related to them.

14.4.3 Intellectual Property Issues

Commercializing traditional knowledge has led to disputes over intellectual property rights. Pharmaceutical companies often seek to patent plant-based remedies and their compounds, which can lead to conflicts with indigenous communities that have used these plants for generations. These communities may not receive fair compensation or recognition for their traditional knowledge, leading to ethical and legal concerns about the appropriation of their cultural heritage.

14.4.4 Lack of Documentation

Much of the traditional knowledge about MPs is passed down orally, which can lead to inaccuracies and loss of information over time. This knowledge may be lost without proper documentation as practitioners and communities disappear. Efforts to document this knowledge often face challenges due to variations in plant usage, preparation methods, and the complexity of traditional healing systems.

14.4.5 Loss of Biodiversity

Overharvesting MPs for commercial purposes, combined with habitat destruction, contributes to the loss of plant species. As biodiversity decreases, the range of MPs available for traditional use diminishes, reducing the pool of knowledge about these plants. This loss can undermine traditional medicine practices that rely on a diverse array of plant species.

14.4.6 Cultural Erosion

Globalization and modernization can erode traditional practices and knowledge. As communities integrate more with global cultures, traditional medicine practices may be abandoned in favor of modern healthcare systems. This shift can lead to losing traditional knowledge as younger generations may not learn or practice traditional methods.

14.4.7 Ethical and Conservation Concerns

There are ethical concerns related to collecting MPs for research and commercial use. In some cases, plants are collected without proper consent or compensation from the communities that hold the traditional knowledge. Furthermore, conservation efforts are often inadequate to protect the habitats of MPs, exacerbating the problem.

To address these challenges, a multi-faceted approach is needed. Collaborations between indigenous communities, researchers, and policymakers can help document and protect traditional knowledge. Ethical guidelines for intellectual property rights must be established to ensure fair compensation and recognition. Conservation efforts should focus on protecting plant habitats and promoting sustainable harvesting practices. Additionally, integrating traditional knowledge with modern science can enhance our understanding and preservation of MPs. By valuing and safeguarding this knowledge, we can ensure that it continues to benefit future generations and contribute to global biodiversity.

14.5 Sustainable Harvesting and Cultivation of Medicinal Plants

14.5.1 Importance of Sustainable Practices for Long-Term Availability

Sustainable practices are essential for maintaining the long-term availability of resources, products, and services, ensuring a healthy planet and a prosperous future. Key benefits include preserving resources like water, minerals, and fossil fuels, protecting the environment, promoting economic viability, and supporting social responsibility (Jhariya et al. 2022). These practices are crucial for ensuring the long-term availability of MPs, which are essential for health and medicine. By implementing sustainable practices, we can protect biodiversity and preserve the delicate ecosystems where MPs flourish (Mateo-Martín et al. 2023). This, in turn, helps to shield their populations from overharvesting and habitat destruction. Sustainable harvesting methods, such as setting quotas and using non-destructive techniques, help prevent the depletion of plant species and ensure their continued availability (Shafi et al. 2021). Additionally, conserving genetic diversity in these plants is crucial for future medicinal advancements and breeding programs. Supporting local communities through fair trade and promoting sustainable cultivation practices also helps preserve MPs. These efforts collectively ensure that MPs remain a viable resource for future generations, fostering ecological balance and supporting environmental and economic stability (Chen ShiLin et al. 2016). MPs are vital for producing pharmaceutical and cosmetic ingredients. Developing and commercializing a single drug involves screening tens of thousands of compounds, taking many years of research and development, and costing over 800 million USD. Almost half of the 100 plant-derived prescription drugs come from tropical countries, requiring approximately 500,000 tons of plant material annually from around 60,000 species. The global herbal medicine market was valued at 84.5 billion dollars in 2019 and is expected to grow significantly in the coming years, reflecting the increasing demand for these plant-based resources (Kurnaz and Kurnaz 2021). The increasing demand for MPs and the growing human population has put significant pressure on existing resources. This has resulted in the depletion and extinction of some wild species and a rapid loss of natural flora. To combat this issue, various conservation strategies have been proposed worldwide. These include in situ measures such as creating preservation areas and cultivating MPs, as well as ex situ efforts like establishing botanical gardens and gene banks. It is crucial to investigate and address the factors that threaten the sustainability of MPs to develop effective preventive measures. Ensuring the conservation and sustainable use of these resources is essential for preserving this valuable heritage for future generations (Mir et al. 2021). The herbal and pharmaceutical industries depend on a consistent supply of medicinal and aromatic plants. However, traditional methods of domestication and propagation are often labor-intensive and not universally applicable. Seed gene-bank conservation is limited, leading to interest in biotechnology. Recent advancements in in vitro techniques and *cryopreservation* show promise for improving conservation efforts. Although cryopreservation is still experimental for MPs, it offers potential for long-term germplasm preservation. An effective conservation strategy should include sustainable production methods for in situ and ex situ conservation practices (Sharma and Pandey 2012). Climate change is causing significant disruptions in the Himalayan ecosystems, particularly impacting MPs in the Sikkim Himalaya. Kumar et al. conducted survey using Maximum Entropy Species Distribution Modelling (SDM), the study assessed the habitat distribution of 163 medicinal plant species under current and future climate scenarios (2050 and 2070). Findings indicate that most species currently thrive in tropical and sub-tropical regions but are expected to shift northward and upward in elevation. By 2050 and 2070, 13–16% of species may lose their habitats. The study identifies elevations between 860 and 2937 m as crucial for conservation. Of the eight Protected Areas (PAs) in Sikkim, only five are effective for current and future conservation, suggesting a need for PA boundary expansions to accommodate shifting species distributions. The study highlights the need for an integrated approach to assess climate change impacts and inform conservation strategies (Manish 2022). A survey conducted by Hassanpouraghdam et al in Iran, with its diverse climatic and topographic conditions, hosts around 8200 vascular plant species, of which approximately 2300 are medicinal or aromatic. The survey identified 180 endemic medicinal and aromatic plants (MAPs) across 10 families and 30 genera, predominantly within Lamiaceae, Fabaceae, and Apiaceae. Most of these plants are concentrated in ten provinces in the Iran-o-Turanian region, which is a major center of MAP diversity. This region, rich in biodiversity due to its varied climate and geography, faces threats from unsustainable harvesting and climate change. To protect these valuable species and ensure their future availability, it is crucial to focus on conservation and propagation efforts, particularly in key areas of endemism (Hassanpouraghdam et al. 2022). Shen et al investigated the impact of climate change on the distribution and quality of *Gentiana rigescens* Franch., a medicinal plant in Asia. Using the MaxEnt model, researchers predict that the plant's highly suitable habitats, currently concentrated in southwest China, may drastically reduce by 2070 under severe climate scenarios (RCP8.5), with a potential loss of 99.22%. Chemical analysis showed that plants from highly suitable areas have higher concentrations of medicinal compounds, indicating that climate-induced habitat shifts could affect the quality of *Gentiana rigescens* Franch. The findings highlight the need for conservation efforts and provide insights into how climate change may influence medicinal plant distribution and quality (Shen et al. 2021).

14.5.2 Examples of Sustainable Harvesting Techniques

Selective Harvesting is a sustainable harvesting method where only specific parts of the plant, such as mature plants, leaves, or flowers, are collected, while the rest of the plant is left intact. This approach allows the plant to continue growing, reproducing, and maintaining its population (Kushwah et al. 2023). Ghimire et al. reported the impact of different harvesting practices on two threatened Himalayan MPs, *Nardostachys grandiflora* DC. and *Neopicrorhiza scrophulariiflora* (Penell) DY Hong., in Nepal's Shey-Phoksundo National Park. Researchers compared selective harvesting by traditional Tibetan medicine practitioners (*amchi*) with unselective, high-intensity commercial harvesting. Experiments showed that low levels of *selective harvesting* improved plant density, but higher harvesting reduced recruitment and survival rates. *N. grandiflora* DC. was found to be more vulnerable to harvesting than *N. scrophulariiflora* (Penell) DY Hong., due to differences in their reproductive strategies. The study highlights the need to tailor sustainable management practices to specific harvesting patterns and plant life forms (Ghimire et al.

2005). Rotational harvesting is a sustainable method that involves cycling plant collection through different areas or populations over time. Instead of continuously harvesting from the same location, different sections are harvested in rotation. This approach allows each area to have time to recover before being harvested again (Plagányi et al. 2015). Rokaya et al. reported the long-term effects of harvesting on the survival of two Himalayan MPs, *Rheum acuminatum* Hook. f. & Thomson and *Rheum australe* D. Don, over 6 years in Nepal. Using matrix modeling, researchers found that while population dynamics were stable across different habitats and years, the plants showed varying sensitivity to harvesting. The study concludes that sustainable harvesting is possible under specific conditions, recommending selective or rotational harvesting strategies, with management practices tailored to species and habitat conditions. These findings can inform sustainable harvesting of other alpine and perennial MPs in the Himalayan region (Rokaya et al. 2017). Harvesting during non-critical periods involves collecting plants when they are least vulnerable, such as after seed dispersal or during dormancy, to safeguard the plant's reproductive cycle and allow future populations to thrive without disruption. Galindo et al. studied the effects of drought stress on pomegranate (*Punica granatum* L.) during the critical period of fruit ripening. Researchers compared fully irrigated plants with those experiencing varying levels of water restriction before harvest. The findings show that irrigation is essential during most of the ripening period to ensure maximum yield. However, a short 6-day irrigation restriction at the end of ripening can reduce water use, accelerate harvest time, and enhance bioactive compounds (like anthocyanins and phenolics) in the fruit, without compromising yield or size. This indicates that brief, controlled water stress can improve fruit quality and market value. Understanding how crops respond to drought stress during different growth stages is crucial for minimizing yield impact during non-critical periods and addressing significant effects during critical periods (Galindo Egea et al. 2017). Agroforestry is the method of combining crops, trees, and livestock on the same land to enhances biomass productivity, sequesters carbon, and ecosystem services, especially in tropical regions. Agroforestry offers solutions to food and nutrition challenges, with significant contributions to timber and fuelwood production. In India, agroforestry covers around 14 million hectares, with potential for expansion. Various agroforestry models (AFM) cater to different socio-economic and climatic conditions, offering options like apiculture and sericulture. Agroforestry improves soil health, linking soil fertility to crop productivity (Raj et al. 2019). Palada et al investigated the role of medicinal and culinary herbs in improving small farm productivity in the Virgin Islands by integrating them into an agroforestry system with medicinal trees. On-farm experiments assessed a range of herbs, including indigenous medicinal plants such as *Verbesina alata* L. and *Eupatorium triplinerve* Vahl, as well as culinary herbs like basil and lemongrass. These herbs were cultivated in alleys formed by hedgerows of Moringa trees. The results indicated that *Moringa oleifera* Lam. was more productive than *Moringa stenopetala* (Baker f.) Cufod. While the growth and yield of the herbs varied by species, lemongrass, and blue verbena proved to be the most productive. Overall, intercropping with hedgerows slightly reduced herb yields, but competition for resources was minimal.

(Palada et al. 2003). By implementing these sustainable harvesting methods, we can preserve medicinal plant diversity while meeting their needs for health and livelihood.

14.5.3 Benefits of Cultivating Medicinal Plants in Controlled Environments

(a) *Supply of High-Quality Medicinal Plants:* The increasing demand for MPs has led to overexploitation and the risk of extinction in the wild. Systematic cultivation offers a sustainable alternative, ensuring a reliable supply of high-quality MPs while reducing pressure on natural populations. Cultivation also provides economic benefits, including livelihood opportunities and export potential. The WHO has set guidelines for sustainable cultivation practices, which can be applied through traditional agricultural methods or advanced plant tissue culture for high-value compounds. Overall, commercial cultivation of MPs is vital for meeting global demand and supporting rural economies (Alamgir and Alamgir 2017). The economic benefits of controlled environments are also significant, ensuring consistent and reliable production, better market stability, increased profitability, and the creation of value-added products. Together, these advantages contribute to medicinal plant cultivation's scientific advancement and economic sustainability (Ragaveena et al. 2021).

(b) *Rich secondary metabolite production:* MPs, essential for various therapeutic compounds, are affected by environmental stresses such as temperature, CO_2 levels, light, ozone, soil water, salinity, and fertility. These factors significantly influence the plants' physiological responses and secondary metabolite (SM) production, which are crucial for drug development. Plants produce SMs to counteract stress, but the impact of environmental variables on SM accumulation is complex and varies by species. They optimize cultivation techniques, ensuring high-quality SM production under varying environmental conditions (Pant et al. 2021). Large-scale cultivation of MPs is essential to meet the growing demand. However, breeding studies are crucial for advancing this cultivation. Despite some progress, challenges persist due to the complexity of defining breeding targets and limitations in traditional and modern breeding methods. This review analyses selection strategies for breeding directions and models, highlighting the importance of breeding research in enhancing medicinal plant cultivation (Wang et al. 2020).

(c) *Reduced Harvesting Pressure on Wild Populations:* Knowledge about cultivating MPs in controlled environments reduces the need for wild harvesting, helping to conserve natural populations and prevent overexploitation. Over-exploitation and destructive harvesting threaten the sustainability of wild MPs (WMP) in Europe and the Mediterranean. This study, reported by Papageorgiou et al on Lemnos Island, Greece, explored local knowledge about WMP harvesting and its ecological sustainability. Interviews with 16 experienced harvesters revealed 144 useful plant taxa, with 81 harvested in the past

4 years, mainly for digestive and respiratory issues. While many sustainable practices were identified, some plant species and areas face pressures from climate change, pollution, and unsustainable harvesting. The study emphasizes the value of local knowledge in assessing and promoting sustainable WMP harvesting (Papageorgiou et al. 2020). Research opportunities can be enhanced by growing MPs in controlled environments. These settings allow for precise study of plant growth, genetics, and compound production, leading to a deeper understanding of medicinal plant biology and improved cultivation techniques (Li et al. 2020). Conservation and sustainable use of MPs involves direct and indirect actions, such as commercial systems, ex situ conservation, and bioprospecting. However, these efforts only contribute to in situ conservation if they improve natural habitats. MPs play a vital role in broader biological conservation due to their significance in health, income, cultural identity, and livelihoods. Challenges like biopiracy and restrictive research policies have gained attention, with the Convention on Biological Diversity emphasizing fair benefit-sharing from bioprospecting. However, regulations to prevent biopiracy must not hinder unrelated scientific research.

14.6 Health Benefits of Medicinal Plants

Medicinal plants (MPs) have been utilized for their health benefits for centuries, providing a natural alternative to conventional medicine. They offer a wide range of therapeutic properties that can aid in treating and managing various health conditions. MPs are rich in bioactive compounds that provide numerous health benefits, including immune system enhancement, inflammation reduction, and even cancer prevention (Leitzmann 2016; Zhu et al. 2018). This section will delve into the health benefits of MPs, emphasizing their role in treating common ailments, promoting overall well-being, and their potential applications in modern medicine (see Table 14.1).

14.7 Common Medicinal Plants and Their Uses

14.7.1 Echinacea

This plant is renowned for its immune-boosting properties. Echinacea is often used to prevent and treat the common cold and respiratory infections. Beyond respiratory illnesses, echinacea may help manage skin conditions like eczema and wounds due to its anti-inflammatory effects. It also shows potential in reducing symptoms of urinary tract infections (UTIs) and may have benefits in alleviating some symptoms of anxiety. Its active compounds, such as echinacoside, are believed to enhance the body's natural defenses by stimulating white blood cell activity. Research also suggests that it may reduce the duration and severity of cold symptoms (Liu et al. 2020).

Table 14.1 Some of the important medicinal plants in the treatment of various diseases

Sr. No.	Medicinal Plant	Botanical Name	Health Benefits	Reference
1.	Echinacea	*Echinacea purpurea* (L.) Moench	Boosts the immune system, reduces the severity and duration of colds, and fights respiratory infections.	Liu et al. (2020)
2.	Elderberry	*Sambucus nigra* L.	It enhances immune function, reduces flu symptoms, and is rich in antioxidants.	Sidor and Gramza-Michałowska (2015)
3.	Garlic	*Allium sativum* L.	It supports immune health, lowers cholesterol, reduces blood pressure, and has antimicrobial properties.	Tesfaye (2021)
4.	Turmeric	*Curcuma longa* L.	Anti-inflammatory, antioxidant, supports cardiovascular health, and may help prevent cancer.	Hewlings and Kalman (2017)
5.	Ginger	*Zingiber officinale* Roscoe	Anti-inflammatory, aids digestion, reduces nausea, lowers blood sugar levels, and alleviates muscle pain and soreness.	Shahrajabian et al. (2019)
6.	Green Tea	*Camellia sinensis* (L.) Kuntze	Rich in antioxidants, supports cardiovascular health, boosts metabolism, may reduce cancer risk, and improves brain function.	Aboulwafa et al. (2019)
7.	Peppermint	*Mentha piperita* L.	Relieves symptoms of irritable bowel syndrome (IBS), eases digestive discomfort, and relaxes gastrointestinal muscles.	Tafrihi et al. (2021)
8.	Fennel	*Foeniculum vulgare* Mill.	Relieves bloating, gas, and indigestion, and supports digestive health.	Badgujar et al. (2014)
9.	Hawthorn	*Crataegus monogyna* Jacq.	Promotes cardiovascular health, dilates blood vessels, lowers blood pressure, and strengthens heart muscle.	Zhang et al. (2022)
10.	Rosemary	*Rosmarinus officinalis* L.	Rich in antioxidants, protects the brain from oxidative stress, and has anti-inflammatory and antimicrobial properties.	Ghasemzadeh Rahbardar and Hosseinzadeh (2020)
11.	Ginkgo Biloba	*Ginkgo biloba* L.	Improves memory and cognitive function, increases blood flow to the brain, may help treat Alzheimer's disease and dementia.	Mohamed (2014)

(continued)

Table 14.1 (continued)

Sr. No.	Medicinal Plant	Botanical Name	Health Benefits	Reference
12.	St. John's Wort	*Hypericum perforatum* L.	Treats mild to moderate depression, improves mood by increasing levels of serotonin and dopamine.	Mohamed (2014)
13.	Chamomile	*Matricaria chamomilla* L.	Promotes relaxation, aids sleep, reduces anxiety, and has anti-inflammatory properties.	Mohamed (2014)
14.	Aloe Vera	*Aloe vera* L.	Heals skin wounds and burns, soothes skin irritations, reduces fasting blood glucose levels, improves lipid profiles, anti-inflammatory and antimicrobial properties.	Mohamed (2014)
15.	Lavender	*Lavandula angustifolia* Mill.	Reduces anxiety, promotes relaxation and sleep, and helps alleviate headaches and migraines.	Kajjari et al. (2022)
16.	Licorice Root	*Glycyrrhiza glabra* L.	Soothes sore throat, supports respiratory health, anti-inflammatory and antioxidant properties.	Alanazi et al. (2023)
17.	Milk Thistle	*Silybum marianum* (L.) Gaertn.	Supports liver health, protects against toxins, has antioxidant and anti-inflammatory effects.	Alanazi et al. (2023)
18.	Valerian Root	*Valeriana officinalis* L.	Promotes relaxation, aids in sleep, reduces anxiety, and can help with insomnia.	Alanazi et al. (2023)
19.	Dandelion	*Taraxacum officinale* F.H. Wigg.	Supports liver and digestive health, acts as a diuretic, rich in antioxidants.	Alanazi et al. (2023)
20.	Sage	*Salvia officinalis* L.	Improves cognitive function, supports oral health, has anti-inflammatory and antimicrobial properties.	Alanazi et al. (2023)
21.	Ashwagandha	*Withania somnifera* (L.) Dunal	Reduces stress and anxiety, supports adrenal health, enhances cognitive function, boosts energy levels.	Alanazi et al. (2023)
22.	Cinnamon	*Cinnamomum verum* J. Presl	Regulates blood sugar levels, has antioxidant properties, supports cardiovascular health, and may reduce inflammation.	Alanazi et al. (2023)

(continued)

Table 14.1 (continued)

Sr. No.	Medicinal Plant	Botanical Name	Health Benefits	Reference
23.	Fenugreek	*Trigonella foenum-graecum* L.	Supports digestive health, regulates blood sugar, and promotes lactation in breastfeeding mothers.	Alanazi et al. (2023)
24.	Holy Basil	*Ocimum sanctum* L.	Reduces stress, supports immune health, reduces blood sugar levels, enhances insulin sensitivity, and has anti-inflammatory and antioxidant properties.	Alanazi et al. (2023)
25.	Neem	*Azadirachta indica* A. Juss.	Supports skin health, exhibits hypoglycemic effects, supports pancreatic health has antimicrobial and anti-inflammatory properties, and supports oral health.	Alanazi et al. (2023)
26.	Moringa	*Moringa oleifera* Lam.	Rich in vitamins and minerals, supports immune health, and has antioxidant and anti-inflammatory properties.	Alanazi et al. (2023)
27.	Thyme	*Thymus vulgaris* L.	Supports respiratory health, has antimicrobial properties, and helps alleviate coughs and bronchitis.	Alanazi et al. (2023)
28.	Cranberry	*Vaccinium macrocarpon* Aiton	Prevents urinary tract infections (UTIs), supports cardiovascular health, rich in antioxidants.	Alanazi et al. (2023)
29.	Ginseng	*Panax ginseng* C.A. Mey.	Boosts energy levels, enhances cognitive function, supports immune health, and has anti-inflammatory properties.	Alanazi et al. (2023)
30.	Yarrow	*Achillea millefolium* L.	Heals wounds, reduces fever, supports digestive health, and has anti-inflammatory properties.	Saeidnia et al. (2011)
31.	Bhringaraj	*Eclipta alba* Hassk.	Promotes hair growth, protects the liver, fights bacteria, and alleviates swelling and inflammation.	Jha et al. (2022)
32.	Patharchatta	*Bryophyllum pinnatum* (Lam.) Oken	Acts as a diuretic, aids in kidney stone removal, reduces acidity, and soothes skin irritation.	Kumar et al. (2019)

(continued)

Table 14.1 (continued)

Sr. No.	Medicinal Plant	Botanical Name	Health Benefits	Reference
33.	Lemongrass	*Cymbopogon flexuosus* (Nees ex Steud.) Stapf	Alleviates respiratory conditions, reduces pain, and inhibits bacterial growth	Shah et al. (2011)
34.	Insulin plant	*Costus pictus* D. Don	Enhances glucose uptake and insulin sensitivity	Selvakumarasamy et al. (2021)
35.	Moringa	*Moringa oleifera* Lam.	Reduces blood sugar levels and provides antioxidant effects.	Pareek et al. (2023)
36.	Bitter Melon	*Momordica charantia* L.	Lowers blood glucose levels and increases insulin secretion	Gayathry and John (2022)

14.7.2 Ginger

The ginger plant (*Zingiber officinale* Roscoe) is a tropical herbaceous plant belonging to the Zingiberaceae family. It is widely recognized for its effectiveness in treating digestive issues. It is commonly used to alleviate nausea, particularly morning sickness during pregnancy and motion sickness. Its anti-inflammatory properties aid in managing osteoarthritis and muscle pain. Ginger also supports digestive health by reducing bloating and indigestion. Additionally, it has antioxidant effects that may benefit cardiovascular health by improving circulation and lowering cholesterol levels. Ginger's potential anti-cancer properties and its ability to regulate blood sugar levels further highlight its broad therapeutic applications (Shahrajabian et al. 2019).

14.7.3 Turmeric

Turmeric (*Curcuma longa* L.) is a flowering plant from the ginger family, Zingiberaceae, and is native to South Asia. The active component in turmeric, curcumin, is known for its potent anti-inflammatory and antioxidant effects. It has been shown to inhibit the activity of inflammatory molecules like cytokines and enzymes like COX-2, which are involved in the inflammatory process. Turmeric is used to manage chronic inflammatory conditions like arthritis, and it may also help improve digestive health, support liver function, and potentially reduce the risk of certain cancers. Its ability to enhance brain function and mood is also gaining attention (Hewlings and Kalman 2017).

14.7.4 Peppermint

Peppermint (*Mentha piperita* L.) is a hybrid plant resulting from the cross between watermint (*Mentha aquatica* L.) and spearmint (*Mentha spicata* L.). It is widely used for its therapeutic properties. Due to its antispasmodic effects, Peppermint effectively alleviates digestive issues like irritable bowel syndrome (IBS) and bloating. It also relieves headaches and migraines when applied topically. Peppermint oil is a versatile remedy for various ailments. For example, it helps ease respiratory conditions, such as sinus congestion and coughs, by acting as a natural decongestant. Its antimicrobial properties further contribute to oral health, helping to combat bad breath and gum issues (Tafrihi et al. 2021).

14.7.5 Chamomile

Chamomile (*Matricaria chamomilla* L. or *Chamaemelum nobile* All.) is a herbaceous plant in the Asteraceae family, recognized for its small, daisy-like flowers with white petals and a yellow center. It is renowned for its calming effects, making it an effective remedy for insomnia and anxiety. Its anti-inflammatory properties also make it useful for soothing digestive discomfort, such as indigestion and stomach cramps. Chamomile tea is often used to relieve menstrual pain and improve overall relaxation (Mohamed 2014).

14.7.6 Lavender

Lavender (*Lavandula angustifolia* Mill.) is a popular aromatic herb in the Lamiaceae family, native to the Mediterranean region. Lavender is celebrated for its ability to reduce anxiety and promote relaxation. Its essential oil is commonly used in aromatherapy to help with stress relief, insomnia, and mood enhancement. Lavender can also be applied topically to minor burns, insect bites, and skin irritations to reduce inflammation and promote healing (Kajjari et al. 2022).

14.7.7 Aloe Vera

Aloe vera (*Aloe barbadensis* miller) is a succulent, perennial plant that belongs to the Asphodelaceae family. Aloe vera is widely known for its skin benefits. It is applied topically to treat burns, cuts, and other skin irritations due to its soothing and moisturizing properties. Internally, aloe vera juice supports digestive health by soothing the gastrointestinal tract and treating constipation. Emerging evidence suggests that Aloe Vera may contribute to glycemic control in diabetic patients by enhancing insulin sensitivity and improving overall glucose metabolism. Cardiovascular health benefits are also observed, with Aloe Vera aiding in reducing serum cholesterol levels, enhancing blood circulation, and potentially lowering blood pressure, thereby mitigating cardiovascular risk factors. In the field of dentistry, Aloe Vera's antimicrobial properties are beneficial in managing periodontal diseases and facilitating the healing of oral ulcers. Additionally, its rich antioxidant profile supports immune function by neutralizing oxidative stress (Mohamed 2014).

14.7.8 Garlic

Garlic is a powerful herb with numerous health benefits, primarily due to its sulfur compounds, such as allicin. It supports cardiovascular health by lowering blood pressure, reducing cholesterol levels, and improving circulation. Regular consumption of garlic has been associated with a reduced risk of certain types of cancer, such as stomach, colon, and esophageal cancers. Garlic's potential anticancer properties are attributed to its ability to enhance DNA repair, reduce cell proliferation, and induce apoptosis (programmed cell death) in cancer cells. It also has antimicrobial and antiviral properties, which may help prevent and reduce the severity of colds and other infections. Consuming garlic regularly is thought to enhance immune function and help the body fight off pathogens (Tesfaye 2021).

14.7.9 Ginseng

There are several types of ginsengs, with the most common being Asian ginseng (*Panax ginseng* C.A. Mey.) and American ginseng (*Panax quinquefolius* L.). Ginseng is an adaptogen that helps the body adapt to stress and maintain balance. Ginseng may also support the immune system and improve physical endurance, making it a popular choice for fatigue and chronic stress management. Ginseng, particularly American ginseng, has been shown to improve blood glucose levels in people with type 2 diabetes. It may enhance insulin sensitivity and help regulate glucose uptake by cells, contributing to better blood sugar control. Some studies suggest that ginseng may have anti-cancer properties, potentially reducing the risk of certain cancers like breast, colorectal, and lung cancer. Ginseng's antioxidant and anti-inflammatory properties may help inhibit the growth and spread of cancer cells. It is often used to enhance cognitive function, including memory, concentration, and overall mental performance. It is believed to increase acetylcholine levels, which is important for memory and learning. It may help improve lung function and reduce symptoms in individuals with chronic obstructive pulmonary disease (COPD) and asthma. It is believed to have anti-inflammatory and bronchodilator effects, which can ease breathing (Alanazi et al. 2023).

14.7.10 *Ginkgo biloba*

Ginkgo biloba L., derived from the leaves of the Ginkgo tree, is a popular herbal supplement known for its potential health benefits. It has been used in traditional medicine for thousands of years and is now commonly used for various health conditions. *Ginkgo biloba* L. is often used to improve memory and cognitive function, particularly in older adults. Some studies suggest that it may enhance mental performance and slow cognitive decline, especially in conditions like Alzheimer's disease and vascular dementia. It may also help reduce anxiety symptoms by regulating neurotransmitter function and improving blood flow to the brain, which can be calming. Its antioxidant properties help protect brain cells from oxidative stress, while its ability to enhance blood circulation supports overall brain health. Ginkgo's anti-inflammatory and antioxidant properties may help reduce inflammation in the airways, potentially improving asthma symptoms (Mohamed 2014).

14.7.11 Holy Basil (Tulsi)

Holy basil, also known as Tulsi (*Ocimum sanctum* L.), is a revered herb in Ayurvedic medicine and is known for its wide range of medicinal properties. It is an adaptogen, helping the body cope with stress and maintain balance. Tulsi has anti-inflammatory and immunomodulatory properties that help reduce inflammation in the airways and improve respiratory function. It can be used to relieve symptoms of asthma, bronchitis, and other respiratory conditions. It also treats coughs, colds, and asthma. Holy basil also has anti-inflammatory and antioxidant effects, benefiting overall well-being. Tulsi can help alleviate digestive issues like indigestion, bloating, and stomach cramps. Its antimicrobial properties may also help in treating infections in the digestive tract (Alanazi et al. 2023).

14.7.12 Milk Thistle

Milk thistle (*Silybum marianum* (L.) Gaertn.) is a flowering herb native to the Mediterranean region. It is known for its distinctive appearance and medicinal properties. Milk thistle is primarily used to support liver health. Milk thistle is used in managing liver diseases such as hepatitis and cirrhosis and promoting detoxification. Silymarin, the active compound in milk thistle, possesses antioxidant and anti-inflammatory properties that safeguard liver cells from damage caused by toxins and oxidative stress. Some research indicates that milk thistle may also help reduce LDL cholesterol levels and enhance overall lipid profiles, thereby supporting better cardiovascular health. Milk thistle also offers neuroprotective effects, which may be beneficial for conditions such as Alzheimer's and Parkinson's disease. Additionally, its anti-inflammatory and antioxidant properties can help alleviate skin conditions like acne, eczema, and psoriasis (Alanazi et al. 2023; Mishra et al. 2023) (Fig. 14.2).

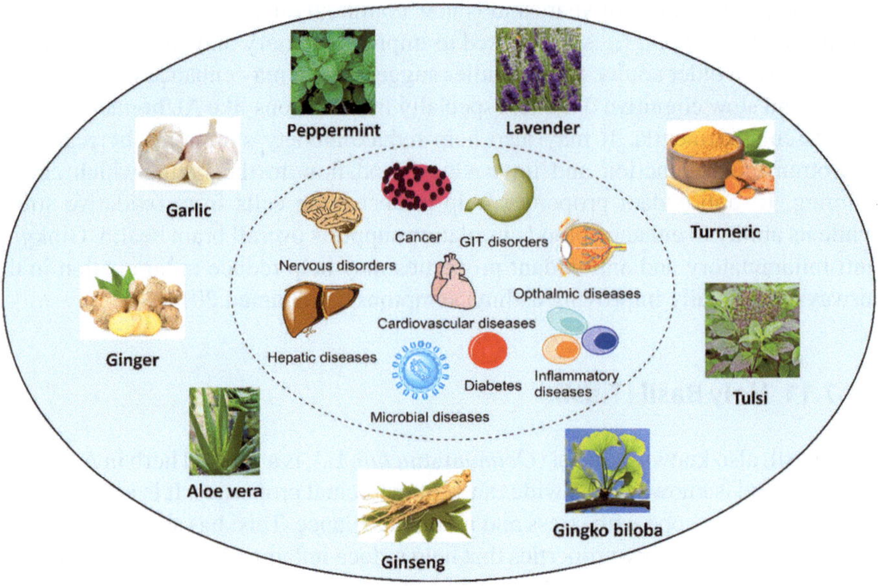

Fig. 14.2 Role of MPs in the treatment of various diseases

14.7.13 Hawthorn

Hawthorn (*Crataegus* spp.) is a genus of shrubs and small trees in the rose family (Rosaceae). This plant is known for its use in traditional medicine, especially for its benefits to heart health. The hawthorn plant's leaves, berries, and flowers are used for medicinal purposes. The vasodilating properties of hawthorn help increase blood flow to the heart muscle, which may reduce the frequency and severity of angina attacks. It helps improve heart function, manage symptoms of heart disease, and reduce high blood pressure. Its antioxidant properties contribute to reducing oxidative stress on the heart and improving circulation. Hawthorn is also used to alleviate symptoms of anxiety and digestive disorders. It also helps reduce cholesterol levels and prevent plaque buildup in the arteries, reducing the risk of atherosclerosis and related conditions such as heart attacks and strokes (Zhang et al. 2022).

14.7.14 Dandelion

Dandelion (*Taraxacum officinale* F.H. Wigg.) is a common flowering plant known for its bright yellow flowers and jagged leaves. It is a versatile plant with various health benefits. It acts as a natural diuretic, helping to manage fluid retention and support urinary tract health. Its liver-supportive properties aid in detoxification and improving digestive function. The diuretic effect of dandelion can help reduce blood pressure by decreasing fluid volume in the body. Some studies suggest that dandelion may help regulate blood sugar levels by enhancing insulin sensitivity and lowering blood glucose levels. Dandelion has anti-inflammatory properties due to its rich content of antioxidants, including beta-carotene, vitamin C, and polyphenols. This can help reduce inflammation and support the immune system (Alanazi et al. 2023).

14.7.15 St. John's Wort

St. John's Wort (*Hypericum perforatum* L.) is a well-known herbal remedy, particularly recognized for its potential benefits in addressing various health conditions, especially mental health issues. It is most used to treat mild to moderate depression, as it is believed to enhance mood by increasing the levels of neurotransmitters such as serotonin, dopamine, and norepinephrine in the brain. Several studies have shown that St. John's Wort may be as effective as conventional antidepressants in some cases, but it generally has fewer side effects. It also helps to treat anxiety. Its calming effect and ability to balance neurotransmitter levels can help reduce symptoms of anxiety and improve overall emotional well-being. Traditionally, St. John's Wort has been applied topically to aid in wound healing. Its anti-inflammatory and antimicrobial properties help reduce inflammation and promote the healing process (Mohamed 2014).

14.8 Scientific Evidence Supporting the Efficacy of Medicinal Plants

Recent research trends are shifting towards a deeper understanding of the pharmacological properties of these plants, emphasizing their roles in traditional medicine and their efficacy against diseases like diabetes and cancer (Mishra et al. 2022b, 2024b). This analysis points to a growing global interest in the therapeutic applications of plant-derived compounds. The use of MPs, which date back thousands of years, forms the foundation of modern medicine. Despite their historical significance, the scientific evaluation of herbal medicines faces challenges due to the variability in plant species, growing conditions, and the complex nature of herbal mixtures. There is a pressing need for systematic approaches to assess these products' quality, safety, and efficacy, as many available herbal medicines lack rigorous scientific validation and quality control (Salmerón-Manzano et al. 2020). A comprehensive review of more than 50 MPs highlights the anticancer potential of MPs, particularly against oral, breast, lung, cervical, and colon cancers. This study underscores the ability of secondary metabolites found in these plants to inhibit cancer cell growth through various mechanisms. The research, which involved extensive literature reviews and in vitro studies, showcases the promising role of phytochemicals in cancer therapy (Kothiyal et al. 2023; Mukonowenzou et al. 2021).

14.9 Role of Medicinal Plants in Preventive Healthcare

MPs play a vital role in preventive healthcare by providing a natural means for disease prevention and health promotion. They contribute to preventing both communicable and non-communicable diseases. While their direct impact on infectious disease prevention might seem limited, certain plants have been shown to boost immune responses, potentially lowering the risk of infections (Sofowora et al. 2013). In the realm of non-communicable diseases (NCDs), MPs are acknowledged for managing modifiable risk factors like unhealthy diets and physical inactivity, which are key components of the WHO's global strategy for NCD prevention. Integrating MPs into the Primary Health Care (PHC) framework aligns with its fundamental principles of accessibility and community involvement. Promoting MPs can engage local communities in health promotion activities, fostering a sense of ownership over their health and well-being (Sofowora et al. 2013).

14.9.1 Challenges and Future Directions

MPs are valuable sources of herbal goods worldwide, yet they are disappearing rapidly. The resources in MPs face ongoing risks of extinction due to factors such as population expansion, overexploitation, environmental degradation, illicit trade, and unsustainable harvesting methods. This section explores the advancements, worldwide patterns, and future possibilities for the strategies and sustainable utilization of MPs resources and approaches in conservation.

14.9.2 Threats to the Availability of Medicinal Plants

The recent release of a World Scientists Warning to mankind emphasized that without strong measures to mitigate or adapt to climate change, it will significantly harm mankind and other species, affecting several parts of existence. This research focuses on the impact of climate change on MPs. These herbs offer several advantages for human well-being, especially in areas where Western medicine is inaccessible. Regarding other species, their populations might face threats due to alterations in temperature and precipitation patterns, disturbance of mutually beneficial connections, and rising pests and infections. Additionally, anthropogenic habitat fragmentation can hinder migration, further exacerbating the situation. In addition, medicinal species are frequently collected in an unsustainable manner, which, when combined with other stresses, can lead to the extinction of many populations (Applequist et al. 2020; Ripple et al. 2017). It is well-recognized that several plant species are currently or will soon be at risk of local or global extinction. A recent study shows over 600 plant species have been extinct during the last 250 years (Humphreys et al. 2019). Human interference, such as habitat degradation and fragmentation, poses a significant threat to wild plant populations worldwide, even without the influence of climate change. These activities lead to the formation of small, isolated populations that are more susceptible to local extinction. Other potential dangers include the arrival and rapid spread of non-native species and foreign diseases and increased plant consumption due to the disappearance of big carnivores (Matthies et al. 2004; Callen and Miller 2015). Highly valuable MPs are at risk of being harvested in an unsustainable manner, which poses an additional hazard to their survival. An instance of this is the significant medicinal plant American ginseng (*Panax quinquefolius* L.), which is utilized for various ailments such as weariness, hypertension, and upper respiratory infections (McElhaney et al. 2011). It is extensively traded to meet the demand in the Chinese market. The high demand has led to a significant issue of illicit harvesting, resulting in a fall in both the population size and average size of the species over time. Additional therapeutic plants with slow growth rates, such as snow lotus (*Saussurea laniceps* Hand.-Mazz.) and goldenseal (*Hydrastis canadensis* L.), also exhibit comparable reductions in size or population (Mulligan 2003; Law and Salick 2005). In the most severe scenario, the combination of commercial harvesting and habitat degradation can lead to the total eradication of a highly prized species, as demonstrated by the instance of the North African plant silphium (likely *Ferula* sp.), which was wiped out during classical times (Kiehn 2007; Parejko 2003). Climate change will modify environmental circumstances in several locales to the extent that they will no longer be optimal—or even viable—for some species that currently occupy them. The projected appropriate range for several species, including MPs, is expected to contract or shift significantly due to anticipated climatic changes (Pompe et al. 2008; Zhao et al. 2018; Abdelaal et al. 2019), while other species may see an extension in their prospective range. The distributions of several creatures are currently undergoing fast shifts toward higher latitudes or elevations (Lamprecht et al. 2018). This phenomenon intensifies the competitive strain on the species already inhabiting these areas. Habitat fragmentation heightens the likelihood that a species cannot migrate and, therefore, face extinction. Phenological change, such as earlier leaf-out or egg hatch date, fruiting patterns and early flowering (Lenoir et al. 2024; Kharouba et al. 2018), can alter the connections between some species and their pollinators and other commensal creatures. Human actions, such as habitat degradation and pollution from pesticides and other chemicals, have significantly diminished insect populations (Sánchez-Bayo and Wyckhuys 2019). The growing effects of climate change will further aggravate the situation.

14.9.3 Need for Regulation and Agricultural Efforts

The agricultural system has effectively provided substantial food and related products to the worldwide market. Implementing resource-intensive farming practices and heavy reliance on foreign inputs has resulted in extensive deforestation, significant loss of biodiversity, and acute water shortages (Kavaliauskas 2008). The primary rationale for allocating land resources for various purposes in emerging nations is the socio-economic demands of rapidly growing populations. The sustainable and prudent utilization of land has become the primary concern for policymakers, government entities, and land users to safeguard resources for current and future generations (Resources and Service 1996). The primary obstacle policymakers face is reversing land degradation patterns in previously cultivated regions by enhancing the conditions and restoring soil fertility. The agroecological zoning approach was created in this context, utilizing sophisticated software packages to address issues of land resources, ultimately promoting sustainable agriculture. The agroecological zoning investigations utilize a Geographic Information System (GIS) to integrate geographical data layers to identify specific areas suitable for crop planning (Nabati et al. 2020). MPs' successful cultivation and economic viability rely heavily on the quality of the harvested crops. Ensuring uniformity is a significant challenge in agriculture, mostly owing to many disruptive biological and non-biological variables. Good agricultural practices (GAP) for MPs are crucial in ensuring the quality of herbal medicine (Bansal et al. 2016). Implementing GAP for MPs is crucial for ensuring the quality of medicinal products made from plants. Discussions were conducted in the early phases, using the work of David Connor, a visiting scientist, as a point of reference to explore the shared principles of GAP. The principles emphasized by GAP focus on utilizing existing technology to promote sustainable agriculture, ensuring safe and healthy food production while achieving economic viability, social responsibility (although social aspects are not adequately addressed), and environmental sustainability. GAP utilizes current knowledge to ensure the sustainable use of natural resources while compassionately promoting the production of safe and healthful food or non-food products. This approach considers economic and social viability issues (Singh and Baldi 2018; Saha et al. 2018; Singh et al. 2022). The World Health Organization (WHO) has produced a set of technical standards for the quality control of herbal medicines. One of the initiatives in this area is the implementation of Good Agricultural and Collection Practices (GACP) guidelines. In 2003, the WHO created GACP for MPs. Furthermore, a resolution on herbal medicine was adopted, and during the 56th session of the World Health Assembly, member states were encouraged to develop national standards and monographs for raw herbal materials to ensure the quality, effectiveness, and safety of herbal formulations (Saha et al. 2018). Many nations, like India, the United States, the United Kingdom, etc., have developed their own GACP recommendations, modelling them after the ones developed by the WHO for MPs. Herbal starting material guidelines on good agricultural and collection practices were approved in 2006 by the European Medicines Agency's Evaluation of Medicines for Human Use group. Quality assurance, education and training, infrastructure, machinery, paperwork, seeds, and propagation materials, growing, collecting, harvesting, processing, packaging, storage, and distribution are all crucial aspects of medicinal plant quality management addressed in Europe's GACP regulations (Zhang et al. 2021). Ayurveda, Siddha, and Unani (ASU), three branches of the Indian medical system, use plant-based ingredients in over 90% of their formulations. While the National Medicinal Plants Board (NMPB) of India has established GACP for the chosen MPs to keep their quality and effectiveness intact, they have also acknowledged that their standards might not address the precise agronomic needs of a given crop in a different agroclimatic zone. Strict collection method rules are necessary to protect unique medical plants and biodiversity, as most MPs are gathered without due process. Critical, major, and minor categories were used to classify the document's vital aspects, such as site selection, compliance with legal criteria, collecting authorization, botanical authenticity, etc. In addition, the NMPB has created the GAP standard necessary for MPs. A framework for creating GAP monographs for specific medicinal plant species was developed. The document addressed important details such as seed and propagation materials, culture, centimeter spacing (row-by-row and plant-by-plant), fertilizers, chemicals, plant protection, pesticide use, and drying procedures (Brinckmann et al. 2020). There is an immense need to improve medicinal plant cultivation while considering farmers' economic sustainability. This can be achieved by integrating knowledge of the ideal growing zone and conditions, conducting a financial feasibility analysis, implementing GAP, and evaluating the quality of plants based on a comprehensive examination of key variables. These types of studies might be used in various regions of the nation to identify potential areas for cultivating different MPs, considering each place's ecological conditions. The need to develop region-specific GAP for certain MPs should be underlined to ensure high-quality commerce and benefit farmers.

14.9.4 Opportunities for Research and Innovation in the Field of MPs

Medicinal and aromatic plants are an important part of the natural biodiversity in many regions across the globe. They play a crucial role in supporting health, local economies, cultural integrity, and overall well-being, particularly for economically disadvantaged and socially vulnerable populations in rural areas, such as the elderly, children, and women. In the past decade, there has been increasing recognition of the significance of these plants, leading to a shift in attitudes toward them and other species that were previously marginalized and overlooked in research and conservation efforts. Simultaneously, species' genetic variety and survival are under heightened risks due to unsustainable extraction and habitat degradation. Advancements in pharmacognosy have not been matched by similar progress in understanding the distribution, genetic diversity, ecology, and conservation of medicinal and aromatic plant species. The capacity to prioritize species selection and understand resource management needs for these species is limited due to inadequate focus on and investment in fundamental research. However, current trends promoting environmentally friendly agriculture and increasing local community involvement in the sustainable conservation and use of natural resources are driving the development of innovative strategies to improve the cultivation and utilization of these plants. These approaches are more participatory and specifically tailored to local needs. The growing number of organizations researching medicinal and aromatic plants, alongside the availability of advanced tools for exploring biodiversity, species characterization, and data analysis, as well as the shift from traditional conservation methods to more utilization-focused initiatives, offer opportunities to reassess research goals and partnerships. This could strengthen national collaborations and foster a more supportive policy environment. The survival of medicinal and aromatic plants hinges on our ability to resolve the conflicts between conservation and use, and on the shift toward agriculture that increasingly relies on natural resources, which is being further tested by the globalization of economies (Singh 2006; Padulosi et al. 2002).

The use of herbal remedies is increasing, but wild harvesting is causing habitat destruction and genetic depletion. Cultivating herbs domestically can address these issues and improve the consistency and safety of herbal extracts. Traditional breeding techniques and molecular markers can enhance agricultural and medicinal traits. However, challenges remain in predicting demand for specific extracts and meeting consumer preferences for naturally produced products (Canter et al. 2005). Plants, animals, and minerals are natural substances used for ages to treat many ailments. Recently, there has been a significant focus on conducting thorough examinations of traditional MPs, namely, in pharmacognosy, phytochemistry, and pharmacology. Furthermore, the biological efficacy of natural remedies has been extensively examined in preclinical and clinical research, uncovering many biological effects shown by a vast array of chemical compounds originating from plants. Most of the natural sources that are now used contain active chemicals that have been traditionally used in ethnomedicine. Consequently, several pharmaceutical firms have revamped their approaches to natural product research, intending to identify promising sources and novel compounds for therapeutic development. The ethnopharmacological knowledge might be advantageous for creating and advancing innovative, secure, and cost-effective medications due to its method that can be reinforced by experimental evidence (Süntar 2020).

14.10 Conclusion

To address the increase in novel infectious illnesses and medication resistance, there is a need for a fundamental change in the approach for designing and developing drugs. Novel approaches for the advancement of pharmaceuticals are required. To accomplish this, using inventive approaches inspired by natural items has facilitated the creation and advancement of several compounds with prospective pharmaceutical properties. Technological advancements have facilitated the study of intricate chemical profiles, leading to the design and synthesis of many compounds. Indeed, several molecules and other very successful medications have previously been synthesized from natural products or their derivatives. Natural products play a crucial role in drug development, and current technical advancements are expected to enhance the success rate of developing novel therapeutic substances. In summary, natural products will continue to play a significant role in medication development and our efforts to address global health concerns and achieve sustainable development goals in the health field. Insufficient evidence is available on the safety and efficacy of native herbal medications. Botanical medications are widely used across many cultures and deemed safe, but they lack sufficient data on their effectiveness, so they are well-suited for treatment outcome studies. These studies might be carried out at nearby healthcare facilities in partnership with the relevant health ministries and social security institutions. Retrospective treatment outcome training provides a dependable way to culturally evaluate traditional medicines, including the psychosocial aspects of healing. There is an opportunity for collaboration between local health clinic medical staff, traditional medicine practitioners, and local health workers to overcome cultural barriers and address medical misunderstandings that impede the acceptance of intercultural healthcare models. It would promote adopting and incorporating diverse medical perspectives and encourage communication among traditional health practitioners, patients, and Western biomedicine-trained health professionals. Enhanced cooperation between biomedical and conventional medical practitioners can enhance the affordability, accessibility, and cultural acceptability of healthcare. Priority should be given to studies that focus on the mechanisms of action, interactions with antibiotics or other MPs or substances, and the pharmacokinetic and pharmacodynamic profiles of MP extracts. This chapter aims to provide valuable insights into the key challenges in this field, which are expected to lead to the development of more efficient, effective, and direct methods for quickly utilizing novel therapeutic MPs against various diseases. Indian traditional medicine has been resilient for many years but faces challenges in integration into mainstream healthcare due to a lack of recognition and excessive regulations. Government underutilization and challenges in implementing existing regulations continue to hinder progress. Successful implementation requires the engagement of all stakeholders, including land-owning communities, private cultivators, traditional practitioners, researchers, policymakers, law enforcement, and others.

References

Abdelaal M, Fois M, Fenu G, Bacchetta G (2019) Using MaxEnt modeling to predict the potential distribution of the endemic plant Rosa arabica Crép. in Egypt. Eco Inform 50:68–75

Aboulwafa MM, Youssef FS, Gad HA, Altyar AE, Al-Azizi MM, Ashour ML (2019) A comprehensive insight on the health benefits and phytoconstituents of Camellia sinensis and recent approaches for its quality control. Antioxidants (Basel) 8:455

Alamgir A, Alamgir A (2017) Cultivation of herbal drugs, biotechnology, and in vitro production of secondary metabolites, high-value medicinal plants, herbal wealth, and herbal trade. In: Therapeutic use of medicinal plants and their extracts: volume 1: pharmacognosy, pp 379–452

Alanazi HH, Elasbali AM, Alanazi MK, El Azab EF (2023) Medicinal herbs: promising immunomodulators for the treatment of infectious diseases. Molecules 28:8045

Alzohairy MA (2016) Therapeutics role of Azadirachta indica (Neem) and their active constituents in diseases prevention and treatment. Evid Based Complement Alternat Med 2016:7382506

Applequist WL, Brinckmann JA, Cunningham AB, Hart RE, Heinrich M, Katerere DR, Van Andel T (2020) Scientists' warning on climate change and medicinal plants. Planta Med 86:10–18

Badgujar SB, Patel VV, Bandivdekar AH (2014) Foeniculum vulgare mill: a review of its botany, phytochemistry, pharmacology, contemporary application, and toxicology. Biomed Res Int 2014:842674

Bai H, Wang R, Li Y, Liang X, Zhang J, Sun N, Yang J (2022) Network pharmacology analysis, molecular docking, and in vitro verification reveal the action mechanism of Prunella vulgaris L. in treating breast cancer. Evid Based Complement Alternat Med 2022:5481563

Balunas MJ, Kinghorn AD (2005) Drug discovery from medicinal plants. Life Sci 78:431–441

Bansal G, Suthar N, Kaur J, Jain A (2016) Stability testing of herbal drugs: challenges, regulatory compliance and perspectives. Phytother Res 30:1046–1058

Bennett BC (2007) Doctrine of signatures: an explanation of medicinal plant discovery or dissemination of knowledge? Econ Bot 61:246–255

Berlowitz I, García Torres E, Maake C, Wolf U, Martin-Soelch C (2023) Indigenous-Amazonian traditional medicine's usage of the tobacco plant: a transdisciplinary ethnopsychological mixed-methods case study. Plants 12:346

Bisht A, Jain S, Misra A, Dwivedi J, Paliwal S, Sharma S (2021) Cedrus deodara (Roxb. ex D.Don) G.Don: a review of traditional use, phytochemical composition and pharmacology. J Ethnopharmacol 279:114361

Brinckmann JA, Fletcher EJ, Das R, Flaster T (2020) 25 years of DSHEA: impact on supply, conservation and sustainability, GACPs and regulatory compliance of botanical ingredients. In: Medicinal and aromatic plants of North America. Springer, Cham, pp 285–323

Callen ST, Miller AJ (2015) Signatures of niche conservatism and niche shift in the North American kudzu (Pueraria montana) invasion. Divers Distrib 21:853–863

Canter PH, Thomas H, Ernst E (2005) Bringing medicinal plants into cultivation: opportunities and challenges for biotechnology. Trends Biotechnol 23:180–185

Chaachouay N, Zidane L (2024) Plant-derived natural products: a source for drug discovery and development. Drugs Drug Candidates 3:184–207

Chen ShiLin CS, Yu Hua YH, Luo HongMei LH, Wu Qiong WQ, Li ChunFang LC, Steinmetz A (2016) Conservation and sustainable use of medicinal plants: problems, progress, and prospects. Chin Med 11:1–10

Chen S-L, Yu H, Luo H-M, Wu Q, Li C-F, Steinmetz A (2016) Conservation and sustainable use of medicinal plants: problems, progress, and prospects. Chin Med 11:1–10

Chumpitazi BP, Kearns GL, Shulman RJ (2018) Review article: the physiological effects and safety of peppermint oil and its efficacy in irritable bowel syndrome and other functional disorders. Aliment Pharmacol Ther 47:738–752

Chung S, Cha S, Lee S-Y, Park J-H, Lee S (2017) The five elements of the cell. Integr Med Res 6:452–456

Dal Cero M, Saller R, Leonti M, Weckerle CS (2023) Trends of medicinal plant use over the last 2000 years in Central Europe. Plants 12:135

Deshmukh R, Jain AK, Singh R, Paul SD, Harwansh RK (2024) Andrographis paniculata and Andrographolide – a snapshot on recent advances in nano drug delivery systems against cancer. Curr Drug Deliv 21:631–644

Eng YS, Lee CH, Lee WC, Huang CC, Chang JS (2019) Unraveling the molecular mechanism of traditional Chinese medicine: formulas against acute airway viral infections as examples. Molecules 24:3505

Ezekwesili-Ofili Josephine O, Okaka Antoinette Nwamaka C (2019) Chapter 10: Herbal medicines in African traditional medicine. In: Philip FB (ed) Herbal medicine. IntechOpen, Rijeka

Frecska E, Bokor P, Winkelman M (2016) The therapeutic potentials of Ayahuasca: possible effects against various diseases of civilization. Front Pharmacol 7:35

Fu J, Wang Z, Huang L, Zheng S, Wang D, Chen S, Zhang H, Yang S (2014) Review of the botanical characteristics, phytochemistry, and pharmacology of (Huangqi). Phytother Res 28:1275–1283

Fuloria S, Mehta J, Chandel A, Sekar M, Rani NNIM, Begum MY, Subramaniyan V, Chidambaram K, Thangavelu L, Nordin R (2022) A comprehensive review on the therapeutic potential of Curcuma longa Linn. in relation to its major active constituent curcumin. Front Pharmacol 13:820806

Galindo Egea A, Girón Moreno IF, Corell González M, Moriana A, Torrecillas Melendreras A, Hernández F (2017) Water stress at the end of the pomegranate fruit ripening stage produces earlier harvest and improves fruit quality. Sci Hortic 226:68–74

Garcia MK, Cohen L (2020) Acupuncture. In: Gellman MD (ed) Encyclopedia of behavioral medicine. Springer International Publishing, Cham, pp 29–30

Gayathry KS, John JA (2022) A comprehensive review on bitter gourd (Momordica charantia L.) as a gold mine of functional bioactive components for therapeutic foods. Food Prod Process Nutr 4:10
Ghasemzadeh Rahbardar M, Hosseinzadeh H (2020) Therapeutic effects of rosemary (Rosmarinus officinalis L.) and its active constituents on nervous system disorders. Iran J Basic Med Sci 23:1100–1112
Ghimire SK, McKey D, Aumeeruddy-Thomas Y (2005) Conservation of Himalayan medicinal plants: harvesting patterns and ecology of two threatened species, Nardostachys grandiflora DC. and Neopicrorhiza scrophulariiflora (Pennell) Hong. Biol Conserv 124:463–475
Grienke U, Zöll M, Peintner U, Rollinger JM (2014) European medicinal polypores – a modern view on traditional uses. J Ethnopharmacol 154:564–583
Hamilton AC (2004) Medicinal plants, conservation and livelihoods. Biodivers Conserv 13:1477–1517
Hassan H (2015) A short history of the use of plants as medicines from ancient times. CHIMIA Int J Chem 69:622–623
Hassanpouraghdam MB, Ghorbani H, Esmaeilpour M, Alford MH, Strzemski M, Dresler S (2022) Diversity and distribution patterns of endemic medicinal and aromatic plants of Iran: implications for conservation and habitat management. Int J Environ Res Public Health 19:1552
Hawkins J, Baker C, Cherry L, Dunne E (2019) Black elderberry (Sambucus nigra) supplementation effectively treats upper respiratory symptoms: a meta-analysis of randomized, controlled clinical trials. Complement Ther Med 42:361–365
Hewlings SJ, Kalman DS (2017) Curcumin: a review of its effects on human health. Foods 6:92
Humphreys AM, Govaerts R, Ficinski SZ, Nic Lughadha E, Vorontsova MS (2019) Global dataset shows geography and life form predict modern plant extinction and rediscovery. Nat Ecol Evol 3:1043–1047
Jagtap CY, Mishra AK, Nariya M, Shukla VJ, Prajapati PK (2024) Product development and characterization of the Ayurvedic herbo-mineral-metallic compound- Hridayarnava Rasa. J Ayurveda Integr Med 15:100886
Jain S, Sharma S, Paliwal A, Dwivedi J, Paliwal S, Paliwal V, Paliwal S, Sharma J (2024) Discovery of novel fatty acid amide hydrolase (FAAH) inhibitors as anti-Alzheimer's agents through pharmacophore-based virtual screening, molecular docking and experimental validation. Med Chem Res 33:136–150
Jaiswal YS, Williams LL (2017) A glimpse of Ayurveda–The forgotten history and principles of Indian traditional medicine. J Tradit Complement Med 7:50–53
Jamshidi N, Cohen MM (2017) The clinical efficacy and safety of Tulsi in humans: a systematic review of the literature. Evid Based Complement Alternat Med 2017:9217567
Jha U, Singh K, Baghla AS (2022) Phytochemical and pharmacology activity of Bhringraj: a review. Int J Health Sci:11113–11125
Jha SK, Mishra AK, Kumar V, Dane G, Kumari S, Charde V, Saddam M, Jagtap C, Chuhan S, Chaturvedi SK, Narasimhaji CV (2024) Ecological and behavioral impacts of COVID-19 on human existence and potential preventive measures through traditional and alternative medicine – a narrative review. Pharmacol Res Natural Products 3:100042
Jhariya MK, Banerjee A, Meena RS (2022) Importance of natural resources conservation: moving toward the sustainable world. In: Natural resources conservation and advances for sustainability. Elsevier, pp 3–27
Kajjari S, Joshi RS, Hugar SM, Gokhale N, Meharwade P, Uppin C (2022) The effects of lavender essential oil and its clinical implications in dentistry: a review. Int J Clin Pediatr Dent 15:385–388
Kang S, Min H (2012) Ginseng, the 'immunity boost': the effects of Panax ginseng on immune system. J Ginseng Res 36:354
Kavaliauskas P (2008) A concept of sustainable development for regional land use planning: Lithuanian experience. Technol Econ Dev Econ 14:51–63

Kharouba HM, Ehrlén J, Gelman A, Bolmgren K, Allen JM, Travers SE, Wolkovich EM (2018) Global shifts in the phenological synchrony of species interactions over recent decades. Proc Natl Acad Sci 115:5211–5216
Kiehn M (2007) Silphion revisited. Med Plant Conserv 13:4–8
Klemow KM, Bartlow A, Crawford J, Kocher N, Shah J, Ritsick M (2011) Medical attributes of St. John's Wort (Hypericum perforatum). In: Benzie IFF, Wachtel-Galor S (eds) Herbal medicine: biomolecular and clinical aspects. CRC Press/Taylor & Francis Copyright © 2011 by Taylor and Francis Group, LLC, Boca Raton (FL)
Koithan M, Farrell C (2010) Indigenous native American healing traditions. J Nurse Pract 6:477–478
Kothiyal S, Gahlot M, Choudhary A, Palai S, Almeida R, Vasconcelos J, Santos F, Farias P, Coutinho H (2023) Scientific evidences of anticancer potential of medicinal plants. Food Chem Adv 2:100239
Kumar Srivastava A (2018) Chapter 1 – significance of medicinal plants in human life. In: Tewari A, Tiwari S (eds) Synthesis of medicinal agents from plants. Elsevier, pp 1–24
Kumar P, Malik S, Dubey K (2019) Bryophyllum Pinnatum: a review on medicinal benefits and potent bioactive molecules. Curr Bioact Compd 15
Kurnaz ML, Kurnaz IA (2021) Commercialization of medicinal bioeconomy resources and sustainability. Sustain Chem Pharm 22:100484
Kushwah A, Sharma P, Kushwaha H, Sharma B, Carpenter G, Nag RH, Yadav R, Chowdhury M (2023) Innovative selective harvesting technology for cauliflower: a design approach using plant characteristics. Environ Ecol 41:2595–2601
Lamprecht A, Semenchuk PR, Steinbauer K, Winkler M, Pauli H (2018) Climate change leads to accelerated transformation of high-elevation vegetation in the central Alps. New Phytol 220:447–459
Law W, Salick J (2005) Human-induced dwarfing of Himalayan snow lotus, Saussurea laniceps (Asteraceae). Proc Natl Acad Sci 102:10218–10220
Leitzmann C (2016) Characteristics and health benefits of phytochemicals. Forsch Komplementmed 23:69–74
Lenoir J, Svenning J-C, Sheffer M (2024) Latitudinal and elevational range shifts under contemporary climate change. In: Encyclopedia of biodiversity, pp 690–709
Leonti M, Verpoorte R (2017) Traditional Mediterranean and European herbal medicines. J Ethnopharmacol 199:161–167
Li Y, Kong D, Fu Y, Sussman MR, Wu H (2020) The effect of developmental and environmental factors on secondary metabolites in medicinal plants. Plant Physiol Biochem 148:80–89
Liu Z-H, Niu F-J, Xie Y-X, Xie S-M, Liu Y-N, Yang Y-Y, Zhou C-Z, Wan X-H (2020) A review: natural polysaccharides from medicinal plants and microorganisms and their anti-herpetic mechanism. Biomed Pharmacother 129:110469
Longhurst JC (2010) Defining meridians: a modern basis of understanding. J Acupunct Meridian Stud 3:67–74
Manish K (2022) Medicinal plants in peril due to climate change in the Himalaya. Eco Inform 68:101546
Mao Q-Q, Xu X-Y, Cao S-Y, Gan R-Y, Corke H, Beta T, Li H-B (2019) Bioactive compounds and bioactivities of ginger (Zingiber officinale Roscoe). Foods 8:185
Marshall AC (2020) Traditional Chinese medicine and clinical pharmacology. Springer
Mateo-Martín J, Benítez G, Gras A, Molina M, Reyes-García V, Tardío J, Verde A, Pardo-de-Santayana M (2023) Cultural importance, availability and conservation status of Spanish wild medicinal plants: implications for sustainability. People Nature 5:1512–1525
Matthies D, Bräuer I, Maibom W, Tscharntke T (2004) Population size and the risk of local extinction: empirical evidence from rare plants. Oikos 105:481–488
McElhaney JE, Simor AE, McNeil S, Predy GN (2011) Efficacy and safety of CVT-E002, a proprietary extract of Panax quinquefolius in the prevention of respiratory infections in influenza-vaccinated community-dwelling adults: a multicenter, randomized, double-blind, and placebo-controlled trial. Influenza Res Treat 2011:759051

Mikulska P, Malinowska M, Ignacyk M, Szustowski P, Nowak J, Pesta K, Szeląg M, Szklanny D, Judasz E, Kaczmarek G (2023) Ashwagandha (Withania somnifera)—current research on the health-promoting activities: a narrative review. Pharmaceutics 15:1057

Mir TA, Jan M, Khare RK, Bhat MH (2021) Medicinal plant resources: threat to its biodiversity and conservation strategies. In: Medicinal and aromatic plants: healthcare and industrial applications. Springer, Cham, pp 717–739

Mishra AK, Sahoo PK (2022) Characterization of nanophytopharmaceuticals. In: Phytoantioxidants and nanotherapeutics, pp 239–265

Mishra AK, Pandey M, Dewangan HK, Sl N, Sahoo PK (2022a) A comprehensive review on liver targeting: emphasis on nanotechnology- based molecular targets and receptors mediated approaches. Curr Drug Targets 23:1381–1405

Mishra AK, Sahoo PK, Lal G, Bajpai M, Dewangan HK (2022b) Anti-diabetic effect of sprouted Trigonella foenum-graecum L. seed solid dosage form in low-dose Streptozotocin induced diabetic rats. Indian J Pharm Educ Res 56:1156–1163

Mishra AK, Neha SL, Rani L, Jain A, Dewangan HK, Sahoo PK (2023) Rationally designed nanoparticulate delivery approach for silymarin with natural bio-enhancer: in vitro characterization and in vivo evaluations of hepatoprotective effects in a mouse model. J Drug Deliv Sci Technol 86:104580

Mishra AK, Pandey M, Pannu A, Dewangan HK, Sahoo P (2024a) Review on diabetes mellitus: an insight into the current scenarios, the challenges of therapy, and application of traditional drugs. Curr Tradit Med 10:107–128

Mishra AK, Neha SL, Jain A, Jagtap CY, Dane G, Paroha S, Sahoo PK (2024b) Effectiveness of Semecarpus anacardium Linn fruits in cancer and inflammatory diseases: a mini review. Fitoterapia 175:105978

Mishra AK, Singh R, Rawat H, Kumar V, Jagtap C, Jain A (2024c) The influence of food matrix on the stability and bioavailability of phytochemicals: a comprehensive review. Food Humanity 2:100202

Mohamed S (2014) Chapter 10 – Herbs and spices in aging. In: Preedy VR (ed) Aging. Academic Press, San Diego, pp 99–107

Mukonowenzou NC, Adeshina KA, Donaldson J, Ibrahim KG, Usman D, Erlwanger KH (2021) Medicinal plants, phytochemicals, and their impacts on the maturation of the gastrointestinal tract. Front Physiol 12:684464

Mulligan MR (2003) Population loss of goldenseal, Hydrastis canadensis L.(Ranunculaceae), in Ohio. Miami University

Nabati J, Nezami A, Neamatollahi E, Akbari M (2020) GIS-based agro-ecological zoning for crop suitability using fuzzy inference system in semi-arid regions. Ecol Indic 117:106646

Okpako DT (1999) Traditional African medicine: theory and pharmacology explored. Trends Pharmacol Sci 20:482–485

Ottersen OP, Engebretsen E (2020) COVID-19 puts the sustainable development goals center stage. Nat Med 26:1672–1673

Padulosi S, Leaman D, Quek P (2002) Challenges and opportunities in enhancing the conservation and use of medicinal and aromatic plants. J Herbs Spices Med Plants 9:243–267

Palada M, Mitchell J, Becker B, Nair P (2003) The integration of medicinal plants and culinary herbs in agroforestry systems for the Caribbean: a study in the US Virgin Islands. In: III WOCMAP congress on medicinal and aromatic plants-volume 2: conservation, cultivation and sustainable use of medicinal and 676, pp 147–153

Panduro A, Roman S, Mariscal-Martinez IM, Jose-Abrego A, Gonzalez-Aldaco K, Ojeda-Granados C, Ramos-Lopez O, Torres-Reyes LA (2024) Personalized medicine and nutrition in hepatology for preventing chronic liver disease in Mexico. Front Nutr 11:1379364

Pant P, Pandey S, Dall'Acqua S (2021) The influence of environmental conditions on secondary metabolites in medicinal plants: a literature review. Chem Biodivers 18:e2100345

Papageorgiou D, Bebeli PJ, Panitsa M, Schunko C (2020) Local knowledge about sustainable harvesting and availability of wild medicinal plant species in Lemnos Island, Greece. J Ethnobiol Ethnomed 16:1–23

Pareek A, Pant M, Gupta MM, Kashania P, Ratan Y, Jain V, Pareek A, Chuturgoon AA (2023) Moringa oleifera: an updated comprehensive review of its pharmacological activities, ethnomedicinal, phytopharmaceutical formulation, clinical, phytochemical, and toxicological aspects. Int J Mol Sci 24:2098

Parejko K (2003) Pliny the elder's silphium: first recorded species extinction. Conserv Biol 17:925–927

Philippu A, Seifert R (2023) History of pharmacology: 1-the Department of Pharmacology of the University of Tartu (Dorpat): genealogy and biographies. Naunyn Schmiedeberg's Arch Pharmacol 396:5–17

Pimm SL, Russell GJ, Gittleman JL, Brooks TM (1995) The future of biodiversity. Science 269:347–350

Plagányi ÉE, Skewes T, Murphy N, Pascual R, Fischer M (2015) Crop rotations in the sea: increasing returns and reducing risk of collapse in sea cucumber fisheries. Proc Natl Acad Sci 112:6760–6765

Pompe S, Hanspach J, Badeck F, Klotz S, Thuiller W, Kühn I (2008) Climate and land use change impacts on plant distributions in Germany. Biol Lett 4:564–567

Ragaveena S, Shirly Edward A, Surendran U (2021) Smart controlled environment agriculture methods: a holistic review. Rev Environ Sci Biotechnol 20:887–913

Raj A, Jhariya MK, Yadav DK, Banerjee A, Meena RS (2019) Agroforestry: a holistic approach for agricultural sustainability. In: Sustainable agriculture, forest and environmental management. Springer, Singapore, pp 101–131

Rawat H, Bhat SA, Dhanjal DS, Singh R, Gandhi Y, Mishra SK, Kumar V, Shakya SK, Narasimhaji CV, Singh A, Singh R, Acharya R (2024) Emerging techniques for the trace elemental analysis of plants and food-based extracts: a comprehensive review. Talanta Open 10:100341

Resources, A. O. o. t. U. N. S. & C. Service (1996) Agro-ecological zoning: guidelines. Food & Agriculture Org

Ripple WJ, Wolf C, Newsome TM, Galetti M, Alamgir M, Crist E, Mahmoud MI, Laurance WF, S. S. f. C. 15 (2017) World scientists' warning to humanity: a second notice. Bioscience 67:1026–1028

Rokaya MB, Münzbergová Z, Dostálek T (2017) Sustainable harvesting strategy of medicinal plant species in Nepal–results of a six-year study. Folia Geobot 52:239–252

Rudrapal M, Mishra AK, Rani L, Sarwa KK, Zothantluanga JH, Khan J, Kamal M, Palai S, Bendale AR, Talele SG, Pathan VT, Borse LB, Neharkar VS, Sahoo PK (2022) Nanodelivery of dietary polyphenols for therapeutic applications. Molecules 27:8706

Saeidnia S, Gohari A, Mokhber-Dezfuli N, Kiuchi F (2011) A review on phytochemistry and medicinal properties of the genus Achillea. Daru 19:173–186

Saha S, Mandal A, Dutta A (2018) Good agricultural practices: requirement for the production of quality herbal medicines. In: Natural products and drug discovery. Elsevier, pp 607–631

Salmerón-Manzano E, Garrido-Cardenas JA, Manzano-Agugliaro F (2020) Worldwide research trends on medicinal plants. Int J Environ Res Public Health 17:3376

Sánchez-Bayo F, Wyckhuys KA (2019) Worldwide decline of the entomofauna: a review of its drivers. Biol Conserv 232:8–27

Selvakumarasamy S, Rengaraju B, Arumugam SA, Kulathooran R (2021) Costus pictus–transition from a medicinal plant to functional food: a review. Future Foods 4:100068

Sen T, Samanta SK (2015) Medicinal plants, human health and biodiversity: a broad review. In: Biotechnological applications of biodiversity. Springer, pp 59–110

Shafi A, Hassan F, Zahoor I, Majeed U, Khanday FA (2021) Biodiversity, management and sustainable use of medicinal and aromatic plant resources. In: Medicinal and aromatic plants: healthcare and industrial applications. Springer, pp 85–111

Shah G, Shri R, Panchal V, Sharma N, Singh B, Mann AS (2011) Scientific basis for the therapeutic use of Cymbopogon citratus, stapf (Lemon grass). J Adv Pharm Technol Res 2:3–8

Shahrajabian MH, Sun W, Cheng Q (2019) Clinical aspects and health benefits of ginger (Zingiber officinale) in both traditional Chinese medicine and modern industry. Acta Agric Scand Section B – Soil & Plant Sci 69:546–556

Sharma N, Pandey R (2012) Conservation of medicinal plants in the tropics. In: Conservation of tropical plant species. Springer, pp 437–487
Shen T, Yu H, Wang Y-Z (2021) Assessing the impacts of climate change and habitat suitability on the distribution and quality of medicinal plant using multiple information integration: take Gentiana rigescens as an example. Ecol Indic 123:107376
Sidor A, Gramza-Michałowska A (2015) Advanced research on the antioxidant and health benefit of elderberry (Sambucus nigra) in food – a review. J Funct Foods 18:941–958
Singh H (2006) Prospects and challenges for harnessing opportunities in medicinal plants sector in India. Law Env't Dev J 2:196
Singh PA, Baldi A (2018) Good agricultural practices: a prequisite approach for enhancing the quality of Indian herbal medicines. Biom J 2:4
Singh AK, Gupta AK, Manish M, Singh P (2014) Rasayana therapy: a magic contribution of Ayurveda for healthy long life. Int J Res Ayurveda Pharma 5(1):41–47
Singh PA, Bajwa N, Chinnam S, Chandan A, Baldi A (2022) An overview of some important deliberations to promote medicinal plants cultivation. J Appl Res Med Aromat Plants 31:100400
Smith LW (2012) Leigh Whaley, women and the practice of medical care in early modern Europe, 1400–1800. Soc Hist Med 25:563–565
Sofowora A, Ogunbodede E, Onayade A (2013) The role and place of medicinal plants in the strategies for disease prevention. Afr J Tradit Complement Altern Med 10:210–229
Srivastava JK, Shankar E, Gupta S (2010) Chamomile: a herbal medicine of the past with a bright future (review). Mol Med Rep 3:895–901
Sulaiman N, Zocchi DM, Borrello MT, Mattalia G, Antoniazzi L, Berlinghof SE, Bewick A, Häfliger I, Schembs M, Torri L, Pieroni A (2024) Traditional knowledge evolution over half of a century: local herbal resources and their changes in the Upper Susa Valley of Northwest Italy. Plants 13:43
Süntar I (2020) Importance of ethnopharmacological studies in drug discovery: role of medicinal plants. Phytochem Rev 19:1199–1209
Tafrihi M, Imran M, Tufail T, Gondal TA, Caruso G, Sharma S, Sharma R, Atanassova M, Atanassov L, Valere Tsouh Fokou P, Pezzani R (2021) The wonderful activities of the genus Mentha: not only antioxidant properties. Molecules 26:1118
Tainter ML, Marcelli GM (1959) The rise of synthetic drugs in the American pharmaceutical industry. Bull N Y Acad Med 35:387–405
Tesfaye A (2021) Revealing the therapeutic uses of garlic (Allium sativum) and its potential for drug discovery. ScientificWorldJournal 2021:8817288
Thangavelu L, Geetha RV, Roy A, Kumar Subramanian A (2011) Yarrow (Achillea millefolium Linn.) a herbal medicinal plant with broad therapeutic use – a review. Int J Pharm Sci Rev Res 9:136–141
Thomford NE, Senthebane DA, Rowe A, Munro D, Seele P, Maroyi A, Dzobo K (2018) Natural products for drug discovery in the 21st century: innovations for novel drug discovery. Int J Mol Sci 19:1578
Uprety Y, Asselin H, Dhakal A, Julien N (2012) Traditional use of medicinal plants in the boreal forest of Canada: review and perspectives. J Ethnobiol Ethnomed 8:1–14
Veeresham C (2012) Natural products derived from plants as a source of drugs. J Adv Pharm Technol Res 3:200
Vinjamury SP, Vinjamury M, Sucharitakul S, Ziegler I (2011) Panchakarma: ayurvedic detoxification and allied therapies—is there any evidence? In: Evidence-based practice in complementary and alternative medicine: perspectives, protocols, problems and potential in ayurveda, pp 113–137
Wagner C, De Gezelle J, Komarnytsky S (2020) Celtic provenance in traditional herbal medicine of Medieval Wales and classical antiquity. Front Pharmacol 11:105
Wahab S, Annadurai S, Abullais SS, Das G, Ahmad W, Ahmad MF, Kandasamy G, Vasudevan R, Ali MS, Amir M (2021) Glycyrrhiza glabra (Licorice): a comprehensive review on its phytochemistry, biological activities, clinical evidence and toxicology. Plants 10:2751

Wang W, Xu J, Fang H, Li Z, Li M (2020) Advances and challenges in medicinal plant breeding. Plant Sci 298:110573

Wanyenze RK, Alfvén T, Ndejjo R, Viberg N, Båge K, Batte C, Helldén D, Lindgren H, Mayega RW, Ndeezi G, Peterson SS, Nawangwe B, Ottersen OP (2023) Sustainable health—a call to action. BMC Global Public Health 1:3

Will H, Eisenmann-Tappe I (2016) Monastery medicine – what's the story behind it? What's reasonable, what's no good? Dtsch Med Wochenschr (1946) 141:1858–1862

Yin Q, Wang J, Cheng H, Cheng M, Cheng W (2024) Yin-Yang balance concepts for clinical diagnosis and treatment: an integrated view of Chinese medicine, anesthesiology, and quantum mechanics. Transl Perioper Pain Med 11:560–573

Zhang M, Wang C, Zhang R, Chen Y, Zhang C, Heidi H, Li M (2021) Comparison of the guidelines on good agricultural and collection practices in herbal medicine of the European Union, China, the WHO, and The United States of America. Pharmacol Res 167:105533

Zhang J, Chai X, Zhao F, Hou G, Meng Q (2022) Food applications and potential health benefits of hawthorn. Foods 11:2861

Zhao Q, Li R, Gao Y, Yao Q, Guo X, Wang W (2018) Modeling impacts of climate change on the geographic distribution of medicinal plant Fritillaria cirrhosa D. Don. Plant Biosystems 152:349–355

Zhu F, Du B, Xu B (2018) Anti-inflammatory effects of phytochemicals from fruits, vegetables, and food legumes: a review. Crit Rev Food Sci Nutr 58:1260–1270

Ayurnutrigenomics: Ayurveda-Inspired Nutrition from Inception to Evidence Using Omics Platform

15

Nidhi V. Maheshwari, Preeti Jain, Manoj Kumar Tripathi, and Anil Kumar

Abstract

For perpetuation of human race as well as prevention and mitigation of diseases, food and medicine are intertwined as per concept of Ayurveda. Food is consumed in large quantity as compared to any drug. The effect and interaction of nutrition with the genome to understand disease and their management is thus essential. Nutritional Genomics emphasis on the interaction between bioactive food components and the genome, which includes Nutrigenetics and Nutrigenomics. Ayurgenomics is a personalized approach in the predictive, preventive, and curative aspects of medicine. It is the study of interindividual variability due to genetic variability in humans for assessing diagnosis and prognosis of diseases, mainly based on the Prakriti. The amalgamation of nutritional practices as per ayurveda with respect to one's prakriti involving various omics tools for the dietary and therapeutic selection gave rise to the concept of "Ayurnutrigenomics." It is the emerging field of science involving Ayurveda systems biology, where the selection of an appropriate dietary, therapeutic, and lifestyle regime is made on the basis of clinical assessment of an individual maintaining one's Prakriti. This Ayurveda-inspired concept of personalized nutrition is a novel concept of nutrigenomic research for developing personalized functional foods and nutraceuticals suitable for one's genetic makeup with the help of Ayurveda using omics approach.

N. V. Maheshwari (✉) · P. Jain
Somaiya Vidyavihar University, Mumbai, Maharashtra, India

M. K. Tripathi
ICAR- Central Institute of Agricultural Engineering, Bhopal, Madhya Pradesh, India

A. Kumar
Rani Lakshmi Bai Central Agricultural University, Jhansi, Uttar Pradesh, India

A. Kumar et al. (eds.), *Innovations in Ayurvedic Nutrition*,
https://doi.org/10.1007/978-981-95-1213-3_15

Keywords

Ayurveda · Ayurgenomics · Ayurnutrigenomics · Prakriti · Personalized medicine

15.1 Introduction

Even though modern medicine seems successful in treating many dangerous diseases, combining it with ayurveda is expected to pave the path in discovering effective preventative techniques and strategies for personalized care and therapy (Huang et al. 2022). Three doshas, Vata, pitta, and kapha and their relationship with a person's physical, physiological, and psychological functions including metabolism has been described in ayurveda. The expression of different doshas in a particular proportion defines prakriti of an individual, reflected in their nature and body type (Rotti et al. 2014; Gadre 2019). Based on these phenotypes, an ayurvedic practitioner determines an individual's prakriti first before taking decision on the approach of treatment. In contrast to modern medicine, which analyses heterogeneity among individuals based on genome, gene expression and epigenetics, prakriti and doshas serve the basis for variability assessment in ayurveda. Pharmaceutical industries are trying to test different herbal formulations, which can be explicitly applied for disease treatment.

15.2 Concept of Ayurveda

The ayurvedic medicine also known as "Kayachikitsa" mainly consists of the etiopathogenesis, diagnosis, and treatment of diseases. Ayurveda is a vast, natural system of health care that originated in ancient India during the Vedic period. The word "Ayurveda" originates from Sanskrit: "Ayus," which means lifespan or life, and "Veda," which implies science or knowledge. Taken together, Ayurveda means "the science of life," or "the science of lifespan." Knowledge of Ayurveda enables one to understand how to create this balance of body, mind, and consciousness according to one's own individual constitution and how to make lifestyle changes to bring about and maintain this balance. Ahara (diet), Nidra (sleep), and Brahmacarya (abstinence) are recognized as the three Upasthambhas (sub pillars) essential for the smooth running of life. Ahar (Food) is considered as the best sustainer of life. All the dietary articles and our body are composed of Panchamahabhutas [Vayu (Air), Jala (Water), Aakash (Space or ether), Prithvi (Earth), and Teja (Fire)] (Sumantran and Tillu 2011). For sustenance of life, all five Mahabhutas are essential. Tridoshas/ biohumors (Vata, Pitta, Kapha) are the biological derivatives of these five Mahabhuta. Tridoshas control the physiology of each individual." Each dosha has its own set of characteristics and functions (Table 15.1).

Prakriti is the mix of these three doshas that each human is born with.

A proper balance between these three doshas is required for good health (Rotti et al. 2014). The Mahabhutas Akasa (space) and Vayu (air) make up the Vata Dosha.

Table 15.1 Tridoshas with its own characteristics and functions

S. No.	Doshas	Characteristics	Functions	References
1	Vata	Responsible for transfer inside the body Adds to shape manifestation, cell division, signalling, waste elimination, movement, thought	Aids in the transmission of molecules to nerve impulses Normalizes the function of pitta and Kapha	Sumantran and Tillu (2013), Prasher et al. (2017)
2	Pitta	Regulates digestion and various metabolic processes within a cell	Responsible for energy balance, thermoregulation, vision, pigmentation, and host surveillance, among other things	Prasher et al. (2016)
3	Kapha	Oversees the body's structure and cohesiveness	Storage, stability, development, and maintenance of body	Wallace (2020)

Pitta Dosha is made up of the Mahabhutas Tejas or Agni (fire) and Ap (water). Kapha Dosha is composed of the Ap (water) and Prithvi (earth) Mahabhutas. If there is an imbalance in the Doshas, the person is classified as Vata, Pitta, or Kapha dominant. A person can be classified as belonging to a certain Dosha type depending on the attributes that each Dosha bestows upon them (Shilpa and Venkatesha Murthy 2011).

According to Charaka and Sushruta, people can be divided into seven groups based on how common the Doshas are in each group's bodies. The following criteria are used to determine whether someone fits a particular Prakriti or constitution:

Those with a predominant Vata Dosha, sometimes referred to as Vata Prakriti (or constitution). There are individuals with dominant Pitta Dosha/Prakriti, strong Kapha Dosha/Prakriti, dominant Vata-Pitta Dosha combination, strong Vata-Kapha Dosha combination, prominent Pitta-Kapha Dosha combination, balanced Doshas, or a combination of Vata-Pitta-Kapha Doshas.

Every person has a different level of tridosha at birth, which is influenced not just by genetics but also by the environment during foetal development. Given that a person's physiology is governed by their dominant Dosha, Prakriti, and other features, defining prevention and therapy on this basis may aid in identifying the optimal combination of lifestyle changes and pharmaceuticals. Dosha Prakrtiti has been taken into account in Dashavidha Pariksha, the foundation of personalized medicine (Charaka Samhita).

15.3 Concept of Prakriti

The relative proportion of the three Tridoshas, or entities, Vata, Pitta, and Kapha, results in the Prakriti. This is not just determined by genetics (Shukra Shonita) but is also influenced by the environment (Mahabhuta Vikara), particularly by the lifestyle and diet of the mother throughout the development of the foetus, as well as by the parents' ages (Matura Ahara Vihara). In addition to these, it is believed that an individual's ethnicity (Jati), familial traits (Satmya), and place of origin (Desha) all have an impact on how Prakriti develops.

Prakriti and Tridoshas are important concepts in Ayurgenomics, and they help to explain how each person has a distinct constitution known as prakriti. The typical way that each person reacts to drugs, environmental variables, and nutritional considerations is determined by Prakriti (Heinrich et al. 2004). According to Ayurveda, Prakriti is the fundamental clinical denominator that characterizes a person's physical, physiological, and psychological characteristics and serves as the basis for individualized dietary advice, lifestyle counselling, and medical care. The individual's genome is expressed in its entirety as their prakriti. The symptoms, preferences, mental and emotional tendencies, as well as physiological assessments like lab and blood tests, all help to articulate this unique genomic signature (Patwardhan and Bodeker 2008).

The three Doshas—Vata, Pitta, and Kapha—coordinate to maintain an individual's state of health while also regulating one another. A situation in which one or both Mahabhutas are entirely absent cannot exist. For existence of life, all five are necessary.

15.4 Ayurgenomics: Ayurveda and Genomics

Linking ayurvedic parameters, i.e. prakriti and doshas with genetic variability is covered under the branch "Ayurgenomics." Ayurgenomics allows efficient utilization of already discovered medications to target individuals with certain prakriti. Identification of genetic markers underlying these ayurvedic parameters would allow to establish molecular mechanistic detail of the impact of ayurveda on diseases. Numerous genes have been identified to be modulated by these ayurvedic parameters. Prakriti based modulation of CYP2C19, Prothrombin, Cholesterol, human leukocyte antigen, EGLN1 (gene responsible for high altitude adaptation), inflammatory, oxidative stress pathway, Phosphoglucomutase 1 (PGM1), and ESR1(Epigenetic) genes have been reported (Huang et al. 2022). In addition, 52 SNPs (Single Nucleotide Polymorphism) have been suggested as one of the bases for categorising individuals to the groups, Vata, Pitta, and Kapha (Govindaraj et al. 2015). Different Prakritis are found to possess different drug metabolism rates associated with polymorphism of drug-metabolizing enzymes. Reported regulation of DNA methylation pattern in different prakriti subtypes is suggestive of the crucial consideration of epigenetics phenomenon in Ayurveda (Rotti et al. 2015).

The Ayurvedic concept of shatkriyakaal states that disease manifestation occurs after crossing six stages and these stages can be stratified. Attempts to stratify individuals into these stages in a cohort study can be done and their linkage with genes can be deduced (Patwardhan 2014). These stage specific identification of biological markers would allow early diagnosis of disease, even before its manifestation. This branch, not only establishes a link between traditional and modern medicinal approach but also, accelerates the discovery of patient focused wellness systems and pharmacogenomics-based research. Recent efforts have found the relevance of ayurgenomics in the treatment of cancer (Dhruva et al. 2014).

The Ayurgenomics branch shifts traditional ayurveda to evidence based ayurveda. This shifting requires scientific evidence and their systematic documentation. Along with cohort studies, as stated above, Randomized controlled trials (RCT) along with epistemologically sensitive approaches would be the key for this shift (Patwardhan 2014). However, there are many challenges reported in this shift. Lack of suitable biomedical research models, which can test new ayurvedic medicine, is one among the key challenges. To develop better understanding of ayurvedic medicine, discovery of suitable research models is required. Moreover, now the focus is to understand the influence of environmental factors on the genomics of individuals of certain prakriti. These factors can be (1) behaviour and lifestyle (2) Digestion and diet (3) Stress. This understanding can be built by utilizing techniques of advanced genomics and the tools which can differentiate an individual's prakriti. However, these techniques require a large sampling size to prove the results statistically significant.

Ayurgenomics provides a customized approach to molecular variability's predictive, preventative, and curative aspects of stratified medicine, which converges mind and body (Sethi et al. 2011; Patwardhan and Bodeker 2008). It embodies the investigation of interindividual variation resulting from genetic variation in humans (Frazer et al. 2009) for determining diagnosis and prognosis, primarily based on the Prakriti or Prakriti type of an individual (Mukerji et al.2011). Person's Prakriti is taken into consideration while choosing a suitable nutritional, therapeutic, and lifestyle regime based on the results of a clinical assessment of the person (Patwardhan et al. 2005; Patwardhan and Mashelkar 2009).

15.5 Ayurnutrigenomics

Person's prakriti is not only genetically determined (Shukra sonita) but also influenced by environmental factors (maha bhuta vikara) like maternal diet, lifestyle (mathura ahara vihara) and age of the parents (kala 22 garbhasaya) (Phillips 2013). Obesity is reported to be not only influenced by genetic variations in genes such as INSIG2 (insulin induced gene-2), FTO (Fat mass and obesity associated gene) —an obesity susceptibility locus, MC4R (melanocortin-4 receptor gene) but also by the nature, healthy/unhealthy diet intake (Shifa et al. 2022). Similarly, diabetes, cardiovascular and CANCER disease is reported to be influenced by gene-diet interaction (Shifa et al. 2022).

The mechanisms through which nutrient/s influence gene expression are:

1. Their capacity to interfere with the ability of transcription factors to initiate transcription.
2. Their ability to regulate gene expression via nuclear receptors.
3. They regulate molecular signalling pathways such as kappa B (Shifa et al. 2022).

The principle of Ayurveda believes that along with drugs, it is important to incorporate changes in diet (Ahara) for perfect disease management. Ayurnutrigenomics is the branch which considers patient prakriti and his genetic makeup specific identification of personalized functional foods. Nutritional requirements differ among individuals due to variations within the 0.1% of the human genome that differs between individual. This variation of 0.1% is mainly due to SNPs (Single Nucleotide Polymorphisms) (Sales et al. 2014). Green tea is found to contain EGCG, which prevents the occurrence of cancer. People having polymorphism in the gene producing COMT enzyme enhances the biological availability of the compound EGCG, which will help in cancer prevention. So green tea will have a protective effect only in those people who have a polymorphism in the gene producing COMT 20 enzyme (Landis-Piwowar et al. 2010). Similarly, other compounds, i.e. curcumin in turmeric can be tested in stratified prakriti individuals so that its anti-inflammatory nature can be correlated with specific prakriti (Rao 2007). A specific application of ayurnutrigenomics is demonstrated for devising personalized diets for newborn of specified prakriti. It will help in deciding appropriate approaches for disease treatment of newborn of certain prakriti (Dey and Pahwa 2014).

In a number of diseases such as phenylketonuria, galactosemia, and colorectal cancers, diet regulation is taken as a major preventive measure to control the disease (Shifa et al. 2022). Personalized diet is formulated as follows:

1. Measure the influence of an individual's prakriti on nutrient uptake.
2. Understand how nutrient uptake alters individual gene expression and metabolic profile.
3. Enlist the impact of different environmental factors on nutrient regulated gene expression and metabolic profile.
4. Formulate personalized diet based on interaction between prakriti, nutrient, gene expression, metabolic profile, and environmental factors.

The influence of an individual's prakriti on nutrient uptake can be measured by classifying individuals to specific categories of Prakriti and subjecting each group to specific diet. Further, the impact of prakriti on nutrient uptake can be assessed. Juyal R.C et al. put forward the concept of prakriti-based classification of individuals (Juyal et al. 2012).

The understanding of the impact of nutrients on gene expression and metabolic profile can be built based on genomics, transcriptomics, proteomics, and metabolomics techniques. These multiomics techniques allow the nutrient's mechanism of action via identifying cellular targets. Once cellular targets are identified, different drugs can be formulated to correct the nutrient associated diseases. In addition, identification of natural herbal drugs requires multiomics approach (Pandey et al. 2016; Sánchez-Vidaña et al. 2017).

15.5.1 Ayurnutrigenomics: Relatedness of Nutrition and Prakriti with the Disease Treatment

Nutrition plays a major role on both healthy and disease conditions, and also have significance in the prevention and treatment of chronic multifactorial diseases. New biological processes controlling the host's reaction to food may be discovered by nutrigenomic research (Banerjee et al. 2015). By integrating the practical preventative measures of Ayurveda into modern medicine and offering a scientific knowledge of fundamental ideas, ayurgenomics creates a new link between ayurveda and modern medicine. Genomic research and ayurveda can complement one another. As an evidence-based medical system, modern science can support ayurveda and vice versa; particularly through its emphasis on prevention, ayurveda can support modern medicine (Wallace 2020).

Ahara, oushadha, and vihara are chosen in the developing discipline of ayurnutrigenomics based on the clinical evaluation of a person's Prakriti. This novel understanding of nutrigenomic research, which draws inspiration from ayurveda, aims to create personalized functional meals and nutraceuticals that are compatible with one's genetic make-up. The development of personalized nutrition is expected to be strongly supported by the systematic integration of ayurvedic nutritional practises in respect to an individual's Prakriti with data from genomes, proteomics, and metabolomics (Banerjee et al. 2015). In order to advance the fields of food and health sciences and to offer workable answers for current health situations, transdisciplinary research may be crucial. Therefore, this innovative idea of ayurnutrigenomics and its developing study domains may open up future opportunities for smart yet safe medicines.

15.5.2 Diet Balance Health and Disease by Influencing Gene Expression

Nutrients can be thought of as "signalling molecules" that use the proper cellular sensing systems to transmit and convert dietary signals into changes in the expression of genes, proteins, and metabolites (Wellen and Hotamisligil 2005). So, the subject of how food affects our cells when we eat, when we do not eat, or when we eat too much, emerges. Nutrients act as "signatures" on a genetic level through the dietary signals they produce. When metabolic stress and the early stages of organ-specific insulin resistance develop, these dietary "signatures" can be precisely linked to the phenotype (Fig. 15.1).

In addition to being a chemical component needed for a certain metabolic function, a nutrient performs informational or signalling functions in the cell. The "receptor" that receives and transmits this information is transcription factors. The component of the cell that can reprogram the cell to adapt to the changing external conditions must then get this information from the receptors via a transducing process. During this reprogramming, which occurs in the cell's nucleus or cytoplasm,

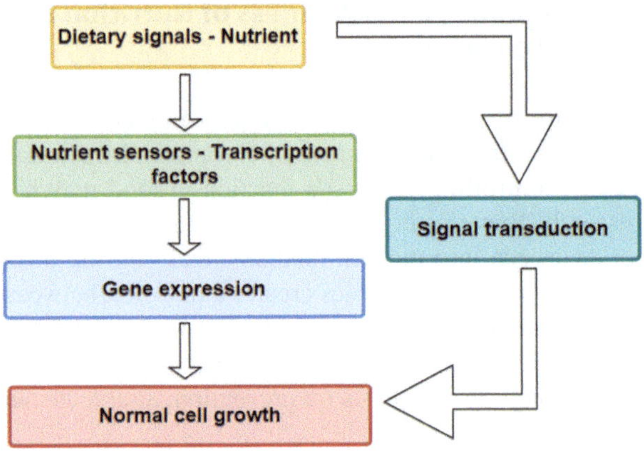

Fig. 15.1 Effect of nutrient on expression of a phenotype

genes' expression, messenger RNA, and protein stability, or protein activity may alter.

Specificity is the underlying idea behind how nutrients regulate gene expression. Each receptor needs to be able to specifically bind a nutrient-signalling molecule (such as carbs, proteins, lipids, carotenoids, vitamins, minerals, flavonoids, and edible phytochemicals) in order to trigger an adaptive change. Thus, through influencing gene expression, common food substances (nutrients) influence the balance between health and sickness.

The nuclear hormone receptor superfamily of transcription factors, with 48 members in the human genome, is the most important group of nutrient sensors. Several receptors in this superfamily bind nutrients and their metabolites, including retinoic acid (retinoic acid receptor (RAR) and retinoid X receptor (RXR)), fatty acids (peroxisome proliferator activated receptors (PPARs), liver X receptor (LXR)), vitamin D (vitamin D receptor (VDR)), oxysterols (LXR), bile salts (farnesoid X receptor (FXR), also known as bile salt receptor), or other hydrophobic food ingredients (constitutively active receptor (CAR) and pregnane X receptor (PXR)) (Zhang et al. 2011).

For instance, nuclear receptors bind with RXR to specific nucleotide sequences (response elements) in the promoter regions of a large number of genes. Nuclear receptors experience a conformational change after ligand binding (nutrient), which triggers the coordinated dissociation of co-repressors and the recruitment of co-activator proteins to facilitate transcriptional activation.

15.6 Prakriti-Based Medicine Using Omics Approach

It is known that different people have varied reactions to certain foods. Some people can consume dairy products without issues. However, those having lactose intolerance experience gastrointestinal discomfort after consuming specific dairy products. Patients with lactose intolerance are those who cannot digest the natural sugars found in milk products. In people with lactose intolerance, the gene that produces lactase is turned off. As a result, symptoms like nausea, bloating, diarrhoea, and abdominal discomfort may appear. This study of how individual's genetic makeup influences their physical response to the ingested nutrients is commonly known as nutrigenetics.

Ayurgenomics is a currently developed scientific discipline that unites genomics with ayurveda. It helps to understand how different individuals respond to treatments for various conditions. Together, ayurveda and omics can create a solid foundation for effective and affordable disease prevention, diagnosis, outcome prediction, and treatment methods (Dhande and Salunkhe 2018). Pharmacogenomics may take a novel direction with the identification of genetic differences underpinning the metabolic diversity in prakriti. Creating a link between DNA and prakriti is the main obstacle for ayurgenomics. Through the successful integration of omics, prakriti-based medicine can assist in transforming the existing state of global health wisdom. This link between DNA and prakriti allows us to comprehend how our genes affect the way we react to foods, beverages, medicines, and supplements. Disease prevention and promotion of health towards longevity with a better quality of life, the base of personalized medicine, could be achieved through these attributes of Ayurveda. The current limitation of clinical heterogeneity in molecular genetic analysis of complex traits can be overcome by prakriti. A disease according to Ayurveda is a perturbation of Vata, Pitta, and Kapha an individual from his or her homeostatic state. Food or medicines including lifestyle factors have been described to enhance or reduce a particular dosha, and therefore, an individual specific treatment is provided.

Thus, the beauty of Ayurveda lies in the fact that an individual, a disease condition, drug, diet as well as environment are described in terms of doshic components and appropriate customizations are provided to balance these states. Ayurveda describes not only the functional attributes of Vata, Pitta, and Kapha but also their contribution on different scales in seven different constitutions (Mukerji and Prasher 2011).

15.7 Multiomics Approach in Ayurnutrigenomics

It refers to integrating multiple "omics" layers—such as genomics, transcriptomics, proteomics, metabolomics, and microbiomics (Fig. 15.2)—with principles from Ayurveda and nutrition to understand the complex interactions between genes, diet, lifestyle, and health outcomes. This integrative approach not only enhances personalized nutrition but also builds a deeper understanding of health, offering opportunities for new Ayurvedic treatments and preventive strategies based on a more precise, individualized, and evidence-based framework.

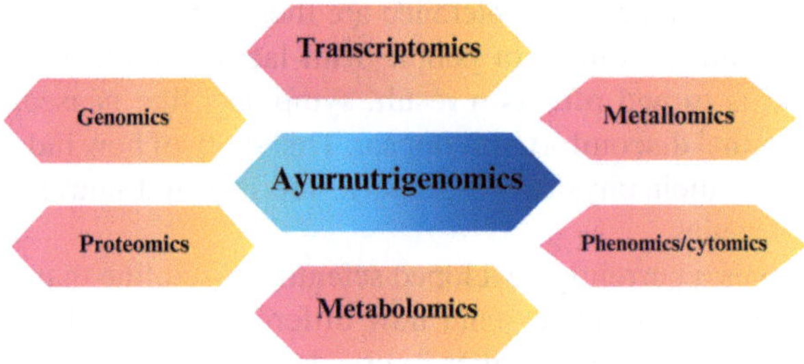

Fig. 15.2 Integration of multiomics approach in Ayurvedic nutrition

15.7.1 Applications of Genomics in Ayurnutrigenomics

The application of genomics has been constantly reported in identifying suitability of nutrients in individuals with specific DNA polymorphisms. DNA chip technologies and DNA barcoding are the two technologies known for the identification of nature of DNA polymorphisms. New advances in genome sequencing methods have been made such as nanoscale DNA sequencing or microsphere-based suspension arrays and mini sequencing. The limitation associated with genomics technologies is that each sequencing reaction is associated with high cost. While epigenomics focuses on identifying nutrient-induced reversible heritable modifications, toxicogenomics is focused on nutrient induced genetic toxicity. In addition, it is important to determine effective dosage of nutrient administration.

15.7.2 Application of Proteomics in Ayurnutrigenomics

Proteomics not only cover the identification of gene products, but also their post translational modifications, i.e. phosphorylation and glycosylation. Numerous analytical techniques, i.e. chromatographic and two-dimensional gel electrophoresis, have been in trend for the isolation of protein of interest from the mixture. In addition, either 2D electrophoresis followed by Mass spectrometry (MS) or isotope labelling, multidimensional electrophoresis followed by Mass spectrometry is used for protein identification. Like genomics, proteomics serves as tools for identification of nutrient-induced changes at the protein level. Chemoproteomics is the term given for the identification of chemical (nutrient)-induced differences in protein structure. The major limitation associated with proteomic techniques is that the samples for proteome analysis cannot be isolated from every tissue of interest.

15.7.3 Application of Transcriptomics in Ayurnutrigenomics

Transcriptomics is a method to assess the expression level of genes at the mRNA level. DNA microarray technology and quantitative Real time PCR have been used to identify nutrient induced changes in gene expression at the mRNA level. While DNA microarray analyses the expression of the whole genome, qRT-PCR is focused on specific genes at a time. Since mRNA is the product studied in transcriptomics, reading this product is difficult to study with clinical samples as mRNA is known as an unstable product.

15.7.4 Application of Metabolomics in Ayurnutrigenomics

Metabolomics is focused on studying changes in small-molecule metabolite profiles of the cell because of added nutrients. Nuclear Magnetic Resonance (NMR) and Mass Spectrometry (MS) are used for studying metabolite profiles. The limitations associated with metabolomics is mainly the reproducibility as small addition or deletion in diet changes the whole metabolic profile. However, in all the techniques of omics, metabolomics seems highly relevant as this study requires minimal experimental design, which allows handling of large numbers of biological samples in one go.

15.7.5 Application of Metallomics in Ayurnutrigenomics

Metallomics is primarily focused on quantitative measurement of mineral composition of the tissue or organism as a response to the external stimuli, namely, nutrient. Minerals serve as cofactor for most of the protein function and physiological processes, i.e. cellular signalling, metabolism, enzymatic activity, and transmembrane transport.

15.7.6 Application of Phenomics/Cytomics in Ayurnutrigenomics

Phenomics deals with identification of expressed traits in a defined population associated with influence of genetic or environmental factors (i.e. introducing new nutrient sources in the diet). Another branch, cytomics covers measurement of expressed traits as a result of added nutrients at the cellular level for understanding of molecular networks.

15.8 Conclusions

Health care system has been trending to shift from generalized medicinal to personalized medicinal approach. It is hypothesized that integration of ayurveda with modern science would enable strategizing personalized therapeutic regimen for individual wellness. Numerous studies have been conducted, which states a correlation between Prakriti and genome. Not only prakriti-genome correlation studies have been conducted, but researchers have been trying to formulate a personalized functional diet for individuals based on their prakriti and genome. This chapter is focused on reviewing studies related to prakriti-genome correlations and estimating the link between diet, prakriti, and genome. Agreeably, the studies relating ayurvedic concepts with modern medicine are sparse and limited. Therefore, collaborative efforts between scientific researchers from Ayurveda and modern medicine is the need of hour. This will help in addressing societal challenges related to healthcare.

References

Banerjee S, Debnath P, Debnath PK (2015) Ayurnutrigenomics: ayurveda inspired personalized nutrition from inception to evidence. J Tradit Complement Med 5(4):228–233

Dey S, Pahwa P (2014) Prakriti and its associations with metabolism, chronic diseases, and genotypes: possibilities of new born screening and a lifetime of personalized prevention. J Ayurveda Integr Med 5(1):15

Dhande S, Salunkhe P (2018) Ayurgenomics. Int J Res Sci Innov 5(4):322–326

Dhruva A, Hecht FM, Miaskowski C, Kaptchuk TJ, Bodeker G, Abrams D, Adler SR (2014) Correlating traditional Ayurvedic and modern medical perspectives on cancer: results of a qualitative study. J Altern Complement Med 20(5):364–370

Frazer KA, Murray SS, Schork NJ, Topol EJ (2009) Human genetic variation and its contribution to complex traits. Nat Rev Genet 10:241–251

Gadre G (2019) Classification of humans into Ayurvedic Prakruti types using computer vision. Master's Projects 710. https://doi.org/10.31979/etd.dmwg-2nee

Govindaraj P, Nizamuddin S, Sharath A, Jyothi V, Rotti H, Raval R et al (2015) Genome-wide analysis correlates Ayurveda Prakriti. Sci Rep 5:15786. https://doi.org/10.1038/srep15786

Heinrich M, Barnes J, Gibbons S, Williamson EM (2004) Fundamentals of pharmacognosy and phytotheraphy, vol No. 615.321 F981f. Churchill Livingstone, Edinburgh

Huang Z, Chavda VP, Bezbaruah R, Uversky VN, Sucharitha P, Patel AB, Chen ZS (2022) An ayurgenomics approach: prakriti-based drug discovery and development for personalized care. Front Pharmacol 13:866827. https://doi.org/10.3389/fphar.2022.866827. PMID: 35431922; PMCID: PMC9011054

Juyal RC, Negi S, Wakhode P, Bhat S, Bhat B, Thelma BK (2012) Potential of ayurgenomics approach in complex trait research: leads from a pilot study on rheumatoid arthritis. PLoS One 7:e45752. https://doi.org/10.1371/journal.pone.0045752

Landis-Piwowar K, Chen DI, Chan TH, Dou QP (2010) Inhibition of catecholO-methyltransferase activity in human breast cancer cells enhances the biological effect of the green tea polyphenol (−)-EGCG. Oncol Rep 24(2):563–569

Mukerji M, Prasher B (2011) Ayurgenomics: a new approach in personalized and preventive medicine. Sci Cult 77:10–17

Pandey R, Tiwari RK, Shukla SS (2016) Omics: a newer technique in herbal drug standardization & quantification. J Young Pharm 8:76

Patwardhan B (2014) Bridging Ayurveda with evidence-based scientific approaches in medicine. EPMA J 5(1):19. https://doi.org/10.1186/1878-5085-5-19. PMID: 25395997; PMCID: PMC4230501

Patwardhan B, Bodeker G (2008) Ayurvedic genomics: establishing a genetic basis for mind–body typologies. J Altern Complement Med 14(5):571–576

Patwardhan B, Mashelkar RA (2009) Traditional medicine-inspired approaches to drug discovery: can Ayurveda show the way forward? Drug Discov Today 14:804–811

Patwardhan B, Joshi K, Arvind C (2005) Classification of human population based on HLA gene polymorphism and the concept of Prakriti in Ayurveda. J Altern Complement Med 11:349–353

Phillips CM (2013) Nutrigenetics and metabolic disease: current status and implications for personalised nutrition. Nutrients 5:32e57. https://doi.org/10.3390/nu5010032

Prasher B, Gibson G, Mukerji M (2016) Genomic insights into Ayurvedic and Western approaches to personalized medicine. J Genet 95:209–228

Prasher B, Varma B, Kumar A, Khuntia BK, Pandey R, Narang A et al (2017) Ayurgenomics for stratified medicine: TRISUTRA consortium initiative across ethnically and geographically diverse Indian populations. J Ethnopharmacol 197:274–293

Rao CV (2007) Regulation of COX and LOX by curcumin. In: The molecular targets and therapeutic uses of curcumin in health and disease. Springer, Boston, pp 213–226

Rotti H, Guruprasad KP, Nayak J, Kabekkodu SP, Kukreja H, Mallya S et al (2014) Immunophenotyping of normal individuals classified on the basis of human Dosha Prakriti. J Ayurveda Integr Med 5:43–49. https://doi.org/10.4103/0975-9476.128857

Rotti H, Mallya S, Kabekkodu SP, Chakrabarty S, Bhale S, Bharadwaj R et al (2015) DNA methylation analysis of phenotype specific stratified Indian population. J Transl Med 13:151. https://doi.org/10.1186/s12967-015-0506-0

Sales NM, Pelegrini PB, Goersch MC (2014) Nutrigenomics: definitions and advances of this new science. J Nutr Metab 2014:202759. https://doi.org/10.1155/2014/202759. Epub 2014 Mar 25. PMID: 24795820; PMCID: PMC3984860

Sánchez-Vidaña DI, Rajwani R, Wong MS (2017) The use of omic technologies applied to traditional chinese medicine research. Evid Based Complement Alternat Med 2017:6359730. https://doi.org/10.1155/2017/6359730. Epub 2017 Jan 31. PMID: 28250795; PMCID: PMC5307000

Sethi TP, Prasher B, Mukerji M (2011) Ayurgenomics: a new way of threading molecular variability for stratified medicine. ACS Chem Biol 6:875–880

Shifa K, Shobhana MC, Raju LV (2022) Ayurnutrigenomics – a step towards personalized nutrition. Indian J Appl Res 12:8–10. https://doi.org/10.36106/ijar

Shilpa S, Venkatesha Murthy CG (2011) Understanding personality from ayurvedic perspective for psychological assessment: a case. Ayu 32:12–19

Sumantran V, Tillu G (2011) Ayurvedic pharmaceutics and insights on personalized medicine. In: Progress in traditional and folk herbal medicine, vol 1. Daya Publishing House, New Delhi, pp 13–55

Sumantran VN, Tillu G (2013) Insights on personalized medicine from ayurveda. J Altern Complement Med 19:370–375

Wallace RK (2020) Ayurgenomics and modern medicine. Medicina 56(12):661

Wellen KE, Hotamisligil GS (2005) Inflammation, stress, and diabetes. J Clin Invest 115(5):1111–1119

Zhang L, Kajiwara H, Kuboyama N (2011) Reduction of CXCR4 expression in rheumatoid arthritis rat joints by low level diode laser irradiation. Laser ther 20(1):53–58

Integrated Approaches for Development of Herbal Medicine

16

Nidhi V. Maheshwari, Swapnil Kadam, Shruti Kakodkar, and S. S. Barve

Abstract

About 75–80% of people worldwide rely mostly on herbal medicine for their primary healthcare needs because of its vast range of biological activities, greater compatibility with the human body, lower risk of side effects, bigger safety margin, and cost-effectiveness. Herbal medicine systems have emphasized a holistic approach to living since the Vedic era. It entails using plants medicinally to treat illnesses and improve overall health and wellness. The medicinal plants constitute 80% of the raw materials used in the herbal medicine preparation. With herbal medicines receiving immense attention in the global market, identification and authentication of the raw material used in herbal formulations requires crucial oversight so that their benefits can reach the consumers. In the contemporary era, technological advancements in the field of molecular biology have led to authentications that are highly efficient and reliable. Such tools are able to detect species-specific genomic differences, thereby enabling researchers to identify and authenticate plant species. Extraction procedures play a significant role in the development of herbal medicines. Advanced extraction methods offer multiple advantages like a faster extraction process and increased selectivity of the desired compound in contrast to the conventional extraction methods. Screening of the bioactive compounds is a crucial step in the development of herbal medicine which needs to be highly sensitive, precise, and specific. Recent technological advances, such as chromatography techniques, affinity techniques, mass spectroscopy, magnetic, optical methods, etc., enable the detection of even low concentrations of bioactive components unlike the conventional screening

N. V. Maheshwari (✉) · S. Kakodkar
Somaiya Vidyavihar University, Mumbai, Maharashtra, India

S. Kadam · S. S. Barve
KET's Scientific Research Centre, Mumbai, India

A. Kumar et al. (eds.), *Innovations in Ayurvedic Nutrition*,
https://doi.org/10.1007/978-981-95-1213-3_16

methods. To enhance the therapeutic effectiveness, majority of herbal formulations in the market are polyherbal or multi-constituent herbal formulations. Such herbal formulations are available in conventional forms, viz., tablets, gels, and ointments as well as unique drug delivery forms like microencapsulated dosages for offering better stability, palatability, patient compliance, and therapeutic benefits.

In order to prescribe herbal medicines to patients in a clinical setting, it is necessary to have a comprehensive grasp of the composition, safety, and efficacy of the active ingredients. To monitor the safety of herbal medical products, however, technical guidelines and international standards in the field of herbal medicine must be developed. In line with the above points, this chapter aims to provide a detailed account of the sequential processes that need to be considered for the development of herbal medicines.

Keywords

Herbal · Fermentation · Genomic · Bioactive · Marker

16.1 Introduction

Growing public knowledge of the advantages of herbal remedies is a key factor driving market expansion worldwide. The need for natural, chemical-free, and reasonably priced herbal medication has increased as a result of the sharp rise in illnesses and disorders. The National Institute of Health, USA, established the Office of Alternative Medicine in 1992 in response to growing recognition of the benefits of using herbal medicines and other non-traditional treatments. When the WHO promoted the use of traditional plant medicine in underdeveloped nations, herbal medicine gained momentum globally as a means of meeting needs not addressed by contemporary medical systems and addressing concerns about the iatrogenic consequences of conventional treatment (Winslow and Kroll 1998).

The World Health Organization has developed standards, recommendations, and strategies for botanical medicines in recognition of the importance of traditional medicine. According to the World Health Organization, traditional medicine, which includes herbal medications, refers to healing methods that have been used for hundreds of years prior to the creation and dissemination of modern medicine and are still in use today. The combination of generations of indigenous medical practitioners' therapeutic experiences is known as traditional medicine. Medicinal plants, minerals, organic materials, etc., are used in traditional remedies. Only traditional medications that predominantly employ medicinal plant extracts for therapy are classified as herbal pharmaceuticals.

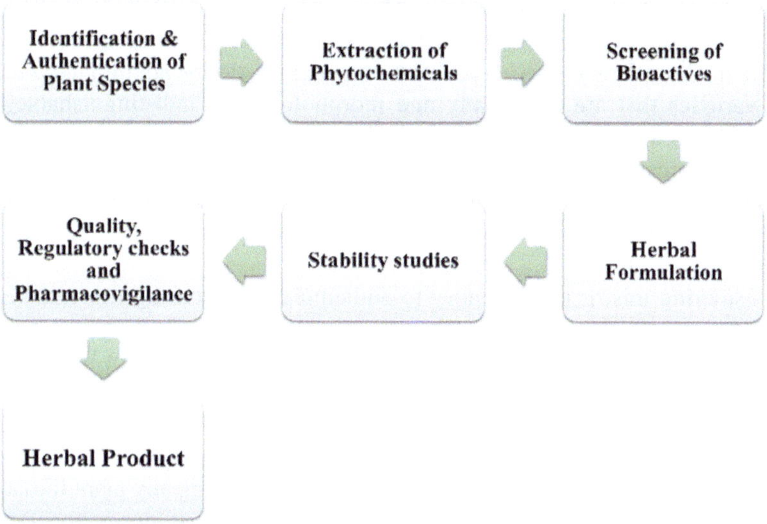

Fig. 16.1 Overview of stages involved in herbal formulation

Accordingly, current biotechnological techniques and proven agro-industrial technologies must be used for the production of herbal medicines as well as for the processing and cultivation of medicinal plants (Akerele 1993). Modern techniques, such as chemical fingerprinting, for the quick, accurate, and precise identification and estimation of active ingredients, are required to bring out consistency of significant constituents in the formulations.

Most herbal formulations available on the market are polyherbal, meaning they contain multiple active ingredients, each of which plays a different role and interacts with others to increase therapeutic efficiency. Herbal medications are produced in a variety of forms, such as tablets, capsules, topical creams, gels, and ointments. Some special drug delivery forms, like microencapsulated dosage forms and extended release, are also produced.

Standardization of herbal medicine, quality control, and phytochemical fractionation guided by bioactivity are crucial for the oversight of the entire drug development process (Fig. 16.1).

16.2 Identification and Authentication of Plant Species

The acceptance of herbal medicine is steeply increasing worldwide (Meena et al. 2010). India is enriched with a plethora of medicinal plants. The herbal formulations that have originated date back to ancient times as per the ethnic culture and geographic locations where such indigenous plant harbor. The methods, properties, and varieties of plants used in herbal medicinal preparations differ according to the plant location. Since different varieties of plants possess different local names, there is always the risk of misidentification (Mattummal et al. 2019). Such misidentifications can affect the quality of the herbal formulations that are designed to perform specific medicinal functions. Also, herbal medicines can be adulterated with other plant varieties that are chemically and morphologically indistinguishable. These counterfeits or adulterants lead to the development of poor-quality formulations that affect the clinical effects of herbal medicine. A study revealed that the same medicinal plants have been allotted different Ayurvedic or Unani names, and in some cases, different medicinal plants have been conferred the same name (Sivarajan and Balachandran 1994).

Considering this, it is mandatory to authenticate the starting raw material, i.e., the medicinal plant to maintain the reproducibility of production and quality of herbal medicines (Peter et al. 2002). According to the guidelines of WHO for traditional medicine research and evaluation, the first step for assuring the quality, efficacy, and safety of traditional medicine is authentication (WHO traditional medicine strategy). Thus, it is of utmost importance that the company purchases authentic plant materials to ensure its purity. Thus, prior to processing any plant into a herbal medicine, an accurate identification of the plant species is necessary. Presently, there is no single "gold standard" method for authenticating various types of medicinal plants. The methods of authentication can be divided into two types based on the level of technology involved in the assessment, viz., conventional methods and modern methods.

16.2.1 Conventional Methods of Authentication

(a) Taxonomic identification

The first step entails taxonomic identification. The botanical and vernacular names of the plant materials are identified (Revathy et al. 2012).

(b) Macroscopic and organoleptic assessment

Macroscopic assessment of plant material is a rapid method that can detect adulterants and provide insights regarding the suitability of the plant for use in medicinal preparations (Upton et al. 2020). In this step, the morphological parameters such as size, shape, color, surface characteristics, odor, taste, and other organoleptic properties of different plant parts are studied and compared to standard reference material (Techen et al. 2004). Both wild and cultivated plants can be studied, and a physical reference sample can be archived for later use. The presence of the requisite characteristics indicates the plant's identity, while the intensity of organoleptic features reflects the plant's quality.

Organoleptic assessment involves evaluation of sensory characters such as color, odor, texture, taste, and mouthfeel (Cooper et al. 1931). For instance, berberine is a yellow colored and extremely bitter bioactive found in medicinal herbs. Thus, berberine-containing herbs can be authenticated by assessing the presence of both color and flavor of the herb. The reduction in the color intensity and bitterness indicates that the herb is improperly dried/stored or the sample is deteriorated (Upton et al. 2020).

(c) Microscopic method

This is a rapid, commonly performed technique of identification. It involves studying the structural, cellular, and internal tissues of the raw material using microscopy (Techen et al. 2004). Botanical microscopy is beneficial in evaluating dried plant materials whose characteristics are drastically altered since drying does not lead to loss of the plant's microscopic features. This method also helps in detecting admixtures of plant materials. However, this method has limitations as it cannot assess finely powdered botanical materials. To overcome the drawbacks of using a light microscope, advanced microscopic methods such as fluorescent microscopy can be used (Revathy et al. 2012).

16.2.2 Modern Methods of Authentication

The conventional methods are simple and quick means for identifying plant species. However, methods such as macroscopic analysis require comparison of reference material with the test material. For this, one requires access to a well-invested and well-maintained herbarium. Storage of reference specimens and macroscopic samples under specific conditions requires big facilities (Techen et al. 2004). Also, such methods, though cost-effective and efficient, cannot be used for analyzing highly processed commercial samples (Ichim et al. 2020). In addition to this, macroscopic methods in some cases lack the ability to distinguish the subtle chemotype and ecotype differences within the plant species. The present advances in technology have led to the development of advanced chemical and molecular biology-based techniques that are able to compensate for these limitations and offer a more precise authentication of plant species. As against the voucher specimens and samples required for macroscopic analysis, these techniques require small quantities of sample for analysis (Ichim et al. 2021). Also, analysis of intra-species differences and multi-taxa identification can be done using appropriate molecular techniques (Techen et al. 2004).

(a) Chemical fingerprinting

Chemical fingerprinting is recommended by several national and international pharmacopeias. It is an excellent and perhaps the most important tool for detecting adulterants/contaminants and identifying plant species (Ichim et al. 2021). Adulteration of commercial herbal medicines is a widespread problem around the world (Ichim et al. 2020). The high percentage of adulterated products can be traced back to century-old Ayurveda (Seepathy et al. 2019). Chemical fingerprinting detects chemical markers that are signature constituents of a plant sample. The chemical markers can be active markers that provide therapeutic benefits or analytical markers that are not involved in the therapeutic activity of the medicinal plant (Srinivasan 2006). Chemical markers can be detected using techniques such as high-performance liquid chromatography (HPLC), thin layer chromatography

(TLC), gas chromatography (GC), HPLC coupled with nuclear magnetic resonance (NMR), gas chromatography–mass spectrum analysis (GC–MS), HPLC-diode array detection (HPLC-DAD), capillary electrophoresis among others (Bansal et al. 2014). In scenarios wherein DNA cannot be adequately extracted, and the raw material has lost its microscopic characteristics, the chemical method can be the only prospect for determining their botanical authenticity. However, chemical method faces limitations in analyzing heterogenous plant materials that cannot be distinguished based on their phytochemical profiles.

(b) DNA markers

Analysis of DNA markers using molecular biology techniques possess more advantages as compared to other authentication methods. They are useful in authenticating raw materials that are adulterated or replaced with phytochemically and/or morphologically indistinguishable plant species/varieties (Balasubramani et al. 2011). DNA markers are unique nucleotide sequences belonging to plant species. These unique sequences can be detected from any part of the plant, at any stage of development since, they are not tissue specific. Despite the advantages that chemical profiling offers, it is not accurate enough to perform precise taxonomic authentication since, a single plant species growing in different regions can produce different metabolite profile based on the environmental factors (Lee et al. 2022).

Molecular markers used for analysis include DNA hybridization methods, restriction fragment length polymorphism (RFLP), random amplification of polymorphic DNA (RAPD), amplified fragment length polymorphism (AFLP), simple sequence repeats (SSR), inter-simple sequence repeats (ISSR), single nucleotide polymorphisms (SNP), or DNA barcoding of rbcL, rpl36-rps8, trnH-psbA, 5S rRNA, trnL-F, matK, and ITS (Ganie et al. 2015; Mattummal et al. 2019). All these techniques target a particular type of nucleotide sequence in the genome. However, these techniques face reproducibility issues. Advanced high-throughput techniques such as microarray-based markers and next-generation sequencing (NGS)-based markers have recently gained momentum due to the high efficiency and accuracy of their results (Ganie et al. 2019). The most widely used method for plant authentication is DNA barcoding (Gerard 2016). However, DNA barcoding faces limitations in providing appropriate resolution for discerning recently diverged species (Delgado-Tejedor et al. 2021). This problem can be overcome by DNA metabarcoding which is an advanced approach that facilitates simultaneous sequencing of DNA barcode amplicons (Wu et al. 2022). Another experimental approach, viz., NGS, provides a scope to study transcriptome, whole genome, epigenome, and exome with superior sensitivity and rapid turnaround time (Ivanova et al. 2016). NGS technology has displayed a promising role in authenticating medicinal plants such as *Echinacea purpurea, Valeriana officinalis, Ginkgo biloba, Hypericum perforatum, and Trigonella foenum-graecum* (Ivanova et al. 2016).

The success of these DNA-based methods entails the extraction of high-quality DNA. This can be a challenge while handling recalcitrant plant material. Also, DNA marker-based methods cannot identify and quantitate the presence of chemical components. Thus, based on the above discussion, it is evident that a single standalone assay cannot be used for the authentication of herbal medicines. Rather, an integrative approach combining conventional methods, chemical profiling, genomic, and metabolomic analysis could be a better strategy for confirming the identity and quality of herbal medicines.

16.3 Extraction Methods for Bioactive Compounds

Bioactive compounds from plants are of important research interest for the development of better herbal medicines. The qualitative and quantitative analyses of bioactive compounds from plant materials mainly rely on the selection of an appropriate extraction method (Fig. 16.2).

16.3.1 Classical Techniques

The conventional extraction methods, including Maceration, Percolation, and Soxhlet extraction, usually use organic solvents and require a large volume of solvents and long extraction time, whereas decoction and hydro-distillation methods use water as a solvent.

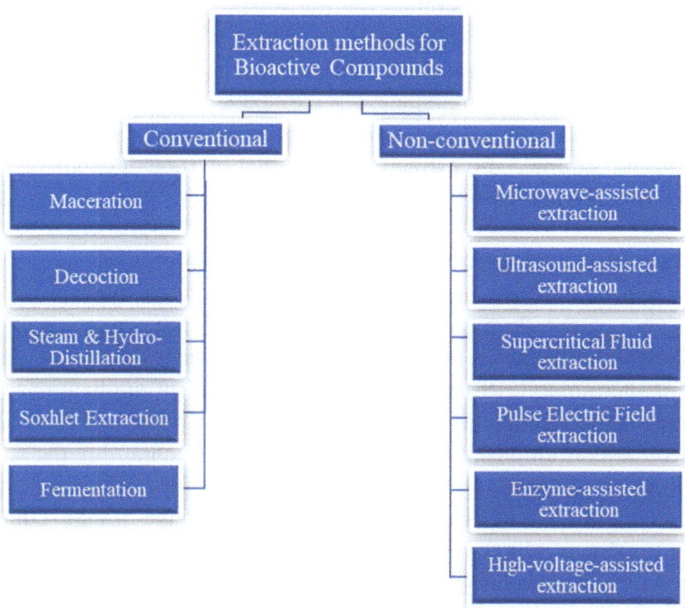

Fig. 16.2 Different extraction methods for bioactive compounds

16.3.1.1 Maceration

Maceration is a well-known traditional method, applied for extraction from powdered solid materials. In this process, the powdered solid materials are placed in a closed vessel and the solvent is added. It is allowed to stand for a long time (varying from hours to days) with occasional shaking. This sufficient time allows solvent to diffuse through the cell wall and to solubilize the sample constituents. After completing the desire time, the solvent is strained off, and the solid residue is pressed to recover maximum solvents. If the solvent is water and the period of maceration is longer, a small quantity of alcohol can be added to stop microbial growth (Rasul 2018).

16.3.1.2 Decoction

Decoction is a water-based extraction method in which plant material is subjected to boiling. Decoction is commonly used for extracting water soluble plant metabolites. In Ayurveda, decoction traditionally known as Kwatha and Yavakuta is a crude drug, small pieces placed in earthen pots or tinned copper vessels coated with clay on the outside (Rasul 2018).

16.3.1.3 Steam Distillation and Hydro-Distillation

Steam and hydro-distillation methods are employed for the extraction of volatile compounds including essential oils and other aromatic or medicinal compounds. This method practiced by generating the hot water vapors to obtain extracts after vapor condensation. Steam distillation is performed at a lower temperature than the boiling point of bioactive compounds. The method is practically applicable to the thermosensitive bioactive compounds, e.g., aromatic compounds. The heat acts to break down in the sample's pores which leads to the release of the targeted compounds from the sample. The extraction or distillation time depends on the type of plant material being processed (Stephane et al. 2021).

16.3.1.4 Soxhlet Extraction

Soxhlet is one of the best methods for the extraction of solids by hot solvent. Basically, it is a glass refluxing unit significantly used for the organic solvent extraction. Soxhlet is a well-known method, comparatively better than other conventional methods for thermolabile compounds and limited field of applications. The powdered sample is placed in a thimble prepared from filter paper and placed inside the Soxhlet. Round-bottom flasks are fitted with apparatus containing the solvent. The gentle boiling of solvent in round-bottom flasks passes the vapors up through the side tube. Condenser condenses the vapors and falls into the thimble containing the sample, and it slowly fills the Soxhlet. When the solvent fills up to the top level of the attached tube, it goes into the flasks. This flows the portion of the sample that it has extracted. The cycle gets repeated until the proper extraction is achieved (Rasul 2018).

16.3.1.5 Fermentation (Aqueous-Alcoholic Extraction)

Fermentation is adopted in a few herbal medicinal bioactive extractions. Fermentation includes the soaking of the samples or powder of the herbs or trees which eases the extraction of active compounds. Fermentation results in the in situ generation of alcohol, which helps in the extraction of the active compounds. The additionally generated alcohol served as a preservative (Stephane et al. 2021).

16.3.2 Innovative (Non-conventional) Technique

16.3.2.1 Microwave-Assisted Extraction (MAE)

Microwaves are the electromagnetic spectrum of light from a range of 300 MHz to 300 GHz, which are used as energy and information carriers. The use of microwave energy results in faster heating compared to other options. Microwave-assisted extraction uses water and alcohol at higher temperatures and controlled pressure levels. This is a feasible green solvent extraction procedure with various benefits like being easy to handle, higher yields, and significantly faster than conventional methods for the extraction of bioactive compounds from medicinal plants.

A few potential advantages of microwave-assisted extraction are given below:

(i) Comparative smaller amount of sample is required
(ii) Short processing time (approx. 15–20 min)
(iii) Yield gets improved
(iv) Thermolabile bioactive compounds or heavy metals can be extracted
(v) By providing stirring in the microwave-assisted extraction, the mass transfer phenomenon gets improved. Microwave-assisted extraction needs special equipment which are equipped with electricity-producing waves.

However, this method leads to higher investment compared to traditional methods (Stephane 2021).

16.3.2.2 Ultrasound-Assisted Reaction (UAE Extraction) or Sonication Extraction

The use of the ultrasound-assisted extraction, i.e., based on the sound frequency mechanism, ranges from 18 to 100 KHz, which is higher than the hearing frequency of the human ear. It is one of the advanced technologies that enhance the mass transfer mechanism and break the cellular matrix. This helps to extract a large amount of targeted bioactive compounds and increase the yield of extraction. The ultrasound generates the acoustic cavitation activity in which microbubbles form when the sample is exposed to ultrasound in the liquid phase. It leads to oscillating rapid changes in the pressure. In case of plant material, ultrasound waves modify the cavitation effect to liberate the extractable bioactive compounds by disrupting plant cell walls.

Ultrasound is repetitively used in the area of plant extraction. Ultrasound can be used for rapid heating and proper mass transfer in the extraction field and employed as a promising choice. Ultrasound extraction enhances the extraction yield when large particles are used or the temperature varies in the range of 70 to 80 °C and higher ultrasound power, respectively. Ultrasound and superfluid extraction show a synergistic effect in increasing the extraction yield up to 1.7-fold for antioxidants and up to threefold for saponin. The combination of different extrication methods is a desirable approach to extract good quality products with a higher yield of extraction (Usman et al. 2022).

16.3.2.3 Supercritical Fluid Extraction (SFE)

SFE is a cutting-edge, eco-friendly extraction technique that produces a wide range of chemicals with significant applications across numerous industries. This method uses supercritical fluids to extract several bioactive compounds. The supercritical phase originally appeared in solvent behavior at a specific pressure and temperature, as noted by Baron Charles. Caffeine from green coffee beans was extracted using supercritical fluid for the first time in Germany.

A few years later, Australia developed the use of liquid CO_2 for oil extraction. In SFE extraction, solid materials are utilized far more often than liquid samples. For solid samples, pre-treated solid plant samples are loaded into columns, which are then filled with supercritical fluid pressure solvent to extract soluble components from the sample matrix. In this process, the extracted compounds are eliminated by diffusion to the separators, where the solvents and extract are separated by either raising the temperature, decreasing pressure, or doing both.

SFE technology overcomes the problem of unwanted chemicals produced during extraction, which may affect the quality of the extract. This can be achieved by coupling multiple separator series and optimizing pressure and temperature according to the equilibrium solubility of targeted bioactive compounds (Uwienza et al. 2020).

16.3.2.4 Pulsed Electric Field (PEF) Extraction

Pulsed electric field (PEF), also known as electroporation, is a non-thermal mechanism that operates on the mechanism of application of an external electric field to a bio cell for nanoseconds or milliseconds. It includes four distinct phases that help ensure proper execution of extraction. It unlocks various applications in food processing on the basis of electroporation interference. The applications depend on two parameters, i.e., the magnitude of the external electric field and the specific energy field. PEF are more employed method because it has a wide scope in solid-liquid extraction at critical speed. PEF becomes more selective and energy efficient in different agro-industries. PEF has the potential to replace the conventional thermal technologies. PEF can mainly accelerate the extraction of pigment or dyes, polyphenols, and secondary metabolites (Usman et al. 2022).

16.3.2.5 Enzyme-Assisted Extraction (EAE)

Phytochemicals are retained in different matrices in the plant cells. Some bioactive compounds present are dispersed in the cell cytoplasm, and some are retained in the polysaccharide-lignin network, which is not accessible to solvent for a routine extraction. Enzyme-assisted extraction helps to release bound bioactive compounds and enhance overall yield. The use of specific enzymes like cellulase, α-amylase, and pectinase enhances the recovery and yield with specific targeted bioactive compounds.

There are two approaches for this extraction method:

1. Enzyme-assisted aqueous extraction (EAAE)
2. Enzyme-assisted cold pressing (EACP)

Both approaches were employed for different targeted extractions. Generally, EAAE is employed for the extraction of oil from different seeds, and EACP is employed for hydrolyzing the seed cell wall. This extraction method has other key factors like particle size of herbs or plant sample, enzyme composition and concentration, soil-to-water ratio, hydrolysis time, etc. The enzyme extraction method is an alternative for agro-based industries for the extraction of bioactive compounds (Azmir 2013).

16.3.2.6 High-Voltage-Assisted Extraction

The principle of this extraction method is similar to pulse electric field, only the difference is that electrical discharge is made through a small point. Needle electrode is used to discharge through this small point in a plate ground electrode. This is a green extraction method and compared to the traditional method has better performance in high selectivity, lower solvent consumption, and short extraction time with high yield. It is also eco-friendly because energy and organic solvents consumption are reduced. The most important advantage of this extraction method is its continuous operability mode, which plays a significant role for commercial extraction and cost-effectiveness (Stephane et al. 2021).

16.4 Screening of Bioactive Compounds

According to the pharmacopeia, the majority of therapeutic herbs in their natural state are not suited for preparation or administration. As a result, a herbal medicine's ability to treat a condition depends on a number of variables, including plant components, crude extract, and extracted active ingredients. The majority of the herbal plant is made up of a number of components that frequently cooperate with one another. The herbal active ingredient is what determines how a herbal medication is prepared. These ingredients either have a well-established medicinal role, are chemically defined substances, or work together to support the therapeutic action of a herbal remedy. Finding pure compounds or crude extracts that are both highly active and non-toxic would be the perfect pharmacological screen for herbal drugs.

Phytochemical screening involves several steps like botanical identification, extraction with suitable methods or solvents, purification, and characterization of the active constituents of pharmaceutical significance. Sophisticated analytical instruments and qualitative chemical examination are employed to detect and isolate the active constituents.

There are various approaches available to screen the herbal active constituent. In the random selection approach of the National Cancer Institute (NCI) in the USA, herbs are randomly selected and extracted, and the extracts are evaluated against different in vitro tumor system, and in vitro cytotoxicity test is performed. The extension of this protocol is to isolate the active metabolite or active compounds from the herbs that show promising activity according to pharmacological tests. In another approach, herbs or plants consisting of specific type of chemical compounds like alkaloids and flavonoids are tested. It is also known as shotgun approach. In this simple test, like a color test on various parts of the plants and assays are carried out in the laboratory. On the cost-benefit ratio, this "shotgun" approaches are considered to be unsatisfactory. In another method, herbs are randomly collected, extracted and subjected to broad screening and pharmacological tests. The success of this method relies on adequate funding, the number of samples assayed, and appropriate bioassay protocols. This method is known as broad-based empirical screening. It is time-consuming, expensive, and not suitable for screening a large number of samples.

Assays for receptor-ligand binding and biochemistry have drawn interest recently in phytochemical screening. This approach makes use of human receptors that are made available through molecular cloning, allowing herbal extracts or other compounds to be evaluated for direct binding to the proteins thought to be therapeutic targets. Molecular biology applications enable the expression of clone receptors as receptor proteins in cells. This screening method is used by international organizations including the Central Drug Research Institute in India and the National Cancer Institute (NCI) in the United States. The screening technologies for herbal medicines have progressed to the point of enzyme isolation. In order to ascertain whether plant extracts can inhibit the activity of the disease-causing enzymes, the enzymes must first be separated. The femtomole concentrations of significant medicinal alkaloids measured by an enzyme immunoassay (Bandaranayake 2006).

Biological Approaches to the Screening and Evaluation of Natural Products
The main purpose of biological screening and evaluation of plant extracts is to find safe compounds with useful pharmacological activities.

There are two primary approaches to accomplish this goal:

(i) Pharmacological approaches: Utilizing several animal models for both in-vivo/in-situ tests and in-vitro experiments.
(ii) Clinical approaches: Plant extract tested on clinical assays, which has a history of traditional uses, after appropriate safety or toxicological investigation.

16.4.1 Pharmacological Approaches

16.4.1.1 Discovery of Bioactive Compounds

The general sequence to determine the biological activity of plant compounds with clinical potential is as follows:

1. Collection of all ethnobotanical or traditional information
2. Taxonomical identification of the plants to be investigated
3. Extraction of herbs or plants active metabolite
4. Pharmacological screening of plant extracts
5. Biological activity-directed fractionation
6. Pharmacological evaluation of biologically active compounds
7. Elucidation of the structure of biologically active compounds
8. Structure modification and synthesis
9. Safety assessment of biologically active principles and synthetic derivatives
10. Clinical evaluation for therapeutic efficacy

16.4.1.2 Pharmacological Models

In-Vivo Model

This model mainly follows the use of intact, non-anaesthetized animals. US Department of Health and Human Services published detailed information about the care and use of laboratory animals. Test extracts can be provided orally, intraperitoneally, or intravenously.

In Situ Model

This model uses anaesthetized animals. Direct injection of test compounds into the target organs is used.

In Vitro Models

The isolated organ technique is used to assess the contraction or relaxation of an organ that is suspended in a tissue bath that is kept at 37 °C and contains a physiological solution. These solitary organs have been shown to be highly efficient in analyzing the behavior of pure substances. They have, however, hardly ever been applied to the plant extract screening process.

The "Culture Method" is the second model. The causative agents of infectious and parasitic disorders are external entities, including bacteria, viruses, fungi, and parasites. Cancer is caused by aberrant cells proliferating. Cultivating these substances in vitro has been made possible by advancements in both basic and applied research. It is feasible to assess the inhibitory effect of plant extract on different external agents using this culture-based assay.

The inhibition of the culture of bacteria, viruses, parasites, and bacteria or cell growth by the addition of the test extract is indicative of biological activity. Plant extracts have been effectively screened using culture techniques to find potential antibacterial, antifungal, antiviral, antiparasitic, and antitumor medications. The "enzyme inhibition and receptor-binding assay" is a third test. Enzyme inhibition quantifies how some plant extracts block particular enzymes throughout a disease's manifestation. The receptor-binding techniques assess a compound's capacity to identify a receptor with selectivity. One technique that has been employed in the hunt for novel medicinal compounds is the enzyme inhibition method.

16.4.1.3 Screening Methods in Pharmacology

To find biologically active compounds, usually three primary screenings are followed.

Simple Screening

This screening technique is used to identify compounds that exhibit a specific kind of activity. This type of screening has been shown to be beneficial for biological activity in traditional medicine.

Blind Screening

This screening aids in the identification of a broad range of biological activities that may indicate the possible activity of plant extracts. In terms of screening techniques, there are two primary tendencies. First, the pharmacological profile of the crude extract is examined using a number of distinct tests. The second trend uses a single technique for screening with numerous goals.

Programmed Screening

This screening process, which consists of a testing program, is necessary to provide details about the extracts that can only yield a battery of appropriate tests.

16.4.2 Clinical Approaches

According to Yangni-Angate, clinical experimentation entails a thorough evaluation of the therapeutic value of conventional medications as well as a crucial scientific method for an extensive repository of information. The present trend of using clinical and preclinical investigations is to evaluate herbal treatments directly. This is typically done following thorough toxicological research as well as after a significant amount of daily plant use. Clinical techniques have the potential to uncover important medications with distinct mechanisms of action. Tests based on biology are important when it comes to finding novel medications made from herbal remedies. These comprise a few experimental techniques that will be used to gauge the herbal medications' potential. Various tests are employed to evaluate the potential and effectiveness of herbal remedies. Among these, some are commonly used: molluscicidal tests (*Bulinus truncatus*), cercaricidal tests (*Schistosoma haematobium*), larvicidal tests (*Culex pipiens*), brine shrimp bioassays (*Artemia salina*), insecticidal tests (*C.pipiens* and *Drosophila melanogaster*), antimicrobial tests (*antibacterial and antifungal*), licicidal and niticidal tests (*Pediculus humanus capitis*), and antiparasitic bioassays (*schistosomiasis*) (Lahlou 2007).

16.5 Herbal Drug Formulations: Multifarious Approaches

Today's pharmaceutical healthcare system treats a wide range of disorders with herbal formulations containing therapeutically active substances such as hepatoprotective agents, anti-diabetics, lipid-lowering medications, and nootropics. To provide specific nutritional or esthetic benefits, these mixes include one or more dried or processed herbs in predetermined amounts. They usually contain an active substance, which could be herbal treatments, chemicals made from herbs, or a combination of both (Adeyi et al. 2015).

Worldwide, there is a considerable demand for herbal medications in basic healthcare because of their broad spectrum of biological activity, lower cost, and higher safety margins. Most herbal formulations on the market are polyherbal, which means that they have multiple active ingredients that collectively combine to enhance their therapeutic efficacy. The active components in the polyherbal mixture have different but related actions. Herbal medication is now available in pills, capsules, topical creams, gels, and ointments. Herbal medicine is also manufactured in a few unique drug delivery forms, such as microencapsulated and delayed release (Katiyar et al. 2012).

Herbal medicines today frequently and extensively use standardized extracts. As herbal medicinal therapies develop, the stability of herbal formulations becomes increasingly important. This is due to the fact that medication molecules or active components are vulnerable to oxidation, hydrolysis, microbial attack, and other environmental deterioration during the manufacturing and extraction of natural goods, generating severe concerns about their stability (Rangari 2008). Similarly, stability can be impacted by a number of variables, such as pH, particle size, properties of the water and other solvents used, kind of container used, and presence of other chemicals due to contamination or intentional mixing of different materials. It is crucial to monitor the quantity and availability of the bioactive components since they have an impact on the quality, efficacy, and shelf life of the natural medicines.

16.5.1 Factors Influencing the Stability of Herbal Medicines

16.5.1.1 Physical Instability

Physical instability is a result of impurity presence and container reactions. The secondary metabolites and chemical makeup of the plants are impacted by microbial infection and insect feeding. Volatile active ingredients in herbal medicines experience reduced activity and volatility with extended storage.

16.5.1.2 Environmental Conditions

Variations in environmental factors like rainfall, soil, altitude, temperature, and storage conditions, as well as different harvesting techniques, time and method of collection, and manufacturing processes like selecting, drying, purifying, and extracting, could all contribute to significant variability in product quality, stability, and concentration of the plant chemicals within different products. Another important component influencing phytoformulations through the production of free radicals is light.

16.5.1.3 Chemical Instability

Herbal medications deteriorate over time due to enzymatic deterioration, hydrolysis, oxidation, crystallization, emulsion disintegration, and chemical reactions with excipients and additives. The two main elements that influence the stability and quality of herbal products are temperature and moisture. A chemical reaction increases by two to three times for every 10 °C increase in temperature. If a solid medicine is hydrolyzable, moisture absorbed on its surface frequently speeds up its degradation. The product's enzyme content accelerates the pace of chemical breakdown as well.

16.5.1.4 Complex Mixtures, Variability, and Inconsistency

It is challenging to determine the stability of the finished herbal preparation based on the activity and stability profile of a single component because herbal formulations are mixtures of multiple components. Every element has a different shelf life, concentration, activity, and consistency.

16.5.1.5 Drug Interactions, Deterioration, Decomposition, and Storage

Herbal formulations contain a variety of active ingredients with varying stability conditions, including alkaloids, glycosides, tannins, and flavonoids. If the moisture level of natural products is determined to be higher than the critical value and mold development occurs, the active components will interact with the packing material. Additionally, interactions between the active ingredient and other chemicals in the formulations cause changes in the unique pharmacological activity. Because of this, the herbal formulation's real stability state differs from that of each of its constituent parts.

A typical procedure for verifying that herbal medicines retain their identity, purity, quality, safety, and efficacy over the course of their shelf life is a stability study.

Aside from providing statistics for determining shelf lives, stability testing is used to assess the quality of herbal products, which varies over time due to environmental factors like temperature, moisture, humidity, oxygen, light, other ingredients or excipients in the dosage form, the drug's particle size, microbial contamination, trace metal contamination, leaching from the container, etc. For the suggested shelf life—typically defined as long-term stability—stability experiments on at least three production batches of the herbal items should be carried out under ambient circumstances.

16.6 Methods to Deal with Natural Product Instability

16.6.1 Determination of the Physical Parameters

In order to prove the identification and purity of the raw material, depending on the type of preparation, sensory qualities, physical constants, moisture, ash content, solvent residues, and adulterations must be examined. Exogenous substances such as heavy metals, aflatoxins, pesticide residues, radiation, and microbial contaminants also need to be tested for. To support the ongoing formulation of herbal treatments and to set relevant standards for consistency, appropriate analytical techniques and the application of various concepts are needed (Natural Health Product Directorate).

16.6.2 Determination of the Impurity Profile

Analytical techniques such as gas chromatography-mass spectrometry (GC-MS), thin layer chromatography (TLC), capillary electrophoresis, spectrophotometry, and high-performance liquid chromatography (HPLC) can be used to identify the presence of contaminants in a new medication or chemical. During the synthesis of a medicine, the chemical in issue may occasionally undergo a recognized degradation process, such as hydrolysis or oxidation.

16.6.3 Non-biased Identification and Quantification of all Metabolites

This is imperative to determine the status and stability of the complex mixtures. Determining the stability and condition of the complicated mixes depends on this. The complete metabolic fingerprint profile of phytoformulations could be obtained using IR spectroscopy in conjunction with chemometric data processing. The method makes it possible to examine materials closely, which permits acceptance or rejection of material classification (Ahmad et al. 2006).

16.6.4 Controlled Storage Conditions

Airtight containers made of materials that won't interact chemically or physically with the material being stored should be kept in ventilated, cool, dry areas for proper storage and protection against deterioration. Additionally, periodic insecticide spraying of the stored area is recommended to stop the spread of infestation. Influence of environmental factors such as light, oxygen, temperature, moisture, additional ingredients or excipients in the dosage form, drug particle size, contamination from trace metals, and microbiological leaching from the container should be considered while storing (Thakur et al. 2008).

16.7 Multifarious Herbal Formulations

Major herbal formulations on the market are polyherbal because they comprise a variety of active components that all operate in concert to enhance the therapeutic effectiveness. Every active ingredient in the polyherbal formulation has a distinct function and is related to all of the others (Parasuraman et al. 2014). Herbs are produced in a variety of contemporary dosage forms (Fig. 16.3), such as topical lotions, ointments, tablets, capsules, gels, and certain special drug delivery forms including microencapsulated and delayed release.

To cope with medicinal instabilities, high bioavailability, ease of administration, and improvement in preparation of these formulations have given rise to a variety of novel products which could be termed as novel herbal formulations. Few of them have been enlisted here:

16.7.1 Novel Herbal Formulations

Formulation of Chewable Tablet Chewable tablets have better dispersion, dissolve more quickly, have a short disintegration time, high bioavailability and stability, good flavor, and are easier to administer in contrast with existing dosage forms of the same constituent (Salunkhe et al. 2009).

Topical Herbal Formulation For the topical treatment of acne and other skin disorders like eczema, aging scars, and psoriasis, this nanoemulsion formulation is

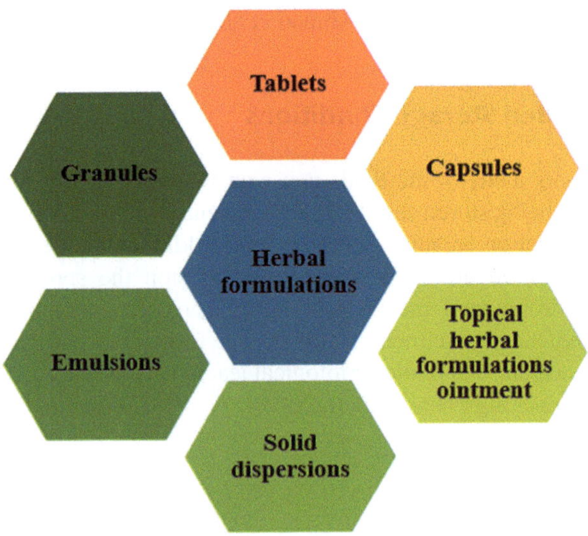

Fig. 16.3 Different types of herbal formulations

made up of an oil phase chosen from one or more essential oils and a therapeutically active aqueous phase. It also exhibits increased efficacy, improved percutaneous penetration, excellent thermodynamic stability ensuring a long shelf life, low skin irritation, and a reservoir effect that promotes drug localization in the skin, aiding in the controlled delivery of the purported therapeutic agents (Chaudhary et al. 2009).

Tablet Formulation for Volatile Liquids The volatile liquid active drug is moistened with colloidal silicon dioxide and combined with β-cyclodextrin to create a visually stable tablet that is damp proof-coated (Shin et al. 1999).

Liquid Preparation Coated with Water-Soluble Cellulose Derivative
Liquid preparation covered in a cellulose derivative that is soluble in water with a water content ranging from 10% to 80% and an active ingredient coated with a substance including a water-soluble cellulose derivative are components of a stable liquid preparation. The liquid preparation can be formed into a hard capsule that can stably retain the water-unstable active ingredient in it and also mask unpleasant taste or smell (Ikeda et al. 2006).

16.7.2 Other Novel Formulations

Numerous other novel formulations have been developed to deal with herbal medicine instability:

- Nanoparticle coating to enhance shelf life
- Semisolid preparations based on supercritical carbon dioxide
- Liquid preparation coated with water-soluble cellulose derivative
- Polymeric plant-derived excipients in drug delivery
- Long-chain fatty acid derivative
- Protein coating substance and use of the plant chaperonin-like Sp1 protein to stabilize therapeutic protein in pharmaceutical use
- Continuous multi-microencapsulation process for biologically active ingredients
- Chelating agents for stabilization of the aqueous plant extracts
- Use of colloidal silicon dioxide in the enhancement of the drying of herbal precipitation with improved storage stability by using β-cyclodextrin as a component

16.7.3 Efficacy Testing of Herbal Formulations

Due to the rise in demand for herbal medicines worldwide, it would be prudent to test and prove the efficacy of these formulations before launching the products to meet the growing demand. Conventional trial methodology adopted for conventional pharmaceutical products can be applied for testing the efficacy of herbal medicine (Ernst et al. 2005). The first crucial step to prove the function of a formulated herbal medicine is to perform preclinical studies involving exhaustive research of the product's preliminary efficacy, pharmacokinetics, toxicity, and safety.

The preliminary efficacy of herbal formulations can be evaluated by in-vitro testing of the product for the activity it is supposed to confer. However, it should be noted that a single bioassay cannot be deemed reliable for understanding the effect of a medicinal preparation on the whole system (Houghton et al. 2007). It is therefore advisable to use a range of tests for assessing different activities which are related to the disease under investigation. For example, the anticancer activity of candidate metabolites like curcumin, quercetin, gallic acid, alliin, ferulic acid, myricetin, and luteolin among others can be evaluated by assessing the cell proliferation and inhibition rates against the desired cancer cell line using in-vitro assays. Similarly, herbal formulations with potential antimicrobial activity against target microorganisms can be evaluated by using suitable microbiological methods such as agar well diffusion method, disk diffusion, broth dilution methods, time-kill test, and flow cytofluorometric methods (Balouiri et al. 2016).

Once the efficacy of a herbal medicine is proven in vitro, the next step would be to assess its efficacy in-vivo studies. It cannot be concluded with full certainty that the efficacy observed in vivo would be the same as that observed in in-vitro tests. This is because in-vitro systems cannot mimic in-vivo absorption and metabolic activities (Laupattarakasem et al. 2003; Houghton et al. 2007). In-vivo studies may not reflect the accurate efficacy of the medicinal preparation since the animal models are subjected to fixed diet models and controlled environmental conditions; unlike what is seen in real-life situations, where conditions are more varied. In-vitro and in-vivo efficacy tests provide crucial information about the dosage concentration that can be effective and free of side effects (Algharably et al. 2022). However, herbal medicines can also lead to adverse effects if not taken in appropriate dosages. Multiple factors such as combinations of plant constituents, contamination by microorganisms or heavy metals, and the presence of concomitant disease can contribute to toxicity. Hence, the most suitable method to establish the efficacy of suitable in-vivo herbal medicine exposures would be to perform well-controlled and appropriate randomized clinical trials. Clinical trials have been performed to study the efficacy of numerous medicinal herbs, and a few of them such as quinine, artemisinin, codeine, morphine, and digoxin have been developed into drugs for treating human diseases (Al Rashid et al. 2020). Keeping in view the potential of medicinal plants in herbal formulations, it is imperative to develop and adopt suitable preclinical and clinical research strategies that will provide clarity regarding their efficacy.

16.8 Monitoring the Safety of Herbal Medicinal Products

Monitoring the safety of herbal medicinal products (Fig. 16.4) is an essential part of ensuring their efficacy and minimizing potential risks to public health. Herbal products are widely used for various health conditions, but like all medicines, they carry

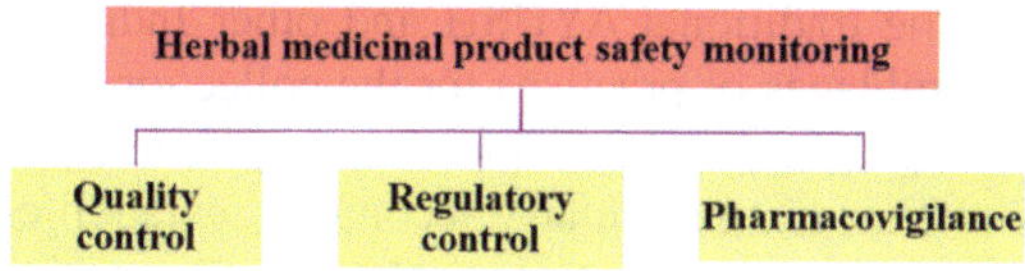

Fig. 16.4 Safety monitoring of herbal medicinal product

the potential for adverse effects, interactions with other drugs, or contamination. Effective safety monitoring helps identify, assess, and mitigate these risks.

16.8.1 Quality Assurance of Herbal Medicine

Regulation of quality and standardization of herbal medicine are crucial for the bioactivity-guided fractionation of phytochemicals, bioprospection utilizing technical standards in accordance with authorized gazette/pharmacopeias, and monitoring the entire process of forming herbal medications (Folashade et al. 2012).

The various factors affecting the quality of herbal drugs are:

- Quality of the raw material and its source of origin, etc.
- Associated variability in wild and non-wild plant varieties
- The harvest conditions (hygrometry, location, etc.) the time that has elapsed between the moment of harvest and that of analysis, and the phenological stage of the plant (beginning, end of flowering, …)
- Complex nature of phytochemicals contributes to the holistic pharmacological response
- Difference in the content of active principle(s) due to various abiotic and biotic factors
- Shortage of standard fingerprints of phytochemicals to analyze efficacy within different batches
- Absence of a wide range of major-minor compounds
- Variability in spectrum of pharmacological potential of species grown naturally vs. chemo varieties/cultivars
- Storage conditions are very important for microbiological quality, the preservation of secondary metabolites, and the conservation of herbal drugs
- Advanced analytical techniques are continuously developed and updated day by day to isolate, identify, and quantify the phytoconstituents responsible for the therapeutic potential of herbs/plants
- Active principle is generally unknown

Effectiveness, safety, and quality are the three cornerstones of rational herbal medicine use. However, there are no formal quality control standards or rules for the herbal medicine used in underdeveloped nations, and thus, there is no way to guarantee uniformity in the quality of various batches. Standardization and optimization procedures of growth conditions, which include not only the collection of medicinal plants but also the time and season of collection, should be taken into consideration in order to improve consumer acceptance and safety for widespread consumption.

The traditional AYUSH and other Indian medical systems offer standardized assemblages of practices for the collection of medicinal plants. In addition to providing data to support the idea that there is variation in the quantity of chemical constituents, particularly secondary metabolites, subject to change in the environment, these practices precisely indicate species location, geographical conditions, ecology, and habitat, the effect of seasonal variation, and occasionally even the stage of plant growth and development. Therefore, it is essential to carefully review our ancient treaties of the Indian classical medical system in order to establish the quality requirements for medicinal plants and to determine a reference standard. When paired with modern scientific knowledge and techniques that make use of advanced analytical instruments, this information will open doors to a more pronounced and sound system.

Research on the relationship between chromatographic fingerprints and the effectiveness of herbal medicines is desperately needed for herbal medicine quality control. Concurrent research should also be done on any contaminants found in herbal products, such as chemical toxins, heavy metals, microbiological contaminants, and excessive or banned pesticides. The research field of quality control of herbal medicines is therefore in fact an interdisciplinary study, a crossover of chemistry, pharmacology, medicine, and even statistics. This is done in order to provide a platform for the quality control of traditional herbal medicines and to encourage the discovery of novel therapeutics composed of multiple chemical compounds.

16.8.2 Regulatory Control

Herbal medicine systems in India include Ayurveda, Siddha, Unani, and homeopathic. All herbal medications are regulated by AYUSH, the Drugs & Cosmetics Act 1940 & 1945 (amendment), and CDSCO (Central Drugs Standard Control Organization). ICMR, CSIR, and the Department of AYUSH collaborate to create novel medications in a safe and efficient manner. In India, the AYUSH system has grouped roughly 8000 herbal medications. The AYUSH department created a certification program for AYUSH pharmaceutical items. Although guidelines for conducting clinical trials on herbal medicines have been developed in India, the registration process is not adequately regulated (Singh and Shukla 2021). A common misperception is that ayurvedic medications don't have any negative side effects. The Charak Samhita explains every cause of a negative medication reaction. The most important aspect of Ayurveda is choosing the right beginning material and using it in formulations to address the negative effects of medications (Thatte and Bhalerao 2008).

These medications are prepared using a strict process. Negative responses may result from carelessness in the production and administration of these medications. Despite this, India has a high incidence of use of these medications. Their long-term safety is called into question by the presence of toxic metals, and there have been instances of negative reactions. "Even a strong poison can become an excellent medicine if administered properly," concludes Charaka. However, if treated improperly, even the most beneficial medication might become poisonous. With 8403 licensed Ayurvedic pharmacies and sales of 4000 crores, it has an effect on the Indian economy and healthcare system. This commercialization makes it more difficult to use ayurvedic medications safely, necessitating the establishment of an official pharmacovigilance program (Thatte and Bhalerao 2008).

16.8.2.1 India

Market Importance and Use of Herbal Medicines

Ordinary people in India have folk knowledge about the traditional usage of herbal remedies. Since the majority of practitioners create and administer their own recipes, it is challenging to gauge the size of the Indian traditional medicine business. The current yearly sales of herbal medicine products produced by major Indian corporations are estimated to be around $300 million USD. Innovative research efforts to improve safety combined with scientifically established efficacy may lead to improved use of traditional herbal medicine.

Legal Status in India

In order to incorporate medications that are derived from traditional Indian medicine, the Indian government revised the Drugs and Cosmetics Act in 1959. Licenses for the production of all traditional herbal medicine products are granted by state drug control authorities.

16.8.2.2 Guidelines for the Regulation of Herbal Medicines in the South-East Asia Region

A drug is considered safe if there is no known or possible damage to users. Three kinds of drug safety are used to determine the type of herbal drug safety.

Category 1: Long-term use establishes safety
Category 2: Safe in certain usage scenarios
Category 3: Uncertainly safe herbal medications

The manufacturer and regulatory agencies share responsibility for ensuring the quality of herbal medicines. Guidelines on many aspects of quality assurance, dossier evaluation, producer data submission, and good manufacturing practices (GMP) compliance were established by national drug regulatory bodies. The manufacturer should follow Good Agricultural and Collection Practices (GACP), Good Manufacturing Practices (GMP), and Good Laboratory Practices (GLP) guidelines in order to create suitable specifications for the product.

16.8.2.3 Who Policy and Activities

The workforce represented by traditional practitioners in poor nations is a potentially significant resource for primary healthcare, according to many resolutions issued by the World Health Assembly (WHA) that highlight traditional medicine. Among other things, the 1978 Alma-Ata Declaration advocated incorporating the use of effective traditional medicines within national drug laws and regulations for the good of society. According to the World Health Organization's 1991 presentation of its policy on traditional medicine to the 44th World Health Assembly, "WHO collaborated with its Member States for the review of national policies, legislation and decisions on the use of traditional medicine in their health systems."

Herbal items are typically regarded as drugs in some nations and are therefore subject to laws. Such laws do not, however, exist in the majority of nations, including the USA, and the majority of botanical products are really sold as dietary supplements. A new regulatory framework for natural health products was created more recently by the Health Directorate of Canada, and it went into force in January 2004. The new regulations require, among other things, better labeling, good manufacturing processes, product and site licensing, and the provision of a wide range of evidence-based health claims. The only legal restrictions that are implemented, even in Canada, are that all products—including natural health products—that are meant for medical use be given a Drug Identification Number (DIN). Bulk herbs and other raw materials don't need these figures. FDA laws limit access to herbal medications in the United States. Research must demonstrate the safety and efficacy of any new chemical or herbal medication before it can be licensed (Wickramsinghe et al. 2006).

16.8.2.4 Regulation and Registration of Herbal Medicines

The legal status regarding the regulation of herbal medicines varies from country to country. There are a higher number of traditionally used herbal medicines in developing countries but very few legislative regulations available in such countries to regulate the process of traditional medicines.

16.8.3 Regulation for a Better Future

Although the ICH guidelines provide international standards for reporting, herbal medicines preparation, and manufacturing, some countries use different formats. Consequently, different formats or reports result to increase the pressure on regulators. It will have a negative impact on data evaluation and final decisions. Therefore, data should be presented in a unified format for a better vision of pharmacovigilance.

16.8.4 Pharmacovigilance

The Ministry of Ayush has launched new schemes for promoting pharmacovigilance of Ayurved, Siddha, Unani, and Homeopathy (ASU&H) drugs. Main objective of the scheme is to develop the culture to undertake safety monitoring and documenting adverse effects of Ayurveda, Siddha, Unani, and Homeopathy drugs. It also aims to surveillance of misleading advertisements appearing in the print and electronic media. All India Institute of Ayurveda, New Delhi, designated the role as National Pharmacovigilance Centre. Technological advancements like innovations, automations, and artificial intelligence will play a significant role in filling the gaps and solving the current problems in Pharmacovigilance.

16.8.4.1 Automation of Pharmacovigilance

Compared to manual collection of data, there is a strong need for automation to handle large and complex data for analysis. This will eventually lead to an increase in the speed of clinical trials. In the post-marketing studies, automation will be helpful to capture the data through mobile applications and electronic health records.

Impact of Cloud Technology on Pharmacovigilance

Using Cloud technology for fully integrating databases for healthcare and research institutions will be crucial for advancing drug safety and pharmacovigilance. Nowadays, every company has its own separate database which has a negative impact on the development of pharmacovigilance.

Different Levels of Automation in Pharmacovigilance

There are different levels of automation that can be used to speed up the process of pharmacovigilance

1. Basic Automation in Pharmacovigilance

   It provides automation of task monitoring, tracking, and collection of continuous metrics. In this case, manual intervention is required during data entry and data processing.

2. Robotic Automation in Pharmacovigilance

   Robotic process automation helps to eliminate the previously manual tasks and helps to achieve automatic entry, processing, and analysis of data. Combination of cognitive automation, natural language processing with robotics process automation can help humans to make accurate and fast decisions.

Artificial Intelligence in Pharmacovigilance

Use of artificial intelligence automation (AI) results in diminishing human intervention. A branch of AI, i.e., machine learning, helps data analysts and data scientists make predictions, which is based on large volumes of data. The major goal is to enhance the current processes of artificial intelligence in pharmacovigilance without replacing them.

16.8.4.2 Why Automation Is Necessary for Better Pharmacovigilance Future?

Pharmacovigilance automation can enhance the future of pharmacovigilance:

- It improves the precision, accuracy, and quality of data.
- It decreases human errors, saves time, and cost-effective.
- It guarantees to follow the regulatory guidelines.

In addition, automation will help to handle a massive amount of data in less time.

Through automation, humans would help to perform their herbal medicines pharmacovigilance study effectively. It will also reduce human intervention. Drug adverse events can be tracked inside the human body through smart pill innovation technology. Automation and advancement in technology are the future of pharmacovigilance.

16.8.4.3 Recommendations

There are several recommendations that system can move forward in attempting to embrace pharmacovigilance systems into herbal medicines.

1. Introduce herbal medicines and pharmacovigilance into the Curriculum at undergraduate and postgraduate levels.
2. Encourage studies of case studies on adverse drug safety.
3. Set up the default online drug response system for consumers which will directly record the feedback online.
4. Make reporting of adverse reactions to regulators mandatory for herbal medicines.
5. Provide unbiased and easily accessible drug information. The Government of India launched the Traditional Knowledge Digital Library which is a good example of how ancient knowledge is available and made digitally accessible.
6. Create awareness about the science of pharmacovigilance among ayurvedic physicians, patients, and paramedical staff.
7. Development of human resources is a key feature for the success of this enterprise. It will be necessary to train herbal medicine experts in the science of Pharmacovigilance and include them in the reporting and assessment of the adverse reactions. A strong collaborative effort from experts in pharmacovigilance and herbal medicines together can ensure that this system is useful and functioning (Thatte and Bhalerao 2008).

16.8.4.4 Pharmacovigilance of Herbal Medicinal Products

Just four of the eleven Southeast Asian nations have a national framework monitoring the safety of traditional medicinal products. To gather and evaluate data about adverse drug reactions (ADRs) involving herbal medications, national pharmacovigilance centers are essential. Every ADR report should be carefully considered as a possible herbal medication. The medical community should also encourage people to ask about any negative effects of herbal medications.

16.9 Conclusion

Herbal therapies are becoming more and more acknowledged as successful treatments for a variety of illnesses in the current period. There is constant research into the need to standardize pharmaceutical products and the several ways that bioactive components might be formulated. Every plant or herbal product should be properly identified, taking into consideration any possible contaminants, adulterants, or impurities. Together, Ayurveda, modern medicine, and science will create a true discovery engine that could result in the creation of novel, safer, more economical, and more efficient therapies. One of Ayurveda's unique selling points is the positive worldwide trend toward integrative sciences, holistic health, and systems biology approaches to medicine and treatment development. In order to produce high-grade herbal products with a quick onset of action and good bioavailability, ayurvedic and contemporary medical approaches must be combined.

The production of standardized herbal products that take into account the quantity of active phytoconstituents required for commercialization, precise raw material identification and supply, and to avoid adulteration is the only way to develop herbal medications. In order to further improve the bioavailability of phytoconstituents, new drug delivery systems should also be considered. Therefore, it becomes the main responsibility of the producers of herbal medications to provide sufficient stability for long-term storage and patient safety. Because the phytoformulation is a combination of several active components, care should be taken while evaluating the stability profile for natural medicines. With a consistent formulation, modern patient compliance will rise.

References

Adeyi AO, Nneji L (2015) Ameliorative potentials of medicinal plants on the pathophysiological complications of diabetes mellitus: a review. J Med Plant Res 9(8):262–288

Ahmad I, Aquil F, Owais M (2006) Modern phytomedicine: turning medicinal plants into drugs. WILEY-VCH Verlag GmbH and Co KGaA, Weinheim, pp 29–36

Akerele O (1993) Nature's medicinal bounty: don't throw it away. World Health Forum, Vol. 14. WHO Geneva, pp 390–395

Al Rashid MH, Kundu A, Mandal V, Wangchuk P, Mandal SC (2020) Preclinical and clinical trials of Indian medicinal plants in disease control. In: Sen S, Chakraborty R (eds) Herbal medicine in India. Springer, Singapore. https://doi.org/10.1007/978-981-13-7248-3_9

Algharably EA, Di Consiglio E, Testai E, Pistollato F, Mielke H, Gundert-Remy U (2022) In vitro–in vivo extrapolation by physiologically based kinetic modeling: experience with three case studies and lessons learned. Front Toxicol 4:885843. https://doi.org/10.3389/ftox.2022.885843

Azmir J, Zaidul ISM, Rahman MM, Sharif KM, Mohamed A, Sahena F, Jahurul MHA, Ghafoor K, Norulaini NAN, Omar AKM (2013) Techniques for extraction of bioactive compounds from plant materials: a review. J Food Eng 117:426–436

Balasubramani SP, Goraya GS, Venkatasubramanian P (2011) Development of ITS sequence-based markers to distinguish *Berberis aristata* DC. from *B. lyceum* Royle and *B. asiatica* Roxb. 3 Biotech 1:11–19. https://doi.org/10.1007/s13205-010-0001-5

Balouiri M, Sadiki M, Ibnsouda SK (2016) Methods for *in vitro* evaluating antimicrobial activity: a review. J Pharm Anal 6(2):71–79. https://doi.org/10.1016/j.jpha.2015.11.005

Bandaranayake WM (2006) Quality control, Screening, Toxicity, regulation of Herbal drugs. Modern Phytomedicine. Turning Medicinal Plants into Drug. Chapter 2, pp 25–57. ISBN: 3-527-31530-6

Bansal A, Chhabra V, Rawal RK, Sharma S (2014) Chemometrics: a new scenario in herbal drug standardization. J Pharm Anal 4:223–233. https://doi.org/10.1016/j.jpha.2013.12.001

Chaudhary M, Naithani (2009) Novel herbal topical formulations for treatment of acne and skin disorders. Indian Pat Appl Publ:28

Cooper JW, Denston TC, Riley M (1931) A textbook of pharmacognosy. Sir Isaac Pitman and Sons, Ltd, London

Delgado-Tejedor A, Leekitcharoenphon P, Aarestrup FM, Otani S (2021) Evaluating the usefulness of next-generation sequencing for herb authentication. Food Chem: Mol Sci 3:100044. https://doi.org/10.1016/j.fochms.2021.100044

Ernst E (2005) The efficacy of herbal medicine—an overview. Fundam Clin Pharmacol 19:405–409

Folashade KO, Omoregie EH, Ochogu AP (2012) Standardization of herbal medicines. Int J Biodivers Conserv 4(3):101–112

Ganie SH, Upadhyay P, Das S, Prasad Sharma M (2015) Authentication of medicinal plants by DNA markers. Plant Gene 4:83–99

Gerard D (2016) Advances in food authenticity testing. Woodhead Publishing

Houghton PJ, Howes M-J, Lee CC, Steventon G (2007) Uses and abuses of in vitro tests in ethnopharmacology: visualizing an elephant. J Ethnopharmacol 110:391–400

Ichim MC, Anthony B (2021) Chemical authentication of botanical ingredients: a review of commercial herbal products. Front Pharmacol 12. https://doi.org/10.3389/fphar.2021.666850

Ichim MC, Haser A, Nick P (2020) Microscopic authentication of commercial herbal products in the globalized market: potential and limitations. Front Pharmacol 11:867. https://doi.org/10.3389/fphar.2020.00876

Ikeda Y, Motoune S, Ono M, Mohri Y (2006) Stable liquid preparation/Stable liquid preparation coated with water-soluble cellulose derivative. US Pat App:2006

Ivanova NV, Kuzmina ML, Braukmann TWA, Borisenko AV, Zakharov EV (2016) Authentication of herbal supplements using next-generation sequencing. PLoS One 11(5):e0156426. https://doi.org/10.1371/journal.pone.0156426

Katiyar C, Gupta A, Kanjilal S, Katiyar S (2012) Drug discovery from plant sources: an integrated approach. Ayu 33(1):10

Lahlou M (2007) Screening of natural products for drug discovery. Expert Opin Drug Discov 2(5):697–705

Laupattarakasem P, Houghton PJ, Hoult JRS, Itharat A (2003) An evaluation of the activity related to inflammation of four plants used in Thailand to treat arthritis. J Ethnopharmacol 85:207–215

Lee YS, Woo S, Kim JK, Park JY, Izzah NK (2022) Genetic and chemical markers for authentication of three *Artemisia* species: *A. capillaris, A. gmelinii,* and *A. fukudo.* PLoS One 17(3):e0264576

Mattummal R, Gopi DK, Bobbili E, Narayana SKK (2019) A review on molecular techniques employed for authentication of Indian medicinal plants. Plant Science Today 6(4):465–478

Meena Devi VN, Nagendra Prasad P, Kalirajan K (2010) Infrared spectral studies on Siddha drug-Pavala parpam. Int J Pharma Biosci 1(4):474–483

Parasuraman S, Thing GS, Dhanaraj SA (2014) Polyherbal formulation: concept of ayurveda. Pharmacogn Rev 8(16):73

Peter AGM De Smet (2002) Herbal Remedies. N Engl J Med 347:2046–2056

Rangari VD (2008) Pharmacognosy and phytochemistry, vol 1, 2nd edn. Career Pub, pp 78–100

Rasul MG (2018) Conventional extraction methods use in medicinal plants, their advantages and disadvantages. Int J Basic Sci Appl Comput 2(6):10–14

Revathy SS, Rathinamala R, Murugesan M (2012) Authentication methods for drugs used in Ayurveda, Siddha and Unani systems of medicine: an overview. Int J Pharm Sci Res 3(8):2352–2361

Salunkhe V, Bhise SB (2009) Formulation and stability studies of chewable herbal tablets. Indian Pharma 8:53–58

Seethapathy GS, Raclariu-Manolica AC, Anmarkrud JA, Wangensteen H, de Boer HJ (2019) DNA metabarcoding authentication of Ayurvedic herbal products on the European market raises concerns of quality and fidelity. Front Plant Sci 10:68

Shin HJ, Lee SC, Hahn YH, Ryou HW (1999) Stable tablets containing volatile liquid drugs. Repub Korea

Singh S, Shukla V (2021) Current regulation for herbal medicine in India. International Journal of Drug Regulatory Affair 9(2):30–34

Sivarajan VV, Balachandran I (1994) Oxford and IBH publications co. Ayurvedic Drugs and Their Plant Sources, New Delhi
Srinivasan VS (2006) Challenges and scientific issues in the standardization of botanicals and their preparations. United States Pharmacopeia's dietary supplement verification program—a public health program. Life Sci 78:2039–2043
Stephane FY, Jules BK, Batiha GE, Ali I, Bruno LN (2021) Extraction of bioactive compounds from medicinal plants and herbs
Techen N, Crockett SL, Khan IA, Scheffler BE (2004) Authentication of medicinal plants using molecular biology techniques to compliment conventional methods. Curr Med Chem 11:1391–1401
Thakur AK, Prasad NA, Laddha KS (2008) Stability testing of herbal products. The Pharma Review. Kongposh Publications
Thatte U, Bhalerao S (2008) Pharmacovigilance of ayurvedic medicines in India. Indian J Pharmacol 40:S10–S12
Upton Roy R, David B, Gafner S, Glasl S (2020) Botanical ingredient identification and quality assessment: strengths and limitations of analytical techniques. Phytochem Rev 19:1157–1177
Usman I, Hussain M, Imran A, Afzaal M, Saeed F, Javed M, Afzal A, Ashfaq I, Jbawi E, Saewan S (2022) Traditional and innovative approaches for the extractions of bioactive compounds. Int J Food Prop 25(1):1215–1233
Uwineza PA, Waskiewicz A (2020) Recent advances in supercritical fluid extraction of natural bioactive compounds from natural plant materials. Molecules 25:3847
Winslow L, Kroll D (1998) Herbs as medicines. Arch Inter Med 158(20):2192–2199
Wu HY, Shaw PC (2022) Strategies for molecular authentication of herbal products: from experimental design to data analysis. Chin Med 17:38

Exploring the Potential of Ayurveda in Developing Sustainable and Reliable Treatment Options for the Future

17

Mahendrakumar Mani, Shiny Punalur John, Gayathiri Ekambaram, and Elumalai Kuppusamy

Abstract

Traditional medicine, mainly herbal medicine, has contributed to healthcare systems worldwide, especially in rural and remote areas, despite modern advancements in science, technology, and allopathic medicine. Ayurveda, a traditional healthcare system used in Indian medicine, has been practiced for thousands of years and has a rich history of effectiveness. Modern research has also recognized the importance of Ayurvedic medicine. Many Ayurvedic drugs have been developed and used since ancient times, with some transitioning from tradition to trends in modern times. Among the strengths are the individual focus on the patient, which is inherent in Ayurvedic medicine. In the treatment process, pat, its physical characteristics, mental health risks, environment, and social aspects are combined to formulate an effective treatment plan that will enhance the patient's performance while simultaneously minimizing the side effects that may accompany its use. Thus, the advantages of Ayurvedic medicine must be proven through scientific evidence for its acceptance in conventional medical practice. The therapeutic value of Ayurvedic medicine requires more investigation to be

M. Mani (✉)
Department of Biotechnology, Guru Nanak College (Autonomous), Velachery, Chennai, Tamil Nadu, India

S. P. John
Department of Medical Research, Faculty of Medicine and Health Sciences, SRM Institute of Science and Technology, Kattankulathur, Tamil Nadu, India

G. Ekambaram
Department of Plant Biology and Plant Biotechnology, Guru Nanak College (Autonomous), Velachery, Chennai, Tamil Nadu, India

E. Kuppusamy
Department of Advanced Zoology & Biotechnology, Government Arts College (Autonomous), Nandanam, Chennai, Tamil Nadu, India

A. Kumar et al. (eds.), *Innovations in Ayurvedic Nutrition*,
https://doi.org/10.1007/978-981-95-1213-3_17

determined in all its aspects. However, the increasing importance of the Ayurvedic system of medicine implies that it is necessary to achieve this. When ideas from Ayurveda, a branch of traditional Indian medicine, are incorporated into comprehensive modern medical science, healthcare providers should be able to develop a more comprehensive healthcare system. This is a summary of the significance of the Ayurvedic system, the advantages of an individualized approach to medicine, and the call for Ayurvedic science-based healthcare for pertinent therapeutic discoveries and validations in practice.

Keywords

Ayurveda · Traditional Indian Medicines · Medicinal Chemistry · Biopharmaceuticals

17.1 Ayurveda—Lifeline of Traditional Medicine

Ayurveda is an ancient system of medicine that originated in India more than 5000 years ago. It works under the proclivity that a person's mental, physical, and spiritual health are interdependent, and together these form a balance. The Ayurveda system entails a comprehensive system of deliverance from sickness that looks at the patient in proportion to his physical, mental, and spiritual characteristics. Ayurveda is the life wire of traditional medicine because it has been in practice for over 25 centuries and has been shown to be effective in many ailments. The system involves the use of natural remedies and treatments for organs to assist in regaining balance. The form of treatment is derived from a folk system of healing from India that employs herbs and other natural products (Dwivedi et al. 2020).

The first and most important is the idea of doshas, the three life forces that Ayurveda states regulate human biochemistry. These are Vata, Pitta, and Kapha, which have five subtypes and are related to five elements: earth, water, fire, air, and ether. In Ayurveda, we find the concept of doshas: everyone has three types of doshas, but with different quantities that define our physical and mental characteristics. Ayurveda has numerous treatment procedures and methodologies to pacify doshas and maintain health and physiology (Sharma et al. 2008). (Fig. 17.1) Some of the standard therapies used in Ayurveda include.

Ayurvedic Massage In this therapy, warm herbed oils are used to rub the body with the intention of having relaxing and detoxifying effects.

As for some of the benefits of yoga and meditation, they serve to harmonize the mind, body, and spirit and enhance quality of life.

Herbal Remedies In Ayurveda, treatment is recommended depending on the specific health problem that the patient is suffering from.

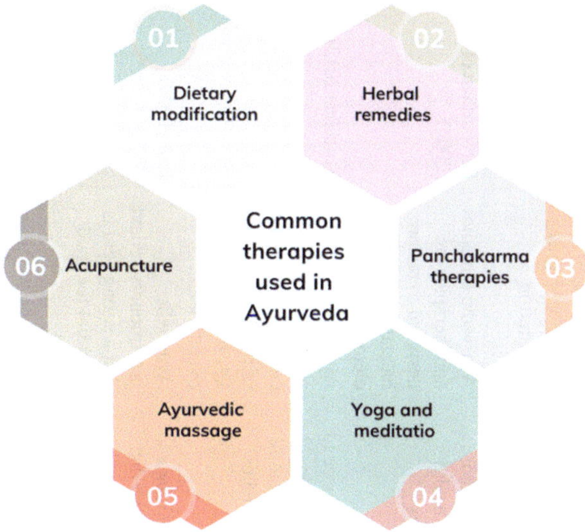

Fig. 17.1 Outline of common therapies used in Ayurveda

Panchakarma This therapy consists of a sequence of treatments aimed at eliminating toxins from the body and balancing dosages.

Ayurveda has received much acceptance globally because of its complete body and soul healthcare system and the inclusion of chronic diseases. It provides relief from several ailments affecting the body, such as digestive disorders, respiratory ailments, skin disorders, and even chronic body pain. It is important to safeguard indigenous forms of knowledge and practice. This has been adopted by different generations and has endured for thousands of years, despite advances in medical practice (Singh et al. 2021). Ayurveda is not merely an art of curing ailments but also a scientific way of living that helps maintain the proper equilibrium in every sphere of life. It is one of the major unique selling propositions of Ayurveda, which makes it a healthcare system that aims at the complete man—physical, mental, and spiritual. It has been in the market for many years and, to date, offers safe and efficient management of various health problems (Table 17.1) (Singh et al. 2021). Ayurveda is not only a system of medicine, but also a complete lifestyle that includes equalization of doshas, building up a healthy body, free from disease, and being happy forever (Fig. 17.2).

17.2 Alchemy of Ayurveda

The term Alchemy of Ayurveda is meant to describe the metamorphosis that occurs in the physical, mental, and spiritual realm of an individual following Ayurveda. Ayurveda is a traditional form of medicine in India and is based on what is

Table 17.1 Fundamentals and therapeutic principles in ayurveda

S. No.	Principle of Ayurveda	Determination	Fundamentals	Therapeutic principles	Other	References
1	Doshas	Unique combination of Vata, pitta, and Kapha	Governing energies of human physiology representing the five elements of earth, water, fire, air, and ether	Restore balance to the doshas and promote health and wellness	Ayurvedic diagnosis and treatment are based on the individual's dosha constitution	Chopra (2002)
2	Panchamahabhutas	Five elements of earth, water, fire, air, and ether	The foundation of Ayurvedic philosophy	Used to diagnose and treat health conditions	Ayurvedic remedies and therapies are designed to restore balance to the five elements	Patwardhan et al. (2004)
3	Dhatus	Seven tissues of the body—Rasa, rakta, mamsa, meda, asthi, majja, shukra	The building blocks of the body	Restore balance to the dhatus through diet, lifestyle, and herbal remedies	Ayurvedic practitioners consider the health of the dhatus to be a key indicator of overall health	Kotecha (2012)
4	Agni	Digestive fire	Essential for the proper digestion and assimilation of food	Restore balance to agni through diet and lifestyle modifications	Ayurvedic practitioners believe that a strong agni is essential for good health	Lad (1999)
5	Ama	Toxins that accumulate in the body due to poor digestion	The root cause of many health conditions, according to Ayurveda	Eliminate ama through panchakarma and other detoxifying therapies	Ama is believed to be the cause of many chronic diseases	Frawley (2001)

6	Prakriti	Individual constitution	Determined by the balance of the doshas at the time of conception	A tailored approach to healthcare based on the individual's prakriti	Ayurvedic practitioners believe that a person's Prakriti determines their susceptibility to specific health conditions	Mishra (2004)
7	Srotas	Channels of the body through which nutrients and waste products are transported	Essential for the proper functioning of the body	Maintain the health of the srotas through diet and herbal remedies	Ayurvedic practitioners believe that blockages in the srotas cause many health conditions	Lad (2002)

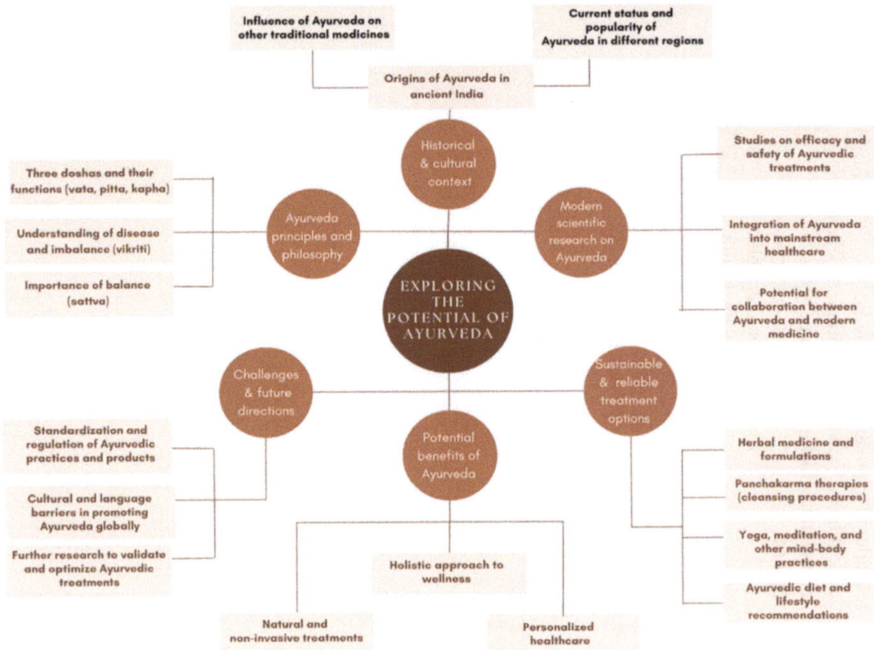

Fig. 17.2 Ayurveda: a holistic approach to sustainable healing

considered a proper balance in all aspects of an individual's life. It is founded on the five basic elements of nature, namely the earth, water, fire, air, and ether, and the three doshas of nature, viz., Vata, Pitta, and Kapha, which prevail over the human body and framework (Singh et al. 2021). Recognizing that Ayurveda is based on the exploration and application of natural resources that must include herbs, oils, and minerals, Ayurveda's experimentation aims at the restoration of the human body and helps restore balance. These remedies are more futuristic because they aim to eliminate the cause of the disease in the best possible way. For instance, if someone is suffering from digestion problems, Ayurveda will ask what could have caused it, probably bad food, stress, etc., and then deal with it through the right food and other correct manners (Kotecha 2018, Sharma 2017, Lad 2012).

These treatments depend on the degree of body dysfunction and constitution, as dictated by the dosha. This intricate form of body and spirit treatment helps bring seven-element harmony and allows the body to achieve the highest level of health. This also entails exercising through the use of yoga, meditation, and pranayama, which act as mind balancers and relieve stress. All these practices are meant to regulate and quiet the nervous system and reduce stress levels and spending, which has a massive influence on physical and psychological well-being (Mishra 2004).

In addition, emotional and spiritual well-being are as important as physical well-being, according to Ayurveda. Ayurveda acknowledges that the physical and mental are one and that the soul undergoing psychological affronts experiences concrete symptoms. Separate spiritual practices, such as meditations and mindfulness, contribute to positive improvement of an individual's emotional and spiritual needs, thus contributing to excellent health and well-being (Lad 1999; Sharma 2011; Tiwari 2017).

In summary, Ayurveda is an effective instrument for changing a human being from the inside to the outside. Ayurveda includes natural approaches to cure a person's diseases or ailments by administering individual therapies and incorporating other holistic procedures into a patient's life. Regardless of whether one is facing gross or more subtle physical, emotional, or spiritual disharmonies, Ayurveda offers a way to obtain the state of health and well-being, as described in Table 17.2.

Table 17.2 Alchemy of Ayurveda: understanding the practices and benefits

S.No	Alchemy of Ayurveda	Description	Practices	Benefits	References
1	Panchamahabhuta theory	Five elements theory that forms the basis of Ayurveda	Understanding the relationship between body and nature	Promotes balance and harmony in the body and mind	Tiwari (2003)
2	Dosha theory	Three doshas (Vata, Pitta, Kapha) govern human physiology	Identifying individual constitution and imbalances	Restores balance to the doshas and promote wellness	Lad (1999); Frawley (2001)
3	Tridosha theory	The interaction of three doshas in the body	Understanding individual imbalances and disease	Helps to identify the root cause of disease and treat it	Lad (1999); Frawley (2000)
4	Rasayana	Rejuvenation therapy that promotes longevity	Herbal remedies, nutrition, yoga, and meditation	Promotes longevity and vitality	Pole (2013); Tiwari (2003)
5	Srotas	Channels of the body through which nutrients flow	Identifying and treating blockages in the channels	Helps to improve digestion and overall health	Lad (2012); Svoboda (1999)
6	Ojas	The vital energy that promotes immunity and vitality	Herbal remedies, nutrition, yoga, and meditation	Promotes life and overall health	Sharma (2011)
7	Agni	The digestive fire that breaks down food and removes toxins	Herbal remedies, nutrition, yoga, and meditation	Helps to improve digestion and eliminate toxins	Lad (2012); Frawley (2000)
8	Ayurvedic diet	A diet based on individual constitution and imbalances	Nutrition based on dosha and digestive strength	Helps to improve digestion and overall health	Chopra (2007)

(continued)

Table 17.2 (continued)

S.No	Alchemy of Ayurveda	Description	Practices	Benefits	References
9	Ayurvedic massage	Body massage with herbal oils for relaxation and detoxification	Use of herbal oils to massage the body	Promotes relaxation, detoxification, and overall health	Saper et al. (2008)
10	Yoga and meditation	Practices to balance the mind, body, and spirit	Yoga postures, breathing techniques, and meditation	Promotes relaxation, mental clarity, and overall health	Khalsa and Cohen (2017)
11	Herbal remedies	Use of herbs and natural substances to treat health conditions	Herbal supplements, teas, and oils	Treats a wide range of health conditions naturally	Petersen and Challem (2008)
12	Panchakarma	A detoxification therapy that involves a series of treatments to remove toxins from the body and restore balance to the doshas	Includes five main treatments: Vamana, Virechana, Basti, Nasya, and Raktamokshana	Removes toxins from the body, improves digestion, strengthens the immune system, and promotes mental clarity	Nayak and Singh (2016)

17.3 History of Ayurveda

Ayurveda, originating from India, is one of the oldest health systems that help people in their treatment all around the globe. Ayurveda has been culled from the two Sanskrit words, Ayus, which translates to life, and Veda, which means science or knowledge. Ayurvedic medicine has its principles that good health and vitality involve thoughts, body, and spirit. The prescription of Ayurveda can be traced back to approximately 3000 BC in India, although the practice was oral. The two earliest documents recording Ayurveda knowledge storage are the Charaka Samhita and the Sushruta Samhita, which were written almost 2600 years ago (Sharma et al. 2017). The Indian system of medicine or Ayurveda was growing and blooming during the Maurya and Gupta empires, covering the period between third century BCE and the sixth century CE. At this time, Ayurvedic texts were expanded and made more sophisticated, and Ayurveda spread throughout India and to adjacent nations. Subsequently, Ayurveda assumed a more permanent place in the culture, and its precepts were put into practice in traditional Indian systems of treating diseases, certain postures, and breathing exercises known as yoga and other related forms of therapy. Conventional Ayurveda also affects other non-conventional systems of treatment, including Chinese medicine, ancient Tibetan medicine, and several others (Chopra, 2014).

17.3.1 Ancient Times

Ayurveda's roots can be traced to over 5500 years, arising from the Indian Vedic civilization. The Ayurveda tradition is said to have written records as early as 3000 BC in ancient Hindu sacred literature called the Vedas. Ayurveda, from the perspective of the Vedas, is a complete science of life or the science of right living in harmony with the self and the environment (Chaudhary 2019). Ayurveda evolved and advanced for centuries by other scholars and practitioners, such as Charaka and Sushruta, who wrote two of the most famous texts on Ayurveda: Charaka Samhita and Sushruta Samhita. These texts discuss Ayurvedic systems of health and disease, drugs, drug action, remedies for specific ailments, hygiene, massage, diet, and regimens to be followed by a healthy man or woman to lead a healthy life. Ayurveda also respects the individuality of a person and stresses on individual approaches to every patient (Vasant Lad 2002).

Ayurveda was practiced during the Mauryan and Gupta dynasties, from the third century BC to sixth century AD. The treatment system was also improved and advanced, and the scope of Ayurvedic medicine expanded across India and neighboring countries. Ayurveda also helped nourish the traditional practices peculiar to Indians, such as yoga and meditation, which are actively used today. Being supreme in almost every aspect of life, Ayurveda traveled across borders as far as it influenced Traditional Chinese Medicine, Tibetan Medicine, and other methodologies of the ancient world. In general, Ayurveda is a science with a very long history dating back to ancient India that has greatly impacted this culture and has had a profound impact on the general consideration of traditional healing and well-being on a global level (Chaudhary 2019).

17.3.2 Medieval Times

The origin and historical development of Ayurveda in India occurred from the sixth century CE to eighteenth century CE, and during this period, Ayurveda continued. Ayurveda's knowledge was synthesized in several texts, and the works, especially the Astanga Hridayam and the Bhava Prakasha, were extensions of Ayurvedic science. In the medieval age, various people, including physicians, scholars, and ordinary people, used Ayurveda. Literature studies also reveal that Ayurvedic works were translated into other languages such as Arabic and Persian, which made their knowledge prevail in other parts of the world (Jha 2018). Another major event during the medieval age was the establishment of colleges to formally educate Ayurvedic treatment systems. The first Ayurveda university was started at Takshashila in modern Pakistan during the Gupta dynasty; however, many more universities were established in the medieval period. The medieval period also brought subspecialization in Ayurvedic treatment systems, such as surgery, pediatrics, and toxicology. In the field of surgery, Ayurvedic surgeons perform various complicated surgeries, such as anesthesia and plastic surgery (Ganguli 2019). The traditional Indian system of medicine for Ayurveda was absorbed into other facets of Indian civilization during the medieval age, incorporated into the arts, literature, religion, etc. As for the life practices of Ayurveda, yoga and meditation started to take hold in this period, and many Ayurvedic practitioners became spiritual figures. During the medieval period, Ayurveda proliferated and developed further, and the Ayurvedic system of medicine continued to progress throughout India and other countries (Jain 2014).

17.3.3 Modern Times

The history of modern Ayurveda dates from the nineteenth century to the contemporary period. At the same time, the Ayurvedic medicine system saw revival and growth in India and received international acclamation and acceptance. During the colonial period, Ayurveda had several vices and drawbacks because of European culture and the introduction of modern medical systems in India. Nevertheless, traditional Ayurveda was practiced by traditional practitioners who passed on their knowledge through generations and word of mouth (Gupta 2017).

During the twentieth century, Ayurveda returned to India as Indian knowledge was actively restored and disseminated worldwide. In 1948, the government of India formed the Central Council for Research in Ayurveda and Siddha organizations that assisted in furthering Ayurvedic research. Ayurveda was also practiced in other countries in the twentieth century; for instance, the first Ayurvedic clinic started in Germany in 1982. Presently, Ayurveda is accepted as a CAM in many countries and is implemented in many aspects of CAM practices, including yoga, meditation, and herbal therapies (Singh 2005).

Over the last few years, Ayurveda has attracted much attention as a system of medicine that also focuses on overall well-being. Today, many people from the Western world are opting for Ayurvedic remedies like Panchakarma, and Ayurvedic specialists are trying hard to adopt Ayurveda in modern systems of medicine. Currently, Ayurveda medicine is considered a CAMs in many nations. They are used in practices such as yoga, meditation, medicine, and food supplements from herbs. In general, the modern history of the Ayurveda period has recorded the incorporation of change along with the progress that Ayurvedic medicine has incorporated in the contemporary period while holding on to the fundamentals of Ayurveda (Narayanaswamy 2010).

17.4 Ayurveda—An Indian Perspective

Ayurveda is a form of healthcare that originated in India. Some people believe that it was developed over 5000 years ago and, to date, it is used at present. The rationale for Ayurveda, which is the cornerstone of effective treatment, is that health is a function of a harmonized body, mind, and spirit. The doshas are also an integral part of Ayurveda and are the principles of the body and mind. According to Ayurvedic principles, there are three doshas: air and ether, fire and water, and earth and water.

The doshas are a blend of the three humors that constitute the bodily type or Prakriti of a person. Traditional Ayurvedic cures are compiled according to date, and the most prevalent Ayurvedic treatments are governed by the patient's prakriti and are intended for the correction of doshas (Rastogi 2018).

The ancient system of medicine that relies on diet and herbal remedies is known as Ayurveda, and takes full advantage of herbs, oils, and spices. Moreover, Ayurvedic cure deals with removing the cause of the disease from the body and balancing the doshas rather than dealing with the signs and symptoms of the diseased state (Birch et al. 2021). Traditional Indian Ayurvedic healers use nourishing modifications, herbals, massage, meditation, yoga, and other lifestyles to rebalance the body and mind. Ayurveda is an integral part of Indians' lives and has always been so for thousands of years. Some people believe that Ayurveda is among the oldest medical systems in the world, and people in India still use it. Ayurveda has influenced almost all facets of Indian culture, such as the arts, literature, and religion. These food habits are compatible with the Indian system of Ayurveda, where yoga and meditation are of prime importance in the day-to-day activities of an Indian (Singh 2005). Today, many people know Ayurveda and are increasingly turning to it for treatment and health promotion. As a result, it has gained popularity among people seeking natural cures for ailments and holistic ways to achieve better health. Today, people in many countries receive Ayurvedic treatments, and in some countries, Ayurveda is being incorporated as part of that country's healthcare system. Nevertheless, it should be highlighted that Ayurveda courses must be conducted by an expert to avoid adverse effects while enjoying the respective treatment (Valiathan 1993).

17.4.1 Pioneers of Ayurveda

Ayurveda is a natural healing science over 5000 years old from the Indian subcontinent. Numerous people have put Ayurveda into practice and growth over the course of many centuries (Rastogi et al. 2018). Some of the pioneers of Ayurveda are as follows.

(i) *Charaka:* Charaka is also known as Ayurveda's father. This was a Greek physician and writer who practiced and wrote at the end of the fourth century or the beginning of the third century BC. Charaka also wrote several other books, the most important of which are known as Charaka Samhita.
(ii) *Sushruta:* Sushruta was another celebrated physician of antiquity who was almost contemporary to Charaka. He has contributed to the field of surgery and is considered to be one of the most prominent surgeons in plastic surgery.
(iii) *Vagbhata:* Vagbhata, whom we know only as a physician, would have been living in the early part of the sixth century CE. He has worked mostly in Ayurvedic pharmacology and wrote about internal medicine.
(iv) *Madhava:* Madhava was a Vedic physician in seventh century CE. He specializes in Ayurveda, particularly the female reproductive system.

Table 17.3 Contributions and accomplishments of Ayurvedic pioneers

S.No	Pioneers of Ayurveda	Contribution	Achievements	Books and writings	References
1	Charaka	Systematized Ayurveda	Wrote Charaka Samhita, one of the foundational texts of Ayurveda	Charaka Samhita, Charaka Nidana, Charaka Chikitsa, Charaka Sutra	Charaka (2003)
2	Sushruta	Contributed to surgical techniques and anatomy	Wrote Sushruta Samhita, one of the foundational texts of Ayurveda	Sushruta Samhita, Sushruta Tantra	Sushruta (2005)
3	Vagbhata	Combined and synthesized the works of Charaka and Sushruta	Wrote Ashtanga Hridaya, a comprehensive text on Ayurveda	Ashtanga Hridaya, Ashtanga Sangraha	Vagbhata (2011)
4	Madhava	Specialized in pediatrics and gynecology	Wrote Madhava Nidanam, a text on the diagnosis	Madhava Nidanam, Sarngadhara Samhita	Madhava (2009)
5	Bhavamishra	Contributed to the field of pharmacology	Wrote Bhavaprakasha, a text on herbal medicine	Bhavaprakasha	Bhavamishra (2012)

(v) *Bhavamisra:* Bhavamisra was a sixteenth-century CE physician. He is best remembered for his collaboration on pharmacopeia in Ayurveda and for his work in toxicology.

These pioneers of Ayurveda have significantly contributed to the development and advancement of Ayurvedic medicine. Their work laid the foundation for Ayurvedic practices that are still in use today (Table 17.3).

17.5 Application of Ayurveda

Ayurveda is a traditional system of medicine that originated in India and has been used for thousands of years. It offers a holistic approach to health and wellness that considers a person's physical, emotional, and spiritual well-being (Fig. 17.3). The following are some applications of Ayurveda.

- *Treatment of ailments:* Ayurveda treats many infections including digestive, respiratory, skin, and musculoskeletal disorders.
- *Promoting wellness:* Ayurveda emphasizes the importance of maintaining balance in the body, mind, and spirit to promote overall health and wellness.
- *Managing stress:* Ayurvedic practices, such as yoga, meditation, and massage, effectively reduce stress and promote relaxation.

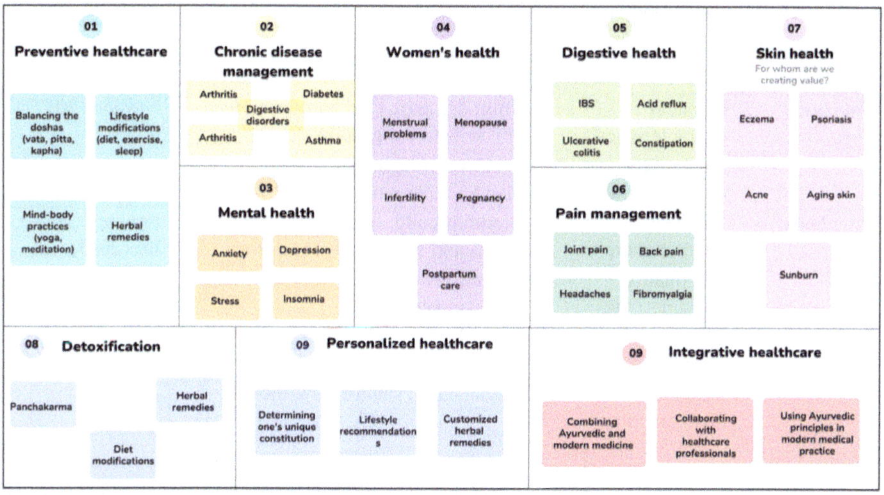

Fig. 17.3 Key applications of Ayurveda

- *Improving digestion:* Ayurveda offers dietary guidelines and herbal remedies to improve digestion and alleviate digestive problems.
- *Boosting immunity:* Ayurveda uses natural remedies and lifestyle changes to boost the immune system and prevent illnesses.
- *Supporting women's health:* Ayurveda offers a range of treatments and practices to support women's health including menstrual issues, fertility, and pregnancy.
- *Management of chronic conditions:* Ayurveda can be a complementary therapy for managing chronic diseases such as diabetes, hypertension, and arthritis.
- *Enhancing beauty:* Ayurvedic treatment and remedies enhance beauty and promote healthy skin, hair, and nails.

It is essential to consult a qualified Ayurvedic practitioner before using Ayurvedic remedies or treatments (Table 17.4).

17.5.1 Folklore

Ayurveda is deeply rooted in Indian culture and often intertwined with folklore and traditional practices. Many Ayurvedic remedies and treatments have been passed down through generations and have become part of Indian folklore (Panda 2019). Here are some examples:

- *Turmeric:* Turmeric is used in the Ayurvedic complaints list of ingredients and is a spice used in Indian cuisines. In India, turmeric is used in their legends to fight evil because it is regarded as a symbol of an empowering magical entity.

Table 17.4 Ayurvedic body types and their characteristics

Ayurvedic body types	Vata, Pitta, Kapha	Information	Reference
Vata body Type	Physical characteristics	Thin, dry skin, cold hands and feet, and sensitive digestion	Naveen (2017)
	Personality characteristics	Creative, imaginative, easily distracted, anxious	
Pitta body Type	Physical characteristics	Medium build, oily skin, warm hands and feet, strong digestion	Frawley (2001), Ito (2013)
	Personality characteristics	Ambitious, confident, competitive, easily angered	
Kapha body type	Physical characteristics	Large build, thick, oily skin, cold hands and feet, and slow digestion	Tiwari (2004)
	Personality characteristics	Loyal, calm, stable, slow-moving	

- *Neem:* Neem is a popular herb used in Ayurvedic remedies and treatments. Neem has been thought of as an element with purification effects and is used to clean oneself and the surroundings.
- *Oil pulling:* Oil pulling is a method of Ayurveda in which coconut oil or sesame is held in the mouth and moved gently for approximately 20 min for various oral diseases. According to ancient Indian culture and customs, pulling oil is said to cure many diseases.
- *Ayurvedic massage:* Generally known as Abhyanga in India, it is a popular practice for Ayurvedic massage to be capable of improving one's health in many ways. Writers synthesizing Ancient Indian legends indicate that massage, according to the rules of Ayurveda, enhances blood circulation, has a calming effect, and can cure some diseases.
- *Yoga:* Yoga was originally from India and is very much connected to Ayurveda. As per the Indian tradition, yoga has many health advantages and is used to enhance the body, mind, and soul.

In general, Ayurveda is closely connected to Indian folk tales and traditions. Most of the cures and treatments practiced in Ayurvedic medicine have been inherited over time and form part of the Indian tradition.

17.5.2 Diagnosis

Mainstream medicine does not easily accept Ayurveda's concept of disease diagnosis and treatment, which revolves around the principles of individual treatment. According to the Ayurveda medical concept, diagnosis of a disease entails the consideration of the body's governing forces in analyzing the causative power of a problem as well as the physical, mental, and emotional state of an individual.

The following are some ways in which Ayurveda is used in disease diagnosis:

17.5.2.1 Pulse Diagnosis

Ayurvedic doctors employ pulse examination to diagnose the general well-being of the client and detect dysfunctions in his body. The practitioner then examines the quality and rhythm of the pulse to determine which doshas (Vata, Pitta, or Kapha) are imbalanced and, therefore, identify what has led to the disease.

17.5.2.2 Observation

The outward appearance of the face, including the skin, tongue, and nails, was examined by Ayurvedic doctors to determine the manifestations of the disease. It also tracks behavior, emotions, and lifestyle habits concerning the overall health of a particular person.

17.5.2.3 Questioning

In Ayurveda, practitioners seek information that includes the symptoms of ailment, past medical history, diet and lifestyle, stress levels, etc., to determine the cause of the ailment.

17.5.2.4 Diagnosis Through Ayurvedic Tools

Ayurvedic examination also includes so-called eye diagnosis, where the Ayurvedic physician looks at the patient's tongue, face, and other manifestations of the disease, and uses stool and urine examinations to determine the nature of the disease.

17.5.2.5 Dosha Imbalance Diagnosis

Based on imbalances in dosha (Vata, Pitta, or Kapha), Ayurvedic physicians can diagnose diseases. They then prescribe specific treatments that seek to balance the doshas and the personal health of the person.

In general, Ayurveda is more comprehensive and defines disease in relation to not only physical, but also mental and spiritual aspects. From this perspective, Ayurveda takes an accurate approach by getting to the cause of the affliction and then equalizing the body (Gupta 2018).

17.5.3 Treatment

Ayurveda differs from standard medicine because it treats diseases due to an imbalance between body, mind, and spirit. According to Ayurveda, the approach toward a disease is built around an individual and the cause of the disease.

Ayurveda is used for the treatment of various diseases:

17.5.3.1 Herbal Remedies

The Ayurvedic system of medicine has many herbal and natural remedies to manage diseases. These remedies are based on the dosha imbalance of the individual and are used to help restore body normalcy.

17.5.3.2 Lifestyle Changes

There are cases where an Ayurvedic practitioner will prescribe certain changes in lifestyle that as diet and exercise, etc., to enable the body in its natural way to correct the imbalances that are the root cause of the ill health. They may also teach stress-relieving activities, including yoga, meditation, and other practices that would increase relaxation.

17.5.3.3 Ayurvedic Massage

Massage itself, as an ancient procedure, belongs to Ayurveda; massage is a common practice in India that helps to relax the body, improve circulation, and fight stress. This technique is one of the popular complementary treatments that are used to treat different diseases.

17.5.3.4 Panchakarma

Panchakarma is an ancient method of detoxification, which is part of the Ayurveda system of healing used for cleansing the body. Ayurveda therapy is a course of specific treatments fitted to individual dosha dysfunction.

17.5.3.5 Acupuncture

Acupuncture is an exotic Chinese treatment employed occasionally in Ayurveda to treat ailments. According to this therapy, a practitioner uses thin needles to penetrate the skin at certain locations for treatment and restoration.

Overall, Ayurveda proposes a more individualist strategy for disease cure, influenced by a return to the equilibrium of a physical, psychic, and even spiritual entity. Ayurvedic treatment is holistic and seeks to establish a state of health and balance by harnessing the principles of noninvasive remedial measures.

17.5.4 Cosmetics

According to the study, Ayurveda offers free and unique cosmetic treatments using natural remedies to balance the body's natural bio energies. Cosmetics in Ayurveda are considered part and parcel of general health and beauty and are selected depending on the dosha. The following are some ways in which Ayurveda is used in cosmetics:

17.5.4.1 Herbal Cosmetics

Ayurvedic cosmetics are prepared from natural products, such as herbs, fruits, and flowers. All these ingredients are selected based on their pharmacological action and are used to restore the body to its normal state.

17.5.4.2 Skincare

Ayurvedic skin care products are formulated to be helpful to both the outer layers of the skin and the entire body. Some are based on the dosha imbalance of the individual and are constantly tailored to meet their requirements.

17.5.4.3 Hair Care

Ayurvedic hair care products can be used to fulfill the purposes of nourishing the hair and scalp, and at the same time to enhance hair well-being. Many are derived from the dosha imbalance of the concerned person and, therefore, suit their peculiar characteristics.

17.5.4.4 Aromatherapy

Ayurvedic cosmetics tend to infuse aromatherapy into their formulas because they help customers become more relaxed. Fragrances are made of essential oils for therapeutic purposes to enhance health and wellness.

17.5.4.5 Cosmetics for Beauty Treatments

Ayurvedic facial and body packs are aimed at the overall restoration of the pleasantness of the human body and face. Many of these procedures involve the use of natural products, including honey, turmeric, and sandalwood, to enhance skin health.

In conclusion, Ayurveda provides updated and integral cosmetology comprising balanced and healthy elements. Ayurvedic cosmetics aim at the well-being of individuals and their beauty, while AU offers natural cosmetics and individual treatment plans.

17.6 Limitations of Ayurveda in Treating Diseases

Many Ayurvedic drugs are used to treat infectious diseases ranging from simple colds to serious ailments. Some commonly used preparations include Triphala churna, Hareetaki churna, Dashmula churna, Manjistadi churna, Sukhsarak churna, Ajmodadi churna, Shivkshar pachan churna, Mahasudarshan churna, Swadisht Virechan churna, and Piplamool churna (Tambekar et al. 2011) (Table 17.5).

17.6.1 Bacterial Diseases

Some Ayurvedic formulations that serve as antibacterial agents consist of medicinal plants. Some plants are being studied to treat oral bacterial infections in diabetic patients, as listed in Table 1 (Rafey et al. 2021). Good antibacterial activity was observed in some of the selected plant parts and extracts, including Juglans regia, Syzygium aromaticum, Eruca sativa, Myristica fragrans, Punica granatum, and Azadirachta indica. Researchers also came out with the verdict that the potency of this activity was due to some of the following identified important constituents of the essential oil: eugenol and phenylethyl isothiocyanate. Tambekar et al (2011). noted that some minor bacterial infections, such as bacterial vaginal, urinary tract, and skin infections, can also be managed with formulations such as Triphala churna, Hareetaki churna, and Dashmula churna. Mahasudarshan churna is used to control bacterial infections such as typhoid fever, intestinal diseases, urinary infections, and respiratory infections. Holarrhena antidysenterica was used as an active antibacterial agent against S. aureus, S. flexneri, S. typhosa, and B. subtilis. Laung and

Table 17.5 Common Ayurvedic churnas used for various health conditions

S.No	Churna name	Key ingredients	Indications	Dosage	Side effects	References
1.	Triphala churna	Amla, Haritaki, Bibhitaki	Detoxification, digestive issues, eye problems, respiratory problems	1–3 g along with water before bed	Diarrhea, abdominal discomfort	Lad (1998)
2.	Hareetaki churna	Haritaki	Digestive issues, constipation, skin problems	1–3 g along with water before bed	Diarrhea, abdominal discomfort	Lad (1998)
3.	Dashmula churna	A blend of 10 herbs, including bilva, agnimantha, shyonaka, gambhari, and others	Joint pain, respiratory problems, digestive issues	1–3 g, along with water or honey	None known	Tiwari (2004)
4.	Manjistadi churna	Manjistha, triphala, and other herbs	Skin problems, detoxification	1–3 g, along with water or honey	None known	Tiwari (2004)
5.	Sukhsarak churna	Fennel, cumin, coriander, and other digestive herbs	Digestive issues, gas, bloating	1–3 g, along with water after meals	None known	Tiwari (2004)
6.	Ajmodadi churna	Ajmoda (celery seeds), ginger, and other herbs	Joint pain, arthritis, gout	1–3 g, along with water or honey	None known	Tiwari (2004)
7.	Shivkshar pachan churna	Hing (asafoetida), ginger, and other digestive herbs	Digestive issues, gas, bloating, acidity	1–3 g, along with water after meals	None known	Tiwari (2004)
8.	Mahasudarshan churna	A blend of 50 herbs, including neem, tulsi, guduchi, and others	Fever, cold, flu, respiratory problems	1–3 g, along with water or honey	None known	Tiwari (2004)

(continued)

Table 17.5 (continued)

S.No	Churna name	Key ingredients	Indications	Dosage	Side effects	References
9.	Swadisht Virechan churna	Haritaki, trivrit, and other herbs	Constipation, detoxification	1–3 g, along with water or honey before bed	Diarrhea, abdominal discomfort	Tiwari (2004)
10.	Piplamool churna	Long pepper, black pepper, and other herbs	Joint pain, digestive issues, respiratory problems	1–3 g, along with water or honey	None known	Singh (2012)

Dashmula churna, with the active ingredient Aegle marmelos of zoo plaksh, were effective against V. cholerae. E. coli and Shigella sp. (Mazumder et al. 2006). The star-shaped herb, which is available in many Asian countries, possesses antiviral, anti-inflammatory, insecticidal, spasmolytic, and anti-nociceptive effects. An example of the usefulness of this herb is that the precursor molecule of the commonly used drug oseltamivir for the treatment of Influenza A and B is derived from shikimic acid (Sharafan et al. 2022) (Table 17.6).

Some lifestyle disorders are on the rise, including obesity, diabetes mellitus, cardiovascular diseases, hypertension, and dyslipidemia. These have become the cause of an approaching reason for death on Earth. According to Ayurveda, it has a major role in managing the condition, illness, and preventing and treating it. Ayurveda contains five groups of treatments that clean and purify the body, called Panchkarma, which has an impact on the rejuvenation of the body, called Rasayana, and the daily routine that should be introduced in human life, called Sadvritta and Dinacharya. These are good regimens for tackling lifestyle-related diseases (Chandola 2012). One sub-branch of Ayurveda, Rasa Shastra, has been found to be very effective in handling such diseases. Diabetes can be treated with the following formulations: Arogyavardhini vatti and Swarna makherdhwaj Rasayan. Preparations include Hirdyarnava Rasa for heart ailments and Laxmi Vilas Rasa for Respiratory tract disorders (Jaiswal et al. 2017). In Ayurveda, several formulations are used cosmetologically and in diseases with lepa called lepakalpana (Hari Anand Tripathi et al 2020).

17.7 Different Types of Ayurvedic Therapies

17.7.1 Shamana Therapy

Shukla et al. (2013), studied the effect of Shamana therapy in managing hypertension. The treatment comprised two groups, Virechana and Basti, both of which were subjected to Arjuna Ghanavati (Shamana therapy), and the diastolic and systolic

Table 17.6 Ayurvedic principles, treatment, and prevention for various pathogens

S No.	Pathogen	Ayurvedic principles	Ayurvedic treatment	Ayurvedic prevention	References
1	Bacteria	Balance of Doshas	Use of herbs and spices with antibacterial properties, such as neem, turmeric, and garlic	Maintain hygiene, avoid sharing personal items, and consume a balanced diet	Sharma (2017)
2	Fungi	Balance of Doshas	Use of antifungal herbs such as neem, turmeric, and tulsi	Avoid wearing tight clothing, maintain hygiene, and consume a balanced diet	Thosar et al. (2013)
3	Virus	Balance of Doshas	Use of antiviral herbs such as tulsi, licorice, and ashwagandha	Maintain hygiene, avoid close contact with infected individuals, and consume a balanced diet	Sharma (2017)
4	Protozoa	Balance of Doshas	Use of herbs with anti-protozoal properties, such as neem and clove	Maintain hygiene, avoid contaminated water and food, and consume a balanced diet	Thosar et al. (2013)
5	Parasite	Balance of Doshas	Use of herbs with anti-parasitic properties, such as neem, ginger, and garlic	Maintain hygiene, avoid raw or undercooked meat, and eat a balanced diet.	Tiwari (2014)
6	MRSA	Balance of Doshas	Use of herbs with anti-MRSA properties, such as tea tree oil and turmeric	Maintain hygiene, avoid sharing personal items, and consume a balanced diet	Tiwari (2014)
7	Candida	Balance of Doshas	Use of antifungal herbs such as neem, turmeric, and tulsi	Avoid wearing tight clothing, maintain hygiene, and consume a balanced diet	Jadhav et al. (2019)
8	Influenza	Balance of Doshas	Use of antiviral herbs such as tulsi, licorice, and ashwagandha	Maintain hygiene, avoid close contact with infected individuals, and consume a balanced diet	Prakash et al. (2014)
9	Malaria	Balance of Doshas	Use of herbs with anti-malarial properties, such as neem, holy basil, and ginger	Avoid mosquito bites, use mosquito nets, and consume a balanced diet	Shankar et al., (2012)

(continued)

Table 17.6 (continued)

S No.	Pathogen	Ayurvedic principles	Ayurvedic treatment	Ayurvedic prevention	References
10	Tuberculosis	Balance of Doshas	Use of herbs with anti-TB properties, such as garlic and ashwagandha	Maintain hygiene, avoid close contact with infected individuals, and consume a balanced diet	Manohar et al. (2015)
11	Dengue	Balance of Doshas	Use of herbs with anti-dengue properties, such as papaya leaf and neem	Avoid mosquito bites, use mosquito nets, and consume a balanced diet	
12	E. Coli	Balance of Doshas	Use of herbs with anti-E. coli properties, such as neem and clove	Maintain hygiene, avoid consuming contaminated food and water, and eat a balanced diet	

pressures were monitored. Patients who received Virechana therapy with Shamana showed better relief after treatment.

17.7.2 Pathya Vyavastha

A well-planned diet based on Ayurveda's principles is believed to prevent health problems. This is a holistic planning of diet, considering factors such as the environment, food preparation, age, health status, and the habitat of a person. Pathya Vyavastha is prescribed in cases of digestive system disorders and other lifestyle disorders (Bhat and Lavekar 2005). Pathya Apathya has also been used to treat inflammatory diseases, such as rheumatoid arthritis. Overall, the same Pathya Vyavastha, which helps prevent the accumulation of amavata, is effective in treating problems that arise from it, such as stiffness in the bones and joints, pain, and tenderness.

17.7.3 Nidan Parivarjan

Nidan Parivarjan is two-sided medicine, being in great use for preventive healthcare and curative healthcare. In their clinical research, Kulkarni et al. (2020) studied patients diagnosed with 'Urdhwaga Amlapitta,' giving them either Nidanparivarjan treatment or no Nidanparivarjan. The findings of this study have proven that with this treatment modality, patients are relieved of the disease for an extended period. Another report states that Rasayana Chikitsa and nidan parivarjan could effectively prevent several lifestyle disorders by addressing the hetu (Kandikattiwar 2021).

17.7.4 Satvavajaya

The human mind plays an important role in the human body, and psychotherapy performed by Ayurveda aims to save the mind from stress. This treatment emphasizes three factors: trivargas, mental health support, and increasing awareness of spiritual entities (Murthy et al. 1987). It includes using yoga techniques, such as Astanga Yoga and Manonigraha. A study of 102 healthy young volunteers was performed to study the effects of Satvavajaya Chikitsa. The authors found that this treatment resulted in better memory (Amin and Sharma 2015). This therapy, done by Adravya and Dravya, has found importance in treating depression by helping one attain insight, awareness, understanding, and coping abilities to overcome unintentional events (Ashwini and Rajashekhar 2019).

17.7.5 Rasayana Therapy

A parallel increase in the occurrence of diseases has been observed, even with an increase in medicine and healthcare management systems. As the primary underlying principle of Ayurveda lies in preventing diseases and maintaining a healthy lifestyle, Rasayanas is the best way to achieve this. It is believed to contain concoctions responsible for supplying nutrients by rejuvenating the body and the mind. According to Table 17.7, several herbs such as Guduchi (*Tinospora cordifolia* (Willd.) Hook. f. and Thoms.), amalaki (*Emblica officinalis* Gaertn.), ashwagandha (*Withania somnifera*), and Guduchi and Pippali (*Piper longum*) are often recommended for patients with pre-diabetic and allergic conditions (Goyal 2018). Lifestyle and exposure to harmful conditions increase free radicals in our bodies. A study involving 30 volunteers was conducted to analyze the effect of Rasayanas, such as Ashwagandha and Guduchi, on combating oxidative stress. By monitoring the levels of SOD and MDA, the formulation was found to be helpful in preventing oxidative stress and premature aging (Kuchewar et al. 2014).

17.8 Ayurvedic Formulations

Ayurveda deals with a wide variety of herbal, mineral, and herbal-metallic formulations; it is essential to understand the behavior of these drugs. These formulations can be prepared using various techniques to develop the necessary therapeutic amount. When taken, the drugs go through digestion, assimilation, absorption, metabolism, and elimination. This constitutes the pharmacological behavior of the drugs without understanding the pharmacological behavior of the drugs the treatment is not complete (Iyer 2018).

Table 17.7 Properties of commonly used Ayurvedic herbs

S.No	Ayurvedic herbs	Properties	Reference
1.	Triphala	A blend of three fruits used to cleanse and rejuvenate the body	Tiwari (2004)
2.	Ashwagandha	Used to balance Vata dosha and reduce stress	Tiwari (2004)
3.	Turmeric	Anti-inflammatory and antioxidant properties	Tiwari (2004)
4.	Brahmi	Used to improve memory and cognitive function	Tiwari (2004)
5.	Ginger	Helps with digestion and is anti-inflammatory	Singh (2015)
6.	Holy basil (Tulsi)	Used to relieve stress, improve respiratory function, and promote cardiovascular health	Ashok (2013)
7.	Neem	Used to treat skin conditions, boost immunity, and detoxify the body	Parihar et al. (2002)
8.	Amla	Rich in vitamin C and antioxidants, used to support the immune system and improve digestion	Mathur et al. (2011)
9.	Guggulu	Used to reduce inflammation and support healthy cholesterol levels	Thakur (2017)
10.	Shankhapushpi	Used to improve memory and cognitive function and promote relaxation	Parihar et al. (2002)
11.	Licorice	Used to soothe sore throats and coughs and to support healthy digestion	Singh (2015)
12.	Haritaki	Used to improve digestion, detoxify the body, and support respiratory health	Ashok (2013)
13.	Shatavari	Used to balance hormones, support fertility and lactation, and promote vitality	Ashok (2013)
14.	Vidanga	Used to support healthy digestion, relieve constipation, and promote weight loss	Singh (2015)
15.	Kutki	Used to improve liver function and treat liver disorders	Singh (2015)
16.	Punarnava	Used to reduce inflammation, support healthy kidney function, and promote detoxification	Tiwari (2004)

17.8.1 Pharmacokinetics

Predominantly, a drug's efficiency expressed in the pharmacokinetic parameter is viewed as an essential characteristic; however, in the case of herbal remedies, this characteristic can be considered rather complicated. Because herbal products are used to treat different diseases, it is important to identify these herb-drug interactions, which may cause adverse effects. The effect of Trikatu on the concomitant administration of diclofenac sodium was studied by Lala et al. 2004; Wele (2006) showed the pharmacokinetics and pharmacodynamics of Piper nigrum in many Ayurvedic formulations. It is used in compounds such as Trikatu, Suvarna, Mallika, Vasa, and Shwasakuthara rasa and possesses various pharmacological activities. The active ingredients were found to enhance the bioavailability of other compounds and nutraceuticals. Because of the importance of plant-based medicines, advanced techniques such as nanotechnology have been used to enhance the pharmacological properties of these drugs. Nanocapsules, nanoemulsions, liposomes, nanoparticles, colloidosomes, and microspheres are used for improved bioavailability, targeted delivery, protection from acidic environments, and sustained delivery (Shankar et al., 2012).

17.8.2 Pharmacovigilance

Several thousand Ayurvedic formulations and herbal extracts are currently available. Although there is a misconception about the adverse effects of Ayurvedic drugs, it is mentioned by early founders that several factors play a vital role in drug preparation. As the use of alternative medicines has increased, adverse effects have not been adequately recorded. If Indian policymakers establish a rigorous routine for such registration, European countries and the FDA, which are keen to process new drugs from the Investigational New Drug (IND), would take it worldwide (Nampoothiri 2016). Several challenges exist in the systematic pharmacovigilance regulations for Ayurvedic drugs. The factors include:

1. Creating awareness among the doctors about identifying and reporting adverse reactions
2. Establishing an accessible library with complete information about the drugs
3. Improve the quality check and assurance for herbal formulations
4. Prevent illegal and counterfeit drugs
5. Focus more on the Pharmacokinetics, pharmacodynamics, and toxicity of the drugs
6. Consumer awareness about reporting plausible adverse reactions
7. Stringent regulations are followed by industries and agencies to monitor safety analyses and reporting (Thatte and Bhalerao 2008). If these factors are considered, Ayurvedic formulations would be restructured and could have a global impact.

17.9 Role of Ayurveda in the Indian Economy

Ayurveda, the ancient Indian system of medicine, is not only a traditional healing system but also a significant contributor to the Indian economy. Ayurveda is believed to have originated over 5000 years ago and has since been a part of the Indian way of life. The Ayurveda industry in India is estimated to be worth approximately USD 5 billion, and it is expected to grow at 16% per annum. This growth can be attributed to the increasing interest in Ayurveda both domestically and globally. Ayurveda has gained popularity worldwide because of its holistic approach to health and wellness, and its ability to cure chronic diseases. Ayurveda significantly impacts the Indian economy as it employs many people, particularly in rural areas. The Ayurveda industry provides jobs for farmers, manufacturers, practitioners, and retailers. The industry also contributes to the development of rural infrastructure, as many Ayurveda manufacturing units are in rural areas, providing employment opportunities to the local population (Sharma 2011). The Indian government has recognized the potential of Ayurveda and has taken steps to promote and develop the industry. The government has established the Ministry of AYUSH, which is responsible for developing, promoting, and regulating Ayurveda, Yoga, Naturopathy, Unani, Siddha, and Homeopathy systems of medicine. The government also established the National Ayush Mission to promote the integration of Ayurveda with the national health system (Ministry of AYUSH 2022).

Promoting Ayurveda has also led to increased tourism in India, as many people come to the country to experience the benefits of Ayurveda treatment. Ayurveda resorts and spas have become popular tourist destinations, particularly in Kerala, where the state government has implemented a tourism policy to promote Ayurveda tourism. Therefore, Ayurveda has great significance in the Indian economy through employment generation, rural development, and the development of the tourism industry. Ayurveda is expected to play an ever-growing role in the global market for healthcare services in recent years because of the growing trend for natural systems of medicine (Sahoo et al. 2019).

17.10 Conclusion

Ayurveda was not only an ancient system of medicine but also a highly effective participant in the construction of the future of medicine. It is an Indian form of medicine that deals with life science and has the capability of medical treatment of a man in totality, not just the body, but the mind and the spirit as well. Yoga, meditation, and herbal remedies are some of the practices that have received worldwide attention because of their efficiency in enhancing health. The Ayurveda industry in India is 5000 crores and with an annual growth rate of 16% and employment opportunities at large. Ayurveda has tremendous opportunities to become a serious player in the global healthcare market and provide people with good and safe treatment options for many conditions. The integration of Ayurveda on one hand and modern medicine on the other hand, holds a promising future for an enhanced form of healthcare which will offer patients with safer, simpler, and more comprehensive form of treatment. Therefore, it is necessary to guarantee that the development and introduction of Ayurveda are produced carefully and with less harm to consumers, keeping in mind the need for safety, efficacy, and quality. With the present trend toward the use of less synthetic and more natural ways to treat sickness, it is imperative that Ayurveda be marketed and practiced ethically, responsibly, and efficiently. Ayurveda is an area with important prospects for the future development of medicine. It is useful in modern medicine because it employs a more comprehensive healthcare approach, has efficient practice, and demand is rising. If done sensibly and without hype, Ayurveda could be a good option for patients as part of modern medicine, and this would create a healthier future in the healthcare business.

References

Amin H, Sharma R (2015) Nootropic efficacy of Satvavajaya Chikitsa and Ayurvedic drug therapy: a comparative clinical exposition. Int J Yoga 8(2):109–116. https://doi.org/10.4103/0973-6131.158473

Ashok PK, Upadhyaya K (2013) Therapeutic potential of neem (*Azadirachta indica*) and its limonoids. J Phytochem Pharmacol 2(2):96–102. https://doi.org/10.13140/2.1.4571.9681

Ashwini A, Rajashekhar CV (2019) Role of Satvavajaya Chikitsa in the management of depression in current scenario. J Ayurveda Integr Med Sci 4(4):275–278.https://doi.org/10.21760/jaims.v4i04.675

Bhat S, Lavekar GS (2005) Ayurvĕdic approach to pathya (ideal diet planning)—an appraisal. Bulletin of the Indian Institute of History of Medicine (Hyderabad) 35(2):147–156

Bhavamishra (2012) Bhavaprakasha. Retrieved from https://www.wisdomlib.org/hinduism/book/bhavaprakasha-english

Birch J, Wujastyk D, Klebanov A, Parameswaran M, Rimal M (2021) Further insight into the role of Dhanvantari, the physician to the gods, in the Suśrutasaṃhitā. Academia Letters

Chandola H (2012) Lifestyle disorders: Ayurveda with lots of potential for prevention. AYU 33(3):327. https://doi.org/10.4103/0974-8520.108814

Charaka (2003) Charaka Samhita. Retrieved from https://www.wisdomlib.org/hinduism/book/charaka-samhita-english

Chaudhary A, Singh N (2019) Ayurvedic medicine: an introduction. J Tradit Complement Med 9(2):158–161. https://doi.org/10.1016/j.jtcme.2018.11.006

Chopra D (2007) Perfect health: the complete mind/body guide, Revised and updated edn. Harmony

Chopra A, Doiphode VV (2002) Ayurvedic medicine: core concept, therapeutic principles, and current relevance. Med Clin North Am Ther Nova 86(6):75–89

Chopra A, Doiphode VV (2014) Ayurvedic medicine—Core concept, therapies, and evidence-based practice. Med Clin North Am 98(6):945–958. https://doi.org/10.1016/j.mcna.2014.07.005

Dwivedi R, Dwivedi S (2020) Ayurveda: introduction and history. J Pharm Res Int 32(6):49–57. https://doi.org/10.9734/jpri/2020/v32i630526

Frawley D (2000) Ayurvedic healing: a comprehensive guide. Lotus Press

Frawley D, Ranade S (2001) Ayurveda, nature's medicine. Lotus Press

Ganguli SC (2019) History of medicine in India. In: History of medicine in India. Springer, Singapore, pp 1–15

Goyal M (2018) Rasayana in perspective of the present scenario. Ayu 39(2):63–64. https://doi.org/10.4103/ayu.AYU_300_18

Gupta AK (2017) History of Ayurveda. In: Textbook of Ayurveda: volume one (fundamental principles). Chaukhambha Publications, pp 1–6

Gupta S, Gupta S (2018) Ayurveda and folklore medicine: a perspective. J Ayurveda Integr Med 9(4):303–305. https://doi.org/10.1016/j.jaim.2017.06.008

Ito T (2013) The encyclopedia of Ayurvedic massage. Singing Dragon

Iyer R, Mishra L (2018) Ayurveda: a comprehensive guide to traditional Indian medicine for the West. Singing Dragon

Jadhav S, Kumar S, Gupta S (2019) In vitro evaluation of the antibacterial activity of turmeric and tea tree oil against methicillin-resistant *Staphylococcus aureus* (MRSA). Int J Curr Microbiol App Sci 8(2):2687–2692. https://doi.org/10.20546/ijcmas.2019.802.314

Jain N, Gupta VK (2014) A review of medicinal uses and pharmacological effects of *Vateria indica* (L.) Roxb. and its bioactive compounds. J Appl Pharm Sci 4(7):113–120

Jaiswal YS, Williams LL (2017) A glimpse of Ayurveda—The forgotten history and principles of Indian traditional medicine. Journal of Traditional and Complementary Medicine, 7(1):50–53https://doi.org/10.1016/j.jtcme.2016.02.002

Jha V (2018) Medieval India and the history of Ayurveda. Anc Sci Life 38(2):56–60. https://doi.org/10.4103/asl.ASL_26_18

Kandikattiwar P (2021) A prevention of lifestyle disorder through Ayurveda (Nidan Parivarjan, Rasayan). Ayurline 5(01). https://doi.org/10.52482/ayurline.v5i01.479

Khalsa SBS, Cohen L (2017) Principles and practice of Ayurvedic medicine. Elsevier

Kotecha P (2018) Ayurveda: the alchemy of life. J Tradit Complement Med 8(3):387–392. https://doi.org/10.1016/j.jtcme.2018.03.006

Kotecha M, Hirpara K (2012) The concept of Malas in Ayurveda. Ayu 33(4):414–417

Kuchewar VV, Borkar MA, Nisargandha MA (2014) Evaluation of the antioxidant potential of Rasayana drugs in healthy human volunteers. Ayu 35(1):46–49. https://doi.org/10.4103/0974-8520.141919

Kulkarni PV, Thamake MJ (2020) To assess the importance of Nidana Parivarjan in the treatment of Urdhvag Amlapitta with Guduchi Satva. J Ayurveda Integr Med Sci 5(4):16–20. https://doi.org/10.21760/jaims.v5i04.938

Lad V (1998) The complete book of Ayurvedic home remedies. New York, NY: Three Rivers Press

Lad V (1999) The complete book of Ayurvedic home remedies. Harmony Books

Lad V (2002) Textbook of Ayurveda: fundamental principles of Ayurveda, vol 1. The Ayurvedic Press

Lad V (2012) Textbook of Ayurveda: fundamental principles. Ayurvedic Press, Albuquerque, NM

Lala LG, D'Mello PM, Naik SR (2004) Pharmacokinetic and pharmacodynamic studies on the interaction of "Trikatu" with diclofenac sodium. J Ethnopharmacol 91(2–3):277–280. https://doi.org/10.1016/j.jep.2003.12.027

Madhava (2009) Madhava Nidanam. Retrieved from https://www.wisdomlib.org/hinduism/book/madhava-nidana-english

Manohar V, Ingram C, Gray M, Talpur NA, Echard BW, Bagchi D, Preuss HG (2015) Antifungal activities of origanum oil against *Candida albicans*. Mol Cell Biochem 402(1–2):145–152. https://doi.org/10.1007/s11010-014-2256-6

Mathur R, Sharma A, Dixit VP, Varma M (2011) Hypolipidemic effect of Guggulu (*Commiphora mukul*) extract. J Phytochem Pharmacol 2(1):28–32. https://doi.org/10.13140/2.1.3674.6884

Mazumder R, Bhattacharya S, Mazumder A, Pattnaik AK, Tiwary PM, Chaudhary S (2006) Antidiarrhoeal evaluation of *Aegle Marmelos* (Correa) Linn. root extract. Phytother Res 20(1):82–84. https://doi.org/10.1002/ptr.1804

Ministry of AYUSH (2022) About us. https://www.ayush.gov.in/about-the-ministry/

Mishra LC (2004) The scientific basis for Ayurvedic therapies. CRC Press

Murthy ARV, Singh RH (1987) The concept of psychotherapy in Ayurveda with special reference to Satvavajaya. Ancient Science of Life, 6(4):255–261

Nampoothiri MR (2016) Ayurvedic medicine: an overview and review of case reports. Complement Med Res 23(5):275–283. https://doi.org/10.1159/000452758

Narayanaswamy V (2010) History of Ayurveda—a brief account. J-AIM 1(3):167–170. https://doi.org/10.4103/0975-9476.72628

Naveen KV, Chopra A (2017) Ayurvedic approach to the management of obesity. In: Integrative medicine for obesity. Springer, pp 45–54. https://doi.org/10.1007/978-3-319-60177-6_4

Nayak S, Singh V (2016) Panchakarma: a review. Ayu 37(3):143–146. https://doi.org/10.4103/ayu.AYU_63_16

Panda S, Jena S (2019) Ayurvedic medicine: a review of its historical and philosophical evolution, cultural and social influence, and current status. J Ethnopharmacol 244:112129. https://doi.org/10.1016/j.jep.2019.112129

Parihar MS, Hemnani T, Bhutani KK (2002) Investigation into the mechanism of action of *Withania somnifera* (Ashwagandha): identification of N-trans-feruloyl tyramine as the active ingredient. J Phytother Res 16(7):640–646. https://doi.org/10.1089/107628002760092922

Patwardhan B, Vaidya AD, Chorghade M (2004) Ayurveda, and natural products drug discovery. Curr Sci 86(6):789–799

Petersen A, Challem J (2008) The encyclopedia of healing foods. Atria

Pole S (2013) Ayurvedic medicine: the principles of traditional practice. Singing Dragon

Prakash B, Singh P, Kedia A, Dubey NK, Upadhyay G (2014) Antifungal, anti aflatoxin, and antioxidant potential of chemically characterized *Boswellia carterii* Birdwood essential oil and its in vivo practical applicability in preserving *Piper nigrum* L. fruits. LWT-Food. Sci Technol 55(1):346–352. https://doi.org/10.1016/j.lwt.2013.09.012

Rafey A, Amin A, Kamran M, Haroon U, Farooq K, Foubert K, Pieters L (2021) Analysis of plant origin antibiotics against oral bacterial infections using *in vitro* and *in silico* techniques and characterization of active constituents. Antibiotics 10(12):1504. https://doi.org/10.3390/antibiotics10121504

Rastogi S, Kumar R (2018) Comprehensive review of Ayurvedic perspective on wound healing, part 1: terminologies and traditional concepts. J-AIM 9(4):291–296. https://doi.org/10.1016/j.jaim.2017.12.005

Sahoo J, Pattanayak S (2019) Ayurveda: the traditional medicine system in India and its role in the Indian economy. J Emerg Technol Innov Res 6(4):309–312. https://doi.org/10.11648/j.etir.2019.0604.27

Saper RB, Phillips RS, Sehgal A, Khouri N, Davis RB, Paquin J, Thuppil V, Kales SN, Burns RB (2008) Lead, mercury, and arsenic in US- and Indian-manufactured Ayurvedic medicines sold via the Internet. JAMA J Am Med Assoc 300(8):915–923. https://doi.org/10.1001/jama.300.8.915

Shankar R, Deb S, Sharma BK (2012) Antimalarial plants of northeast India: An overview. Journal ofAyurveda and Integrative Medicine, 3(1):10.https://doi.org/10.4103/0975-9476.93940

Sharafan M, Jafernik K, Ekiert H, Kubica P, Kocjan R, Blicharska E, Szopa A (2022) *Illicium verum* (star Anise) and trans-anethole as valuable raw materials for medicinal and cosmetic applications. Molecules 27(3):650. https://doi.org/10.3390/molecules27030650

Sharma H (2011) Ayurvedic healing: contemporary maharishi Ayurveda medicine and science. Singing Dragon

Sharma H, Clark C (2017) Ayurvedic medicine for the treatment of dementia: mechanistic aspects. Evid Based Complement Alternat Med 2017:2481078. https://doi.org/10.1155/2017/2481078

Sharma A, Mittal A (2017) Ayurvedic management of infectious diseases: a review. J-AIM 8(4):256–261. https://doi.org/10.1016/j.jaim.2017.02.008

Sharma H, Chandola HM, Singh G, Basisht G, Sharma R (2008) Utilization of Ayurveda in health care: an approach for prevention, health promotion, and treatment of disease. Part 1–Ayurveda, the science of life. J Altern Complement Med 14(5):569–576. https://doi.org/10.1089/acm.2007.0754

Sharma H, Chandola HM, Singh G, Basisht G, Mishra RK (2011b) The concept of Ojas in Ayurveda. J-AIM 2(3):115–120

Sharma P, Yadav CR, Jolly N, Chouhan DC (2020) A literary review of Pathya and Apathya W.S.R to Aamvata. Int Res J Ayur Yoga 03(12):105–111. https://doi.org/10.47223/IRJAY.2020.31204

Shukla G, Bhatted SK, Dave AR, Shukla VD (2013) Efficacy of Virechana and Basti Karma with Shamana therapy in the management of essential hypertension: A comparative study. AYU (J of Research inAyurveda), 34(1):70–76. https://doi.org/10.4103/0974-8520.115455

Singh RH (2005) Ayurveda in the 21st century. Altern Ther Health Med 11(6):42–44

Singh B, Rastogi S (2012) Ayurvedic herbs: a clinical guide to the healing plants of traditional Indian medicine. John Wiley and Sons

Singh S, Majumdar DK (2015) Evaluation of the anti-inflammatory potential of a standardized aqueous extract of *Ocimum sanctum* (Holy Basil) in rats. Phytother Res 29(5):747–751. https://doi.org/10.1002/ptr.5318

Singh SK, Rastogi S (2021) Ayurveda: a traditional system of medicine. Int J Pharm Sci Res 12(3):1297–1305

Sushruta (2005) Sushruta Samhita. Retrieved from https://www.wisdomlib.org/hinduism/book/sushruta-samhita-volume-1-english

Svoboda RE (1999) Prakriti: your Ayurvedic constitution. Lotus Press

Tambekar DH, Dahikar SB (2011) Antibacterial activity of some Indian Ayurvedic preparations against enteric bacterial pathogens. J of Advanced Pharmaceutical Technology and Research, 2(1):24–29.https://doi.org/10.4103/2231-4040.79801

Thakur CP, Thakur B (2017) The Ayurvedic pharmacopoeia of India, part I, vol VI. Government of India, Ministry of AYUSH

Thatte U, Bhalerao S (2008) Pharmacovigilance of ayurvedic medicines in India. Ind J Pharmacol 40(Suppl 1):S10–S12
Thosar N, Basak S, Bahadure R, Rajurkar M (2013) Antimicrobial efficacy of tea tree oil and clove oil against methicillin-resistant Staphylococcus aureus (MRSA). J Indian Soc Pedod Prev Dent 31(1):26–30. https://doi.org/10.4103/0970-4388.112408
Tiwari M (2003) Ayurveda: secrets of healing. Motilal Banarsidass Publishers
Tiwari M (2004) The Ayurvedic encyclopedia. Satmarga Publications
Tiwari R, Tiwari G (2014) Modern and ayurvedic concept of pathogenesis of infectious diseases and their management: a review. J Pharm Bioallied Sci 6(1):2–14.https://doi.org/10.4103/0975-7406.124313
Tiwari M (2017) Ayurveda: secrets of healing. Lotus Press
Tiwari R (2014) Modern and ayurvedic concept of pathogenesis of infectious diseases and their management: a review. J Pharm Bioallied Sci 6(1):2–14. https://doi.org/10.4103/0975-7406.124313
Tripathi HA, Nayak JD, Sathyanarayana B (2020) A comparative pharmaceutico-analytical study of Bhagandharahara lepa with its modified form as a hydrogel. International Ayurvedic Medical J, 4(4):2309–2318.http://dx.doi.org/10.46607/iamjp040472020
Vagbhata (2011) Ashtanga Hridaya. Retrieved from https://www.wisdomlib.org/hinduism/book/ashtanga-hridaya-samhita-english
Valiathan MS (1993) History of Ayurveda: an overview. Ind J Hist Sci 28(3):205–221
Vasant Lad (2002) Textbook of Ayurveda. In: Fundamental principles, vol 1. The Ayurvedic Press, Albuquerque
Wele A (2006) Research Methodology and Statistics Evident in Ayurveda Treatises

MIX
Papier aus verantwortungsvollen Quellen
Paper from responsible sources
FSC® C105338

If you have any concerns about our products,
you can contact us on
ProductSafety@springernature.com

In case Publisher is established outside the EU,
the EU authorized representative is:
Springer Nature Customer Service Center GmbH
Europaplatz 3, 69115 Heidelberg, Germany

Printed by Libri Plureos GmbH
in Hamburg, Germany